Foundations of Professional Personal Training

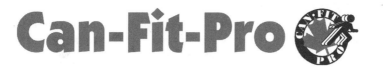

Can-Fit-Pro

Gregory Anderson

Mike Bates

Stéphane Cova

Rod Macdonald

EDITORS

Human Kinetics

Library of Congress Cataloging-in-Publication Data

Foundations of professional personal training.
   p. cm.
  Includes bibliographical references and index.
  ISBN-13: 978-0-7360-6910-6 (soft cover)
  ISBN-10: 0-7360-6910-0 (soft cover)
  1. Personal trainers--Handbooks, manuals, etc. 2. Personal trainers--Vocational guidance--Handbooks, manuals, etc. 3. Physical fitness.
  GV428.7.F68 2007
  613.7'1--dc22

                2007023794

ISBN-10: 0-7360-6910-0
ISBN-13: 978-0-7360-6910-6

The Web addresses cited in this text were current as of February 28, 2007, unless otherwise noted.

Acquisitions Editor: Michael S. Bahrke, PhD; **Managing Editor:** Lee Alexander; **Copyeditor:** Alisha Jeddaloh; **Proofreader:** Julie Marx Goodreau; **Indexer:** Bobbi Swanson; **Permission Manager:** Dalene Reeder; **Graphic Designer:** Nancy Rasmus; **Graphic Artist:** Denise Lowry; **Cover Designer:** Gavin Fung; **Photographer (cover):** Claus Andersen; **Photographer (interior):** Claus Andersen; **Photo Asset Manager:** Neil Bernstein; **Visual Production Assistant:** Joyce Brumfield; **Photo Office Assistant:** Jason Allen; **Art Manager:** Kelly Hendren; **Illustrator:** Alan L. Wilborn; **Printer:** United Graphics

Printed in the United States of America   10 9 8 7 6 5 4 3 2 1

Human Kinetics
Web site: www.HumanKinetics.com

United States: Human Kinetics, P.O. Box 5076, Champaign, IL 61825-5076
800-747-4457
e-mail: humank@hkusa.com

Canada: Human Kinetics, 475 Devonshire Road Unit 100, Windsor, ON N8Y 2L5
800-465-7301 (in Canada only)
e-mail: orders@hkcanada.com

Europe: Human Kinetics, 107 Bradford Road, Stanningley, Leeds LS28 6AT, United Kingdom
+44 (0) 113 255 5665
e-mail: hk@hkeurope.com

Australia: Human Kinetics, 57A Price Avenue, Lower Mitcham, South Australia 5062
08 8372 0999
e-mail: info@hkaustralia.com

New Zealand: Human Kinetics, Division of Sports Distributors NZ Ltd., P.O. Box 300 226 Albany, North Shore City, Auckland
0064 9 448 1207
e-mail: info@humankinetics.co.nz

CONTENTS

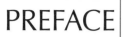

PREFACE

Stéphane Cova
Erin Andersen

About Can-Fit-Pro

Founded in 1993, Can-Fit-Pro was established to assist all fitness professionals in their quest for on-going education and continued professionalism. As an organization, we meet the needs of Canadian fitness professionals and consumers through our professional fitness certification offerings, conference and tradeshow events, Can-Fit-Pro branded fitness education workshops, and diverse membership offerings.

Our Mission

United as members, Can-Fit-Pro takes today's fitness professional challenges and creates tomorrow's solutions through increasing opportunity, ongoing relative knowledge, and personal enrichment.

Our Vision

To move away from the survival mode of just meeting basic needs and into a relationship that demonstrates value and excellence. We believe that growth and education is complete when we are able to provide for all fitness professionals.

Purpose and Goals of Can-Fit-Pro's Certification Program

Launched in 1998, Can-Fit-Pro's certification program was created to provide a high quality nationally recognized fitness certification creating qualified professionals. Starting with the two programs fundamental to fitness, group fitness instruction and personal training, Can-Fit-Pro's certification program portfolio has grown to include specialized certifications to meet the increasingly discriminate needs of fitness consumers. Led by our network of qualified course instructors and examiners called PRO Trainers, Can-Fit-Pro's certification programs are designed to meet the certification needs of all fitness professionals across Canada by being accessible, attainable, and affordable to all who wish to take them.

Complimentary to our certification offerings, Can-Fit-Pro hosts North America's largest fitness professional conference and tradeshow in Toronto in August every year. Can-Fit-Pro also hosts a series of regional conference events which allow our certified members to keep their practical skills and knowledge up to date. Can-Fit-Pro will continue to expand our conference offerings to provide for the always growing need for continuing education opportunities for fitness professionals.

As a Can-Fit-Pro Professional Member you will benefit by becoming part of the largest member-driven fitness organization in Canada, you will receive discounts on Can-Fit-Pro certification and conference event registration fees, you will receive our informational industry magazine and you will have access to discounts with many fitness and non industry-related vendors.

Can-Fit-Pro Certification: A Statement of Excellence

Can-Fit-Pro certified fitness professionals demonstrate **commitment to the fitness industry** and show a **high standard of competency and ability.**

As a leader in the future of Canadian fitness, Can-Fit-Pro certified fitness professionals provide a reliable source of **fitness knowledge** and **safe, effective exercise** for all levels of exercisers.

Achieving this **standard of excellence** makes Can-Fit-Pro certified fitness professionals **competitive** and **in high demand for employment** across the country.

Continuous training shows a dedication to **self improvement** and a commitment to **providing motivation and information** for all participants.

Known for **quality** and **enthusiasm**, Can-Fit-Pro certified fitness professionals establish a **benchmark for excellence and education** in the fitness industry.

Thank you for being a part of the leading edge of fitness training in Canada. Together as fitness professionals, we will Educate, Communicate, and Motivate fitness enthusiasts everywhere toward a healthier and more active lifestyle.

The Can-Fit-Pro Personal Training Specialist Certification

With the tremendous growth of the fitness industry, there is increased opportunity for certified personal trainers. This growth has resulted in a greater need for knowledgeable, mature and qualified individuals. The fitness profession is continually challenged to maintain consistent and quality leadership and educational programs. The availability of an adequate supply of qualified personal trainers helps to standardize the services clubs are able to offer and helps maintain the credibility of the industry as a whole.

The Personal Training Specialist certification has been developed to provide the participant with the opportunity to become better educated about personal fitness training in a fun, adult learning atmosphere. This program will enhance your confidence and motivation to lead and motivate your clients to be active, feel great and get results!

An important goal of this program is to have a positive impact on the activity level of Canadians. The Government of Canada's *Integrated Pan-Canadian Healthy Living Strategy* sets healthy living targets and seeks to obtain a 20% increase in the proportion of Canadians who are

1. physically active,
2. eat healthily, **and**
3. are at healthy body weights by 2015.

This initiative's target on which requests for government grants for health promotion and disease prevention are measured sets the stage for a link between allied health professionals and fitness professionals to provide education and services for those Canadians who want a lifestyle change toward increased physical activity.

From working in a club to starting your own business, the opportunities for certified personal trainers have never been greater. Can-Fit-Pro is proud to be working alongside the Government of Canada and several non-government organizations to get Canadians moving toward improved health.

Our Commitment to You

Can-Fit-Pro and our PRO Trainers promise to:

1. **Educate** you to learn the skills to help you provide safe, effective client sessions.
2. **Motivate** you by providing a learning environment that is educational and fun.
3. **Communicate** with you so that you are directly involved in your own learning process mentally, verbally and physically.

Your Commitment to Yourself

You need take responsibility for your own learning—be accountable for your own success and enjoyment. To do that you should:

1. Commit to attending and actively participating in the entire certification preparatory course.
2. Complete review assignments and projects as required for you to solidify the theoretical concepts and practical concepts you are learning.
3. Network with others to share feedback about this experience and gather information.
4. Set realistic goals for yourself so that you meet your deadlines for certification completion.
5. Ask questions if you do not understand a concept. We can all learn from each other.
6. Give your best effort. Do the best you can both physically and mentally.

What You Need to Know to Become Certified

Eligibility

Certification as a Can-Fit-Pro Personal Training Specialist is open to persons 18 years or older. Candidates must hold a current Cardiopulmonary Resuscitation (CPR) certificate.

Importance of Theoretical Concepts and Practical Competencies

To be a certified Can-Fit-Pro Personal Training Specialist is to have a solid foundational knowledge of theoretical fitness concepts as well as sound practical competencies to be able to provide safe, effective workouts for your clients and provide yourself with a stable, viable income-earning opportunity. You must know and be comfortable with the following.

Required theoretical concepts:

- The benefits of physical activity
- Wellness or holism
- Active living
- Exercise physiology (energy systems, oxygen transport, exercise response)
- Human anatomy (musculoskeletal and cardiovascular)
- Biomechanics (joints, levers, modifications, types of contractions)
- Relevance and interpretation of results of fitness assessments
- Principles of conditioning (FITT and SMART)
- Training program design
- Injury prevention and safety
- Basic nutrition (based on *Canada's Food Guide*)
- Healthy weight management

Required practical competencies:

- Act ethically and in the best interests of the client at all times
- Ability to recommend a variety of exercises and training programs for healthy adults
- Provide safe, effective and enjoyable workout delivery
- Demonstrate strong leadership and communication skills
- Demonstrate competent administration of a limited number of fitness assessments
- Demonstrate proper technique of exercises
- Create a client centred environment
- Educate clients about how their body responds to exercise
- Monitor client progress and ability
- Self evaluation of training effectiveness
- Ability to put theoretical knowledge into practice
- Present a professional appearance

Recommendations

In order to improve your chance for successful certification, we recommend that you prepare for the theory and practical certification exams by attending the Personal Training Specialist preparatory course. The course will help clarify the theory and practical requirements necessary to be a successful personal trainer and will prepare you for the exams.

To ensure that you are aware of the key theoretical and practical concepts being examined, we recommend that you purchase a copy of the Personal Training Specialist course manual, Can-Fit-Pro's *Fundamentals of Professional Personal Training* and the companion Study Guide.

In order to improve your chances of success, we recommend that you attempt the theory exam approximately three to four weeks after taking the Personal Training Specialist preparatory course. This time frame is designed to help you synthesize the course information while it is still top of mind.

To properly prepare for the practical exam, we recommend you practice working through the personal training client life-cycle process. In order to ensure you are ready to demonstrate all of the practical competencies required of a Can-Fit-Pro certified personal trainer we recommend that you invest approximately twenty hours honing your professional skills. If prepared, you may attempt the theory and practical exams on the same day, based on the availability of your PRO Trainer for the two examinations.

About Being a Can-Fit-Pro Personal Training Specialist

The Can-Fit-Pro Personal Training Specialist certification meets or exceeds all national standards for certification in Canada. To maintain a consistent standard of quality and excellence from all of our certified professionals, each must observe the *Can-Fit-Pro Certified Fitness Professional Code of Ethics* and the *Scope(s) of Practice* related to the designation(s) that they hold.

Can-Fit-Pro Certified Fitness Professional Code of Ethics

As a Can-Fit-Pro Certified Fitness Professional, I commit to:

- Educate others to perform safe and effective exercise.
- Motivate others to pursue a healthy, happy and balanced lifestyle.

- Communicate in a genuine, honest, and professional manner to all individuals.
- Continually strive to learn more about new research and exercise techniques.
- Protect and respect the confidentiality of all my professional fitness relationships at all times.
- Maintain annual CPR training and regular First Aid training.
- Respect business, employment and copyright laws.
- Secure liability insurance to properly protect myself and all the individuals who are involved with professional fitness services that I provide.
- Work within my Scope of Practice and refer individuals to more qualified professionals in the health care industry when necessary.
- Promote a fit and healthy lifestyle as a positive Can-Fit-Pro role model.

Can-Fit-Pro Personal Training Specialist Scope of Practice

A certified Can-Fit-Pro Personal Training Specialist is qualified to:

- Evaluate client needs in physical activity and nutrition based on the counseling foundations in the Personal Trainer Specialist program and provide the client with a safe and effective exercise plan based on their needs, abilities and goals.
- Confirm that clients have completed the Physical Activity Readiness Questionnaire (PAR-Q developed by Health Canada), and then provide an individualized training session to apparently healthy individuals who have no known major medical conditions.
- Monitor client resting and exercise heart rate and blood pressure regularly.
- Develop a client specific exercise plan within your level of ability and progress to more advanced training techniques with clients once the proper competency has been achieved.
- Modify all client exercise technique as needed to strive for optimal individual biomechanical effectiveness.
- Promote the benefits of regular physical activity and a balanced lifestyle combined with a healthy diet using Canada's Physical Activity Guide as a reference.
- Provide generalized advice on nutrition based on Canada's Food Guide. Individuals who require more specific advice on diet and supplements must be referred to a qualified nutrition professional.
- Answer general questions for participants on injuries or discomforts related to exercise. All injuries must be diagnosed and treated by a qualified medical professional.
- Provide emergency care based on the participant needs (contact EMS, provide Emergency First Aid or CPR).

As a certified Can-Fit-Pro Personal Training Specialist, I agree to provide a safe and effective individual exercise program that provides appropriate exercise selection and intensity to meet the individual needs of each adult client.

As a certified Can-Fit-Pro Personal Training Specialist, I agree to respect my role, abide by the Code of Ethics and work within my Scope of Practice at all times.

I recognize that failure to follow this Scope of Practice can result in immediate removal of my PTS certification designation.

Please note that the Can-Fit-Pro Personal Training Specialist Scope of Practice and Professional Code of Ethics are fluid documents that do evolve over time. Can-Fit-Pro will always post up to date versions of these documents when changes are made.

INTRODUCTION

Mike Bates, MBA

The fitness industry is consistently ranked as one of the fastest growing industries in the world. At present, there is a major need for personal trainers because most fitness clubs do not have enough trainers to meet the needs of their members. This is a great time for anyone considering the fitness industry as a full-time or part-time career.

What Is Personal Training?

A personal trainer is any certified person who works with clients in a one-on-one or group setting where the goal is to improve the client's level of fitness or health.

There are many benefits to working as a personal trainer. Some of the benefits include the following:

- Provides the opportunity to help people reach their goals and do things they didn't think they could do.
- You can set your own hours and decide how much you want to work.
- Once you have a clientele built up, your business will grow or sustain itself almost exclusively from referrals.
- An unlimited amount of educational material and support allows you to expand your knowledge base whenever you want.
- Has high income potential.

- Has low startup costs compared with many other careers and businesses.

As a Personal Trainer you can choose to work with many different types of populations or focus in on one type of clientele. Regardless of the audience you are attracting you will be judged on your professionalism, knowledge base, the results your clients get, and the consistent level of service you offer these clients. Whether you are working with clients at 6am or 10pm the expectations are the same. Successful trainers consistently show up with a peak attitude and that positive energy plays a role in motivating their clients to keep exercising. This is what clients expect.

As the populations continues to get older we can expect to see a greater emphasis placed on physical activity and its many benefits. Personal trainers have the potential to play a critical role in changing the lifestyle habits of many people in our society today. The fitness industry offers some unbelievable opportunities for anyone that enjoys fitness and is passionate about working with people. The information in this book will prepare you for your career in the field of Personal Training. This course is just the beginning of your educational journey. One of the keys to your long term success as a Personal Trainer is your willingness to constantly be educating yourself on the various changes and different approaches to working with clients. If you embrace this challenge we have no doubt you will be successful. Good luck!

PART I

Fitness Theory and Application

CHAPTER 1

Principles of Fitness, Health, and Wellness Concepts

Mike Bates, MBA
Rod Macdonald, BEd

CHAPTER OBJECTIVES

After completing this chapter, you will be able to

1. understand the difference between the primary components and the secondary components of fitness,

2. understand the concept of health and wellness and list the non-physical benefits,

3. list at least 5 benefits for each of the primary components of fitness,

4. understand the difference between the Health Canada and ACSM physical activity guidelines, and

5. understand each of the 9 principles that fall within the Can-Fit-Pro Personal Training Specialist Scope of Practice.

Fitness, Health, and Wellness

There are many ways to define or express physical fitness. One definition is that physical fitness is an improved physiological state that leads to improved health and longevity. Fitness is a complex concept that is easier to understand if it is broken down into various components.

Primary Components of Fitness

The four primary components (also known as the components of health related fitness) that are important to improved physical health are as follows:

- **Cardiorespiratory capacity** is the ability of the body to take in oxygen (respiration), deliver it to the cells (circulation), and use it at the cellular level to create energy (bioenergetics) for physical work (activity). In fitness, we also refer to cardiorespiratory capacity as *aerobic capacity*. This capacity includes aerobic endurance (how long), aerobic strength (how hard), and aerobic power (how fast). Some of the long-term adaptations of cardiorespiratory training are: decreased resting heart rate, decreased risk of cardiovascular disease, improved endurance, increased stroke volume and cardiac output.

- **Muscular capacity** refers to the spectrum of muscular capability. This includes muscular endurance (i.e., the ability to apply force over a long period of time or to complete repeated muscle contractions); muscular strength (i.e., the ability to generate force, or the maximum amount of force that a muscle can exert in a single contraction); and muscular power (i.e., the ability to generate strength in an explosive way). Some of the long-term adaptations of improving muscular capacity are increased strength, improved muscular endurance, increased basal metabolic rate, improved joint strength, and overall posture.

- **Flexibility** is the range of movement or amount of motion that a joint is capable of performing. Each joint has a different amount of flexibility. Some of the long-term adaptations of improved flexibility are decreased risk of injury, improved range of motion, improved bodily movements, and improved posture.

- **Body composition** is the proportion of fat-free mass (muscle, bone, blood, organs, and fluids) to fat mass (adipose tissue deposited under the skin and around organs). Some of the long-term adaptations of improving body composition are decreased risk of cardiovascular disease, improved basal metabolic rate, improved bodily function, and improved BMI.

Secondary Components of Fitness

The secondary components of fitness (also known as the components of performance based fitness) are involved in all physical activity and are necessary for daily functioning. Athletes experience different levels of success depending on how well these secondary fitness components are developed. Although the primary components of fitness are thought to be the most important, we should not ignore the secondary components because of their importance in the completion of daily tasks. The secondary components include the following.

- **Balance** is the ability to maintain a specific body position in either a stationary or dynamic (moving) situation.

- **Coordination** is the ability to use all body parts together to produce smooth and fluid motion.

- **Agility** is the ability to change direction quickly.

- **Reaction time** is the time required to respond to a specific stimulus.

- **Speed** is the ability to move rapidly. Speed is also known as *velocity* (rate of motion).

- **Power** is the product of strength and speed. Power is also known as *explosive strength.*

- **Mental capability** is the ability to concentrate during exercise to improve training effects as well as the ability to relax and enjoy the psychological benefits of activity (endorphins).

Health and Wellness

Health is a dynamic process because it is always changing. We all have times of good health, times of sickness, and maybe even times of serious illness. As our lifestyles change, so does our level of health.

Those of us who participate in regular physical activity do so partly to improve the current and future level of our health. We strive toward an optimal state of well-being. As our lifestyle improves, our health also improves and we experience less disease and sickness. When most people are asked what it means to be healthy, they normally respond with the four components of fitness mentioned earlier (cardiorespiratory ability, muscular ability, flexibility, and body composition). Although these components are a critical part of being healthy, they are not the only contributing factors. Physical health is only one aspect of our overall health.

The other components of health (Greenberg, 2004, p. 7) that are just as important as physical health include the following:

- **Social health**—The ability to interact well with people and the environment and to have satisfying personal relationships.

- **Mental health**—The ability to learn and grow intellectually. Life experiences as well as more formal structures (e.g., school) enhance mental health.

- **Emotional health**—The ability to control emotions so that you feel comfortable expressing them and can express them appropriately.

- **Spiritual health**—A belief in some unifying force. It varies from person to person but has the concept of faith at its core.

Wellness is the search for enhanced quality of life, personal growth, and potential through positive lifestyle behaviours and attitudes. If we take responsibility for our own health and well-being, we can improve our health on a daily basis. Certain factors influence our state of wellness, including nutrition, physical activity, stress-coping methods, good relationships, and career success.

Each day we work toward maximizing our level of health and wellness to live long, full, and healthy lives. The pursuit of health, personal growth, and improved quality of life relies on living a balanced life. To achieve balance, we need to care for our mind, body, and spirit, as demonstrated in figure 1.1.

If any of these three areas is consistently lacking or forgotten about, we will not be at our optimal level of health. We are constantly challenged with balancing each of these three areas throughout life.

As fitness professionals, we have a responsibility to guide and motivate others to improve their level of health and wellness. We can promote a holistic approach to health (mind, body, and spirit), not just encourage physical activity. As good role models, we should demonstrate positive health behaviours that assist in improving our own health

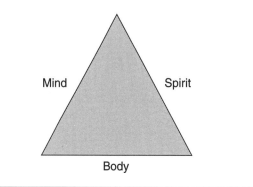

Figure 1.1   Mind-body-spirit balance.

and the health of others. If our focus is strictly on the physical benefits of exercise, we are doing a disservice to our clients and we are not fulfilling our professional obligation.

Benefits of Physical Activity

As fitness professionals, we spend a great deal of time inspiring and assisting others in their pursuit of improved health. Education is an important aspect of this. We must promote the benefits of regular activity and help people understand why they should be active.

Figure 1.2 will help you educate your clients about the benefits of activity and why each of these benefits is important to long-term health.

Activity Guidelines

Health Canada introduced *Canada's Physical Activity Guide to Healthy Active Living* to help Canadians make wise choices about physical activity as a way to improve health. Scientists say you should accumulate 60 minutes of physical activity every day to stay healthy or improve health. The recommendations in the Physical Activity Guide are as follows:

- Endurance—On 4 to 7 days a week, perform continuous activity for your heart, lungs, and circulatory system. Time required for improvements depends on effort.

- Flexibility—On 4 to 7 days a week, perform gentle reaching, bending, and stretching to keep muscles relaxed and joints mobile.

- Strength—On 2 to 4 days a week, perform resistance exercise to strengthen muscles and bones and improve posture.

Benefit	Effect on health
Reduces the risk of premature death.	Active people live longer with a better quality of life.
Reduces the risk of cardiovascular disease.	Strengthens the heart, cardiovascular system, and respiratory system to help fight cardiovascular disease.
Decreases resting heart rate.	Reduces the daily wear and tear on the cardiovascular system.
Keeps resting blood pressure normal.	Lessens the stress on the walls of the veins and arteries in the vascular system and reduces the risk of a coronary event or stroke.
Improves heart efficiency.	Improves the ability to perform daily activities at higher intensities with greater ease.
Decreases body fat.	Reduces the risk of major life-threatening diseases, such as cardiovascular disease and diabetes.
Increases HDL (good) cholesterol and decreases LDL (bad) cholesterol.	Reduces the risk of cardiovascular disease and atherosclerosis (hardening of the arteries).
Lowers the risk of developing diabetes.	Keeps body fat in control, increases cellular sensitivity to insulin, and helps regulate blood sugar levels.
Promotes joint stability.	Increases strength of all connective tissue, decreasing susceptibility to injury.
Increases muscular strength.	Improves ability to perform daily activities with less effort.
Strengthens bones.	Helps reduce the risk of osteoporosis and reduces the chance of injury and broken bones.
Increases muscle mass and decreases body fat.	Improves physique with more toned appearance, and the body burns more calories at rest and during exercise to sustain increased muscle.
Increases resting metabolism.	More calories are required by the body at rest, which helps with weight management.
Improves core strength.	Develops strong abdominals and back muscles for better posture and less chance of back pain.
Improves balance, coordination, and agility.	All movements in daily life become easier and safer when the body has better control.
Improves body image and self-esteem.	Exercisers experience improved mental health and self-image.
Reduces depression and anxiety.	An improved outlook on life makes all activities more enjoyable.
Assists in stress management.	Everyday life becomes more enjoyable because the person has a positive way to deal with stress.

Figure 1.2   Health benefits of regular activity.

The American College of Sports Medicine (ACSM) has also developed activity guidelines for improving health:

- Perform 30 minutes or more of moderate-intensity physical activity on most days of the week for cardiovascular health. The 30 minutes need not be continuous.

- Performing 1 set of 8 to 12 repetitions of resistance training for the entire body is necessary to maintain and develop muscular strength and endurance.

- Flexibility training should be performed daily, including stretches for all major muscle groups, in order to maintain mobility.

Can-Fit-Pro's Training Principles

When designing a program for a client, a personal trainer must be aware of the following collection of training principles. While these principles are not new, they have been adapted and assembled to fit within the scope of practice of a Can-Fit-Pro Personal Training Specialist.

As each component of fitness is examined in this text, these principles will be referred to again where appropriate.

- **FITT:** This principle suggests that when designing a personal training program, the Frequency, Intensity, Time and Type of exercise must be considered. Specifically, Frequency is how often the client should be performing a component of their program. Intensity is the difficulty level of the component of their program (as measured by load, reps, watts, etc.) Time is how long each component should last and how much rest the clients should have (usually measured in minutes or seconds). Type is the choice of exercise used for a given component of their program (usually defined as an exercise, piece of equipment or activity).

- **Individualization:** This principle suggests that programs and modifications to programs must be made to accommodate every person's individual needs. For example, two people with the same goal may require very different programs to achieve this goal. These differences may be due to a variety of variables including available training time, starting fitness level, experience, and virtually any other variable.

- **Specificity:** This principle suggests that if clients want to improve an aspect of their performance, they have to train that aspect. For example, if a client wants to be a better runner, strength training will probably deliver measurable improvements, but the client will still have to continue to run to optimize their results.

- **Progressive overload:** This principle suggests that to improve, clients must continually challenge their fitness. For example, if the client's fitness is not progressively challenged (through increased intensity, duration or complexity), the client will "plateau", or cease to make improvements. It is recommended that any progressive overload is in fact progressive and errs on the side of caution rather than too hard to ensure the client does not become discouraged, or worse, injured.

- **Recovery:** This principle becomes increasingly important as the clients' workouts become more successful. Recovery should not be seen as optional, but as a mandatory principle of training that must be considered for every program. For example, every program must consider other activities the client is engaged in, the type of work they perform, etc. The recovery must allow for the client to return to the next workout at least as fit as the previous workout, if not more fit. If your client does not have enough recovery, he will eventually become ill or injured and discontinue training altogether.

- **Structural tolerance:** This principle suggests that structural tolerance (the strengthening of tendons, ligaments, etc.) will result in the ability to sustain subsequently greater stresses in training, with a greater resistance to injury. While structural tolerance is a positive side effect of most exercise, some clients may require specific activities or exercises that improve structural tolerance. For example, a client who has a goal of running a marathon should have some exercises included in his program that specifically targets the ankles, knees, hips and back, as these areas will be stressed with marathon training.

- **All-around development:** This principle suggests that people who are well developed through all components of fitness are less likely to sustain injury and more likely to perform better in sport and in life. For example, a client who only wants to train cardio and dismisses flexibility and strength training is more likely to become injured should they ever need to call on their strength (i.e. changing a tire, shoveling snow, etc.)

- **Reversibility:** This principle suggests that once training ceases, the body will gradually return to a pre-training state. While at times frustrating to clients when faced with unexpected absences, the principle of reversibility should serve as a cautionary principle in that if the client (and trainer) is not consistent with their adherence to exercise they will lose the benefits and return to their pre-training state.

- **Maintenance:** This principle suggests that once a level of fitness has been achieved, it is possible to maintain it with less work than was needed to attain it. For example, to prevent the reversal of adaptation to exercise, your client could train as little as one third the volume, at the same intensity, for up to 12 weeks (Brooks, 2004)

Common Questions Personal Trainers Are Asked

1. **In order to lose weight around the abdominals, should I do exercises that focus on that region?**

   Research does not support spot reducing as an effective tool for reducing body fat in a particular region of the body. In order to lose body fat, the best option is to exercise large muscle groups that burn more calories. You will eventually see a decrease in body fat in the regions you would like. Ultimately, a large percentage of our figures are genetically determined. This is not to say that we cannot affect this shape, but our goals must be realistic and based on our individual capabilities. Doing 100 crunches will only improve the muscular endurance of the muscle groups in the abdominal region.

2. **Will I get big bulky muscles if I strength train?**

   For the majority of people, the answer to this is a definite no. Males have a significant advantage over females when it comes to building muscle due to the fact that their testosterone levels are 10 to 30 times higher than females. Beyond this, our potential to build muscle is largely determined by our genes and the percentage of fast-twitch and slow-twitch fibres we have. We can all improve our overall strength and muscle mass, but few people have the genetics and time needed to develop a high level of musculature. This is a common question that trainers get from female clients who are not interested in large muscles. The majority of these people who are concerned about this will never need to worry about it for the reasons just stated.

3. **How do I get muscle definition?**

   This is another area where genetics play a major role. As mentioned, we can all improve our health and physique, but we are also limited by our genetics. The best way to get muscle definition is to do the following:
   - Lose body fat.
   - Strength train.
   - Eat a sensible diet.

4. **Should I get into shape before I start to lift weights?**

   The answer is no. Strength training should be part of everyone's exercise program. People who are severely overweight may need to start strength training before they even step on a treadmill so that they can improve the strength of their joints. If strength training is done with minimal rest between exercises, a cardiorespiratory effect can be seen.

5. **If I want to lose weight, should my main focus be cardiorespiratory activities?**

   All programs should include a balance of cardiorespiratory exercise, strength training, and flexibility. If any of these are missing, clients will not see the full benefits from exercising. Strength training can play a major role in helping to lose weight because it burns extra calories in two different ways. First, you burn extra calories during the actual strength training session. Second, over a period of time you add muscle. Since muscle is an active tissue, it is constantly burning calories. This increases your basal metabolic rate, which is the rate at which you burn calories. By strength training, you will be burning more calories even when you are not exercising.

6. **Should a woman's exercise program differ from a man's?**

   From a purely physiological perspective, it is not true that programs should differ. Our muscle fibres are the same and our bodies will respond in similar ways to exercise. Obviously men and women are different, but a better approach to program design acknowledges that we are all different, and these individual differences are what a program should be based on. There are no legitimate organizations that recommend different standards for men and women.

Case Studies

Within this manual you will find continuing case studies at the end of each chapter. These case studies are based on the profiles of the three people described here. They provide a way for you to apply information as you are learning it and to see how the information can be used with a variety of clients. We hope you will find these examples helpful.

Profile 1: Roger

Roger is a 55-year-old male. He is currently working as a business administrator and is a year away from retirement. He is currently not active and he has just joined the gym. This is the first time he has been a member of a gym, but he is willing to work out at least 2 to 4 times a week for 45 to 60 minutes. Since Roger has been working a desk job for the past 30 years, he is concerned about maintaining joint function and mobility. He is overweight and would like to be able to prevent a heart attack. As a bonus to working out, he would not mind losing 5-7 kilograms (10 to 15 pounds) and gaining some muscle mass. He would like to see changes as soon as possible but trusts that a personal trainer will establish appropriate time frames for his goals.

Roger is not very excited about needing to exercise and has limited time due to his busy work schedule. His major barriers are the perceived young age and fitness level of most gym members. He does not feel that there will be many people like him working out in the gym. He is not likely to get much physical activity outside of the program you design for him. Since he has never worked out in a gym before, he does not have any major preferences in terms of equipment.

With respect to nutrition, Roger is aware that he needs to make some changes and is open to suggestions. He skips breakfast regularly, has two or three coffees per day, brings his lunch to work most days, eats a large meal for dinner, and snacks on high-calorie foods throughout the day.

Roger would like to work with a personal trainer twice a week to achieve his goals and is committed to working out twice more on his own. Roger has no major medical conditions and answered *no* to all the questions on the Physical Activity Readiness Questionnaire (PAR-Q). After a fitness assessment was done, it was found that Roger's resting heart rate (HR) is 81 beats per minute (bpm) and his resting blood pressure (BP) is 137/92 mmHg. Roger's waist girth is 109 centimeters (43 inches), he is 175 centimeters (5 feet, 8 inches) tall, and he weighs 89 kilograms (196 pounds). Roger's $\dot{V}O_2$max is 32 millilitres per kilogram per minute. Roger is able to do 11 push-ups and 19 curl-ups, and his grip strength is 42 kilograms (93 pounds) in the right hand and 39 kilograms (86 pounds) in the left. His trunk forward flexion is 14 centimetres (6 inches).

BMI 29.1—Overweight

Health risk—High

Resting HR—<10th percentile

Systolic BP—35th percentile (borderline hypertensive)

Diastolic BP—15th percentile (stage 1 hypertensive)

Aerobic capacity—30th percentile

Push-ups—30th percentile

Curl-ups—30th percentile

Grip strength—Fair

Trunk forward flexion—Needs improvement

Profile 2: Molly

Molly is a 22-year-old student. She is in her 3rd year at an university studying kinesiology, which takes up almost all of her spare time. She recently decided to join the university gym and take advantage of discounted student rates on personal training. She loves to play sports but is currently not active and is overweight. In high school, she was on the basketball and volleyball teams, which trained 3 or 4 times a week. Molly would like to get back to the way she looked and performed in high school. Her main goals are to improve her skills in sports (mostly basketball and volleyball), lose 7 kilograms (15 pounds), and increase her flexibility and endurance.

She loves exercising and is looking forward to making it a regular part of her lifestyle. Her perception is that she will need to work out for about 1.5 hours, 4 or 5 days per week in order to achieve her goals. She would love to lose 5 kilograms (10 pounds) within the next 2 months because she will be attending friend's wedding at that time. Her preferences are jogging and taking group fitness classes. Outside of her regular fitness routine, she would like to start playing volleyball again once or twice a week. She is committed to the program, but it may be difficult for her to make these drastic changes and stick to the program over the long term.

Her eating habits are fairly good, but she is aware that she needs to drink more water and cut back on alcoholic beverages when she is out with friends on the weekends.

Molly would like to work with a personal trainer once a week to achieve her goals and is committed to working out 4 additional days per week. She has no major medical conditions and answered *no* to all the questions on the PAR-Q. After completing a fitness assessment, it was found that Molly's resting HR is 75 bpm and her resting BP is 115/78 mmHg. Molly's waist girth is 71 centimeters (28 inches), she is 167.5 centimeters (5 feet, 6 inches) tall, and weighs 79.5 kilograms (175 pounds). Molly's $\dot{V}O_2$max is 35 millilitres per kilogram per minute. She is able to do 5 push-ups and 17 curl-ups, and her grip strength is 30 kilograms (66 pounds) in the right hand and 29 kilograms (64 pounds) in the left. Molly's trunk forward flexion measures 35 centimeters (14 inches).

BMI 28.3—Overweight

Health risk—Increased

Resting HR—20th percentile

Systolic BP—45th percentile

Diastolic BP—40th percentile

Aerobic capacity—50th percentile

Push-ups—<10th percentile

Curl-ups—30th percentile

Grip strength—Fair

Trunk forward flexion—Good

Profile 3: Jennifer

Jennifer is a 40-year-old career and family woman. She works full time for a bank and takes care of her family, which includes three young children. She is extremely busy and finds that she is exhausted by the end of the day. She recently joined the gym but can only work out 1 or 2 times a week for 30 to 45 minutes, with possibly a third additional workout. She would like an easy workout to increase endurance, strength, and muscle tone. She would also like suggestions on ways to work out outside of the gym (i.e., at work or home).

Jennifer's major barrier is time, and she has not been able to overcome this in the past. She does not have any other major barriers to exercising on her own or with a personal trainer. She is fairly well read with respect to exercise but is a little confused as to what she needs to do to achieve her goals. She has no major preferences regarding equipment but thinks she would like the elliptical machine for her cardio workouts.

Jennifer has good eating habits and other than following Canada's Food Guide, she does not have any major areas for improvement in this area.

Jennifer would like to work with a personal trainer at least once a week to help reach her goals. She has no major medical conditions and answered *no* to all the questions on the PAR-Q. After a fitness assessment was done, it was found that Jennifer's resting HR is 80 bpm and her resting BP is 120/80 mmHg. Jennifer's waist girth is 66 centimeters (26 inches), she is 155 centimeters (5 feet, 1 inch) tall, and weighs 55.5 kilograms (122 pounds). Jennifer's $\dot{V}O_2$max is 29.5 millilitres per kilogram per minute. She is able to do 10 push-ups and 15 curl-ups, and her grip strength is 27 kilograms (60 pounds) in the right hand and 29 kilograms (64 pounds) in the left. Jennifer's trunk forward flexion measures 13 inches (33 centimetres).

BMI 23.1—Normal

Health risk—None

Resting HR—10th percentile

Systolic BP—35th percentile

Diastolic BP—40th percentile

Aerobic capacity—40th percentile

Push-ups—30th percentile

Curl-ups—32nd percentile

Grip strength—Fair

Trunk forward flexion—Good

CHAPTER 2

Nutrition Concepts for Personal Trainers

Brian Justin, MHK

Gregory S. Anderson, PhD

CHAPTER OBJECTIVES

Upon completion of this chapter, you will be able to

1. list the six basic nutrients and explain their functions in health and activity,

2. explain basic principles in planning a healthy and balanced diet,

3. discuss the role of hydration in exercise and long-term health,

4. describe the concept of supplementation and analyze types of supplements and ergogenic aids, and

5. understand the Scope of Practice for certified Can-Fit-Pro Personal Training Specialists in providing nutritional information.

The science of nutrition has become more prevalent over the past decade. Our obsession with weight, fat, and dieting has led to the creation of a multibillion-dollar diet industry, primarily because the average person eats too much and exercises too little. The search for improved health has led to an increased interest in supplements, which are based on the idea that eating the proper foods is not enough to fight disease and maintain health. Most people now know more about cholesterol, fat, fibre, and the links between nutrition and disease than they did before. It is imperative that personal trainers keep up with current research on nutrition and also refer clients to a registered dietician or naturopathic or medical physician for concerns out of their scope of practice.

What Is Nutrition?

Nutrition is the study of food and how the body uses it. Nutrients are chemical components of foods that are essential for energy, growth, cellular repair, and regulation of metabolic functions.

Scope of Practice for Personal Trainers With Regard to Nutritional Counseling

Research on nutrition and food has evolved tremendously over the past decade. Nutrition is a complicated science. It is recommended that personal trainers team up with a dietician or naturopathic or medical physician to whom they can send clients. Establish a referral system and everyone wins!

We also recommend that personal trainers gain additional education on nutrition through the Can-Fit-Pro Nutrition and Wellness Specialist course. Although you can provide nutritional information to clients, remember that personal trainers are not qualified to prescribe or recommend supplements of any kind. Personal trainers are also not able to perform a client diet analysis. Instead, a competent personal trainer can offer general nutritional advice and information based on Canada's Food Guide. Respect the scope of your abilities at all times. In a later section, we will highlight how you can help clients eat more healthfully within your scope of practice. In the meantime, let's discuss the nuts and bolts of nutrition.

What Are the Essential Nutrients?

The body needs six essential nutrients, or components of food, to function. Carbohydrate, fat, and protein are energy nutrients because they provide energy for the body. They are referred to as *macronutrients*. Energy in food is measured in units called *calories*. The remaining three nutrients are vitamins, minerals, and water. They do not provide energy, but they do play a critical role in health. Vitamins are referred to as *micronutrients* because they are needed in relatively small amounts to support normal health and body functions.

What Is Carbohydrate?

Carbohydrate is an important energy source for working muscles and for the brain and nervous tissue. It also assists digestion by providing dietary fibre. Carbohydrate molecules are composed of chains of carbon, hydrogen, and oxygen and provide the body with its most efficient and accessible source of energy. Carbohydrate breaks down into glucose, which is used in the production of adenosine triphosphate (ATP) for cellular energy.

What Are the Categories of Carbohydrate?

The two primary carbohydrate categories are simple (e.g., sugars like jam, syrup, honey, fruit) and complex (e.g., bread, pasta, cereal, potatoes, vegetables). The best sources of carbohydrate are natural sugars in vegetables, fruit, dairy, and whole grains because they also contain other essential nutrients, such as vitamins, minerals, and fibre. On average, Canadians get slightly more than half of their energy from simple carbohydrate. Much of this simple sugar intake is from added sugars in processed food instead of healthy sources such as fruit. Soft drinks are a common source of added sugar. The average Canadian drinks 100 litres of pop a year. Considering that one can of regular cola contains 10 teaspoons of sugar, 100 litres amounts to 11,320 grams of sugar each year! Other common sources of unhealthy simple sugars are cakes, cookies, pies, fruit punches, and candy. Canadians do not eat enough complex carbohydrate, which is a problem since complex carbohydrate is also a source of dietary fibre. The required intake of fibre is 25 grams for women and 38 grams for men, or 14 grams for every 1,000 calories ingested. Good sources of complex carbohydrate are vegetables, whole grains, and legumes.

How Many Calories Are Found in Carbohydrate?

One gram of carbohydrate equals 4 calories. To estimate the total number of calories from carbohydrate in a particular food, take the total grams of carbohydrate and multiply by 4. For example, if four crackers contain 18 grams of carbohydrate, then the total number of calories from carbohydrate would be 72 (18 grams × 4 calories).

How Much Carbohydrate Should We Consume?

The acceptable macronutrient distribution range (AMDR) for carbohydrate intake as established in 2002 by the Food and Nutrition Board of the Institute of Medicine is 45% to 65% of total caloric intake. No more than 25% of carbohydrate intake should be from simple sugars.

What Are Good Sources of Carbohydrate?

Good carbohydrate sources are vegetables, fruits, whole grains, dairy products, and legumes.

How Is Carbohydrate Used During Exercise?

The higher the intensity of exercise, the greater the reliance on carbohydrate. This relates to anaerobic metabolism, which uses only glucose as fuel. Even low-intensity exercise requires carbohydrate, but to a lesser extent because fat can also be used. Thus, all exercise depends to some degree on carbohydrate. Factors that increase reliance on carbohydrate are high-intensity exercise, long-duration activity, exercise in hot or cold temperatures, exercise at altitude, and age (children require more carbohydrate than adults). Factors that decrease the reliance on carbohydrate are endurance training, good conditioning (because you can use more fat for energy), and temperature adaptation.

Active people need to consume enough carbohydrate because it provides fuel for brain cells, red blood cells, and muscles. When carbohydrate intake is insufficient, body protein is used for energy. In addition, you will have to reduce the exercise intensity so that you can rely more on fat for energy. Ideally, active people should consume mostly complex carbohydrate and should consume simple carbohydrate during and immediately after exercise.

What Is Fat?

Fat is one form of a larger group of substances known as *lipids*. The term *fat* applies to lipids that are solid at room temperature. *Oil* is the term for lipids that are liquid at room temperature. Lipids are not soluble in water. They are a major fuel source because they have a high concentration of calories. Fat provides essential fatty acids needed for cell membranes, production of hormones, healthy skin, feeling of satiety from meals, taste enhancement, and transportation of fat-soluble vitamins (A, D, E, and K). Animal products (meat, butter, dairy) and plant products (oil, margarine, nuts) are common sources of dietary fat. Consumption of saturated fat (i.e., fat that is solid at room temperature) should be limited, and we should consume moderate amounts of unsaturated fat (i.e., fat that is liquid at room temperature).

What Are the Three Types of Lipids in Foods?

The three types of lipids in foods are triglycerides, phospholipids, and sterols. Triglycerides represent 95% of the fat we eat. They consist of three fatty acids attached to a glycerol backbone, and they are classified according to their length, saturation, and shape. There are three types of chain lengths: short (fewer than 6 carbon atoms), medium (6-12 carbon atoms), and long (14 or more carbon atoms). Longer chains are found in meat, fish, and vegetable oils, and medium chains are found in dairy products. Fatty acid chain length is important because it determines the method of fat digestion and absorption as well as how fat functions within the body.

Saturation refers to the amount of hydrogen atoms in a fat. If a fat contains a double bond, it will exclude some hydrogen atoms, making it less saturated. Monounsaturated fats contain one double bond and are liquid at room temperature. Sources include olive oil, canola oil, and cashew nuts. Polyunsaturated fats contain more than one double bond and are also liquid at room temperature. Sources include canola oil, corn oil, and safflower oils. Saturated fats contain no double bond and are solid at room temperature. Sources include butter, cream, lard, and beef.

How Many Calories Are Found in Fat?

For every gram of fat, 9 calories are provided. To estimate the total number of calories from fat in a particular food, take the total grams of fat and multiply by 9. For example, if four crackers contain 3 grams of fat, then the total number of calories from fat would be 27 calories (3 grams × 9 calories).

What Are the Essential Fatty Acids?

The essential fatty acids are linoleic (omega-6) and linolenic (omega-3) fatty acids. They are essential because the body cannot make them. Sources of omega-6 fatty acids are safflower oil, peanut oil, vegetable oil, and corn oil. Sources of omega-3 fatty acids are cold-water fish, leafy green vegetables, flaxseed and its oil, fish oil, and canola oil. Omega-3 fatty acids tend to reduce inflammatory responses and reduce blood clotting and plasma triglycerides, thus helping to reduce the risk of a heart attack. It is prudent to include more fish and leafy green vegetables in the diet to increase omega-3 fatty acids because there tends to be an overconsumption of omega-6 fatty acids in the modern diet.

How Much Fat Should We Consume?

The AMDR for fat intake is 20% to 35% of total calories. Good sources include fish, avocados, olive oil, nuts, and seeds. Avoid hydrogenated fats, fast food, and fried foods because they are sources of unhealthy fat. Also, be aware of unhealthy fats in cakes, cookies, and processed foods.

How Are Lipids Used in Exercise?

The lower the intensity of exercise, the greater the proportion of fat burned to satisfy energy needs. As exercise intensity increases, the proportion of fat burned decreases and the proportion of carbohydrate burned increases. Many people believe they should perform lower intensity exercise to burn more fat and thus decrease levels of body fat. However, the proportion of fat burned should not be confused with the total amount of fat burned. As exercise intensity increases, the number of calories burned increases. Although the proportion of fat burned decreases to satisfy the energy needs of the higher intensity activity, the total energy requirement increases and therefore the total volume of fat burned is greater. Therefore, exercise at an intensity that allows for maximum calories burned (minimum of 65% of $\dot{V}O_2$max if possible) and ignore the fat-burning charts on cardio training machines!

It is well known that with endurance training, aerobic metabolism becomes more efficient and can use more fat during physical activity. This spares carbohydrate and improves endurance performance.

What Is Protein?

Protein molecules are large, complex, and found in the cells of all living things. The major role of protein is to build and repair body tissues, such as muscles, tendons, and ligaments. It is not a primary source of energy, except when the body does not get enough carbohydrate or fat due to starving, dieting, or overexercising. Protein is useful for transporting fluids, creating hormones and enzymes, and helping with immune responses.

Protein is made up of chemical structures called *amino acids*. Animal protein (meat, eggs, fish, or dairy) contains all nine essential amino acids and thus is a complete protein. Protein from other sources, like nuts, seeds, beans, and whole grains, is incomplete because it does not contain all essential amino acids. Incomplete proteins must be combined for proper use in the body.

How Many Calories Are Found in Protein?

There are 4 calories in a gram of protein. To estimate the total number of calories from protein in a particular food, take the total grams of protein and multiply by 4. For example, if four crackers contain 2 grams of protein, then the total number of calories from protein would be 8 calories (2 grams × 4 calories).

How Much Protein Should We Consume?

The AMDR percentage of daily protein intake ranges from 10% to 35% of total calories. Another way of calculating protein intake is to use the established recommended dietary allowance (RDA) of 0.8 gram per kilogram of body weight to determine protein needs in grams. However, athletes should increase their protein intake to 1.2 to 1.7 grams per kilogram. The reasoning for this is based on four factors:

1. Athletes have more lean muscle mass, which requires more protein.
2. Athletes lose a small amount of protein in the urine, whereas nonathletes do not.
3. Athletes burn a small amount of protein during physical activity.
4. Athletes require additional protein to recover from muscle damage.

In reality, most athletes consume enough protein to meet these requirements.

How Is Protein Used During Exercise?

If protein is being used as fuel during exercise, then not enough carbohydrate has been consumed. Protein is best used for other functions in the body. High-protein foods have a long gastric-emptying time and so are not recommended immediately before or during exercise. However, consuming a drink with 0.1 gram of protein per kilogram of body weight after heavy resistance exercise does appear to improve muscle protein balance.

What Are Vitamins?

Vitamins are organic compounds that are necessary for good health. The body is not capable of making vitamins, so they must be supplied through diet. Vitamins do not supply energy, but they are necessary for the metabolism of carbohydrate and fat. Some vitamins interact with minerals.

Vitamins are grouped into two categories: water soluble (vitamin B complex and vitamin C) and fat soluble (vitamins A, D, E, and K). Water-soluble vitamins are easily dissolved in water and excess amounts are excreted in urine. Fat-soluble vitamins are absorbed along with fat in the small intestines and excess is stored in the body.

How Can We Maximize Vitamin Intake From Food?

To maximize vitamin intake from your diet, follow these three steps:

1. Eat a variety of colourful fruits and vegetables.
2. Eat fresh fruits and vegetables as much as possible, especially those that are in season.
3. Don't overcook vegetables; keep them a little crunchy.

Dietary Reference Intakes, Functions, Food Sources, and Athletic Requirements for Vitamins

Table 2.1 shows all pertinent information regarding vitamins.

TABLE 2.1 **Vitamins**

VITAMIN	DRI	FUNCTIONS	FOOD SOURCES	DEFICIENCY SYMPTOMS	TOXICITY SYMPTOMS
Vitamin B$_1$ (thiamin)	Male: 1.2 mg Female: 1.1 mg	Carbohydrate metabolism Nervous system function	Whole grains Nuts Legumes	Confusion Weakness Calf pain Heart disease	None known
Vitamin B$_2$ (riboflavin)	Male: 1.3 mg Female: 1.1 mg	Energy metabolism Protein metabolism Skin and eye health	Milk Eggs Dark-green leafy vegetables Whole grains	Inflamed tongue Weakness Fatigue Light sensitivity	None known
Niacin	Male: 16 mg Female: 14 mg	Energy metabolism Glycolysis Fat synthesis	Milk Eggs Turkey Chicken Fish Whole grains	Skin rash Dementia Weakness Lethargy Pellagra	Flushing, burning, and tingling of extremities Gastric ulcers
Vitamin B$_6$ (pyridoxine)	Male: 1.3-1.7 mg Female: 1.3-1.5 mg	Protein metabolism Fat metabolism Glycolysis	Eggs Meats Whole grains	Nausea Mouth sores Impaired immune system Convulsions	Loss of balance and coordination Peripheral neuritis
Vitamin B$_{12}$ (cobalamin)	2.4 μg	Protein metabolism Fat metabolism Glycolysis	Eggs Meats Poultry Cheese	Pernicious anemia Weakness Fatigue	None known

(continued)

Table 2.1   *(continued)*

VITAMIN	DRI	FUNCTIONS	FOOD SOURCES	DEFICIENCY SYMPTOMS	TOXICITY SYMPTOMS
Folic acid	400 μg	Red blood cell development Fetal development	Green leafy vegetables Beans Whole grains Oranges Bananas	Neurological disorders Fatigue Weakness Neural tube defects	None established
Biotin	30 μg	Gluconeogenesis Glucose and fatty acid synthesis	Egg yolks Dark-green leafy vegetables	Muscle pain Dermatitis Depression (these symptoms rarely occur)	None established
Pantothenic acid	5 mg	Energy metabolism Gluconeogenesis	All nonprocessed foods	Unknown	None established
Vitamin C (ascorbic acid)	Male: 90 mg Female: 75 mg	Collagen formation Iron absorption	Fresh fruits and vegetables	Bleeding gums Destruction of muscles and tendons	Kidney stone formation
Vitamin A (retinol)	Male: 900 μg Female: 700 μg	Eye health Immune system health Cell health	Butter Cheese Liver Egg yolks Pigmented fruits and vegetables	Dry skin Headache Blindness Bone pain Irritability	Liver damage Bone malformation
Vitamin D (calciferol)	5 μg	Absorption of calcium and phosphorus Healthy skin	Sun exposure Fish liver oil Eggs	Osteomalacia Osteoporosis	Nausea Loss of muscle function Organ damage
Vitamin E (tocopherol)	15 mg	Antioxidant	Vegetable oils Eggs	Rarely occur	None established
Vitamin K	Male: 120 μg Female: 90 μg	Bone strengthening Blood clot development	Dark-green leafy vegetables Intestinal bacteria	Rarely occur	None established

DRI = dietary reference intake (for adults)

Adapted, by permission, from D. Benardot, 2006, *Advanced Sports Nutrition* (Champaign, IL: Human Kinetics), 39-53.

What Are Minerals?

Minerals are simple but important nutrients that serve a variety of functions. For example, sodium and potassium assist with levels of body fluid, calcium and phosphorus are essential for bone health, iron is important for hemoglobin and the transport of oxygen, and iodine helps regulate metabolism. There are 20 to 30 important minerals, and they are required in small amounts. Most minerals are easily accessible with a balanced diet, so supplementation is rarely recommended.

What Is Hyponatremia?

Hyponatremia occurs from a failure to consume sodium when fluid and sodium losses are high. Sodium levels in the blood become low due to the production of a large volume of sweat. Hyponatremia can also be caused by medications, and clients should check with their doctors regarding the medications they use. This condition is generally only seen in athletes who participate in ultraendurance events.

How Important Is Water Intake?

Water is essential for survival. About 60% of the body is water. Water is used during digestion and metabolism, assisting with chemical reactions, carrying oxygen through blood, regulating body temperature, lubricating joints, removing waste, and assisting with respiration.

The body loses water during both daily life and exercise. The dietary reference intake (DRI) for water as established by the Food and Nutrition Board of the Institute of Medicine is 3.7 litres of total water per day for men (19-50 years) and 2.7 litres for women (19-50 years). This amount can include beverages other than water as long as they do not dehydrate the body. Thirst is the first sign of dehydration, so remind clients to drink water even before they are thirsty. Consuming regular amounts of water throughout the day satisfies the body's need for this important nutrient. Factors that increase water needs are alcohol consumption; physical activity; hot weather; medications; pregnancy; prolonged diarrhea; vomiting; burns; surgery; and increased dietary fibre, protein, salt, or sugar.

Encourage clients to consume 250-500 ml (8 to 16 ounces) of water at least 1 hour before exercise and if possible, 250 ml (8 ounces) of water 20 minutes before exercise. Drink 125-250 ml (4 to 8 ounces) every 10 to 15 minutes during exercise and 500 ml (16 ounces) for every pound of weight lost after exercise. Stay hydrated for good health.

If your urine is dark yellow, you need more water. Ideally, urine should be pale yellow or clear. If you have taken any vitamin supplements, they may alter the color (e.g., B vitamins create yellow urine).

Should We Take Supplements and Ergogenic Aids?

Everyone possesses natural abilities based on genetics, but not everyone has the potential to be Olympic champions. However, we can all enhance our health through physiological and psychological training. Many clients also search for ways to improve their bodies or accelerate their performance through the use of supplements or ergogenic aids.

What Are Ergogenic Aids?

Ergogenic aids are substances or treatments that are designed to improve physiological or psychological functions. *Ergogenic* refers to an increase in the rate of work output.

The policies and rules governing the use of ergogenic aids in the sport world are clear. Amateur athletes must abide by the rules established by the International Olympic Committee (IOC) to be eligible for competition. Many professional sports have strict requirements and suspensions for the use of unapproved substances.

The average client might search for enhanced performance by using some of the same substances that elite athletes use. How should personal trainers advise clients when they ask us about supplements and ergogenic aids? The best approach is education.

If approached by a client regarding a supplement or ergogenic aid, conduct thorough research to determine an educated response.

- Respect the scope of your abilities at all times and refer your clients to a nutritionist for specific advice.

- Remember that our responsibility as personal trainers is to help clients by offering general nutritional advice and information.

- Do not recommend any sport supplements or ergogenic aids. Refer clients to a dietician or naturopathic or medical physician for this information. You do not know the potentially fatal interactions among food, supplements, and individual physiology that could occur.

Table 2.2 is a partial list of available supplements and ergogenic aids. It is a brief resource designed to encourage personal trainers to do additional research in this area.

How Can We Help Clients Eat Better?

The following five points can help you develop a strategy for guiding clients toward healthy eating.

1. Teach clients about *Canada's Food Guide.* However, sometimes the food guide does not fit everyone. At this point, you should refer your client to a dietician or physician to discuss food allergies, intolerances, and other food pyramids that may match their individual physiology.

2. Teach correct portion sizes. The following visual aids of serving sizes may help with this:

- Raw vegetables: size of a salad bowl

TABLE 2.2   **Supplements and Ergogenic Aids**

SUPPLEMENT	CLAIMS	EFFECTIVENESS AND CONCERNS
Caffeine	Stimulates fat utilization.	Must be taken in very large quantities before being effective. Large doses are not recommended for the average population as it increases blood pressure, heart rate, and cardiovascular risk.
Chromium	Believed to enhance insulin sensitivity to reduce body fat and stimulate muscle growth.	Research findings are unclear. Larger doses may accumulate in the body, causing cell damage.
Creatine	Used in an attempt to increase power, speed, and body mass.	Supplementation shows an increase in creatine stored in muscle and an increase in body mass. It is not evident that the increase is muscle because of water gain with creatine. Side effects include excessive thirst and muscle cramping. Long-term effects not known.
Dehydroepiandrosterone (DHEA)	Used in an attempt to decrease body fat and increase muscle mass.	Most studies show that DHEA is most effective after the age of 50 (natural DHEA declines with age) and is not recommended for younger people.
Ephedrine	Used to curb appetite and promote weight loss.	Can have serious side effects, including excessive nervous tension, headaches, and irregular heartbeats.
Protein supplements	Claims to guarantee adequate protein for muscle building.	Most clients can consume adequate protein through natural dietary sources (0.8 g/kg of body weight per day for sedentay adults; 1.2-1.8 g/kg of body weight per day for competitive adult athletes). Most supplements contain only small amounts of protein.
Multivitamin and mineral supplements	Used for health and recovery from exercise.	Each client should be evaluated on an individual basis. Most clients get what they require from a balanced diet. To determine the need for supplements, consult a professional dietician or physician.

- Cooked vegetables: size of a computer mouse
- 90 grams (3 ounces) of protein: size of a deck of cards
- 30 grams (1 ounce) of cheese: size of a computer disk
- Cold cereal: size of a baseball
- Cooked cereal: size of an English muffin

You can also use a scale or measuring cups to measure out food portions so that clients get a glimpse of the real serving sizes.

3. Teach healthy food choices. This will require you to do research beyond this manual to determine the healthiest choices in each food group. For example, brown rice is a better choice than white rice for grain servings because it pos-

sesses nutrients that are removed during the processing of white rice.

4. Teach clients how to read ingredient lists and food labels. Ingredient lists are ordered in most to least by weight (i.e., the largest ingredient is listed first). Look for words that end in -ose, such as fructose, to detect sugar sources. Also, if you can't recognize what is on the list, put it back on the shelf. As for food labels, look at serving sizes, amount of saturated fat, calories from fat, and the percentage of daily value in that serving size.

5. Encourage clients to consume calories evenly throughout the day. Many people consume few calories during the day only to gorge themselves at night because they are so hungry. If calories are consumed evenly throughout the day, it will optimize alertness, energy, and the caloric needs for basic metabolic maintenance and daily physical activity. Encourage clients to eat every 3 to 4 hours.

A Plan for Good Nutrition

Most Canadians believe that they are well informed about proper nutrition. Here are basic guidelines for developing a healthy diet.

- Eat a variety of foods. Follow Canada's Food Guide, consuming the recommended amounts from each food group.
- Choose a diet low in fat and limit saturated fat and cholesterol for heart health.
- Eat plenty of vegetables, fruits, and grains.
- Limit simple sugars.
- Eat a moderate amount of salt and sodium. Choose sea salt more often.
- Drink alcoholic beverages in moderation.
- Balance food intake with physical activity.
- Monitor caloric intake to regulate a healthy weight.

For more information, review Canada's Food Guide. Original copies are available from your local health unit for distribution to clients or online at www.hc-sc.gc.ca/fn-an/food-guide-aliment/index_e.html.

Case Studies

Roger

In order to help Roger reach his goals of losing 5-7 kilograms (10 to 15 pounds) and improve his other fitness parameters, assessing his diet would be a prudent step. It would be advisable for Roger to log 2 weekdays and 1 weekend day of what and how much he eats and drinks. From this log you can then analyze how many servings of each food group Roger is getting and in what quantity. If the amounts from the various food groups are unbalanced, it would then be advisable to present a food guide booklet to Roger and show him the appropriate serving number and size of servings and compare this with his log. He will then see how he needs to be more conscious of what he is consuming. This also needs to be done for hydration. If he is not getting adequate water (8-10 cups, or he reports that his urine is dark yellow), he will need to

be taught the importance of carrying a water bottle with him to sip on throughout the day.

Finally, it is important to teach Roger how to choose healthy foods from each food group. For example, if Roger is eating white bread from the grains food group, you can educate him about choosing whole-grain bread because it possesses more nutritional value. Not all foods in each group are equal in nutritional value. Point out foods that are minimally processed and contain healthy fats, whole grains, and quality proteins, as well as in-season produce. With these suggestions, Roger will be empowered to choose better foods that will supply him with the energy he needs to improve his muscular fitness, lose body fat, and improve his BP. For specific recommendations, Roger should work with a registered dietician.

Molly

In order to help Molly reach her goals of losing 7 kilograms (15 pounds) and improving her other fitness parameters, assessing her diet would be a great first step. You should advise Molly to log 2 weekdays and 1 weekend day of what and how much she eats and drinks. From her log, you can then analyze how many servings of each food group she is eating and in what quantity. If the food group amounts are unbalanced, it would then be advisable to present a food guide booklet to her and show her the appropriate serving size and number and compare this with her log. Since she is a kinesiology student, you may want to share with her the idea that what she eats constitutes the health of the tissues that she uses when exercising. You could even pose the question, "Do you want your tissues to be formed from fast food or from healthy food?" She will then see how she needs to be more conscious of what she eats.

This also needs to be done for hydration. If she is not getting adequate water (8-10 cups, or she reports that her urine is dark yellow), she will need to be taught the importance of carrying a water bottle around campus to sip on throughout the day and to avoid nonnutritious fluids such as soda pop from the vending machines around the school. It is important to let Molly know that dehydration affects physical work capacity and can negatively affect sport performance, so if she is trying to improve her sport skills she needs to ensure good hydration.

Finally, it is important to teach the importance of making healthy choices from each food group.

For example, if Molly is eating white rice from the grains food group, you can educate her about choosing brown rice because it possesses more nutritional value. Not all foods in each group are equal in nutritional value. Point out foods that are minimally processed and contain healthy fats, whole grains, and quality proteins, as well as in-season produce. Additionally, it would be advisable to discuss how she can make quick, healthy meals and snacks that she can take to school to fortify her nutritional intake and avoid buying fast food on an impulse. With these suggestions, you will augment Molly's fitness plan to get in better shape by teaching her how to provide herself with energy-producing food to fuel her workouts and student life. For specific recommendations, Molly should work with a registered dietician.

Jennifer

It sounds like Jennifer has a lot on her plate (no pun intended). As with Roger and Molly, it is important to assess her dietary intake by logging the amounts and types of foods that she eats.

Because she is busy, you may only want to log 1 weekday instead of 2 and 1 weekend day. Supply her with a copy of the food guide and show her what groups she needs to increase and decrease. If her children are old enough, perhaps suggest that the family pitch in on making salads, cutting carrot sticks, helping pack lunches, and so on. A team effort can make it easier to keep the whole family eating healthy foods. As a trainer, you could offer a session with her family to talk about food labels and healthy food choices. This way shopping can be a quicker task because each family member knows what to look for.

A busy mom and employee like Jennifer needs to ensure good hydration to maintain her work capacity. Be sure to educate her on the importance of water intake and minimizing the fluids that do not support good hydration, such as coffee and pop. These suggestions along with her well-designed fitness program will get her on the way to a healthy lifestyle that she will be able to pass on to her children as well. For specific recommendations, Jennifer should work with a registered dietician.

cs Concepts

hD

...er, you will be able to

...nergy for exercise,

...etabolism,

...f ATP,

...ween aerobic and anaerobic production of energy,

...rgy systems produce ATP, and

...nt of the energy systems through interval conditioning.

Definitions

Bioenergetics is the study of how energy flows in the human body. In this chapter, we are concerned primarily with the conversion of food as large molecules of carbohydrate, protein, and fat into a useful form of energy (ATP) for exercise or activity.

Energy can be defined as the ability to do physical work. In daily life we see many forms of energy, such as electrical energy (light), heat (fire), chemical energy (gasoline), and mechanical energy (water to turn a turbine). In examining how the body is capable of performing muscle contraction, we analyze the conversion of chemical energy (food) into mechanical energy (muscle contraction).

Homeostasis is best described as a state of stability or balance where all body functions occur easily and the demand for energy is comfortably met by the supply of available energy. Homeostasis is also called *steady state*, but that does not mean that body functions are stable; instead, they are constantly changing as they adapt to the environment to maintain overall balance.

Metabolism is the sum of all chemical reactions in the body that either use or create energy. In some cases large molecules are broken down into smaller ones (also known as a *catabolic process*, such as the digestion of food), and in other cases the cells build larger molecules from smaller ones (also known as an *anabolic process*, such as the use of amino acids to build muscle). The combination of these catabolic and anabolic processes in the body is collectively called *metabolism*. The energy either used or created from all of the metabolic processes is called *ATP*.

What Is ATP?

Adenosine triphosphate, or ATP, is a chemical compound made up of adenosine and three phosphate molecules. ATP is the energy currency of the body: If you want to perform any activity, you must pay for it in ATP.

The chemical form of ATP looks like this:

Adenosine-P~P~P

*Note: - is a low-energy bond and ~ is a high-energy bond.

When food is broken down, the released energy is captured into the ATP compound to power all cellular needs. How this process is completed is the subject of this chapter.

How Is ATP Created?

The human body has the capacity to create and store its own ATP to use for energy. Whether at rest or exercising at an extreme intensity, the muscles and functions of the body require a specific amount of ATP to accomplish these tasks. Depending on the intensity and the availability of oxygen, the cells of the body can produce ATP using both anaerobic and aerobic metabolic methods.

Introduction to the Energy Systems

The human body uses three systems when forming ATP:

1. ATP–CP (creatine phosphate) system
2. Lactic acid or glycolytic energy system
3. Aerobic or oxidative energy system

The ATP–CP and glycolytic energy systems are both **anaerobic** systems, meaning they operate without the use of oxygen. *Aerobic* means "with oxygen," and the **aerobic** system uses oxygen. The anaerobic systems are limited and inefficient, whereas the aerobic system is very efficient because it uses an abundant supply of fat and carbohydrate to create ATP to fuel activity. While all three energy systems function together at any one time to provide the energy the body requires, there are times when certain systems become more prodominant. For example, the anaerobic systems provide much of the energy at the start of exercise, when intensity increases (i.e., pace increases), and during high-intensity activity (i.e., sprints, agility drills, heavy lifts) (see table 3.1).

Anaerobic Metabolism

As mentioned, in anaerobic metabolism ATP is made through a chemical reaction that does not require oxygen. The activity is so intense that the body cannot get oxygen to the muscles in time to produce ATP oxidatively to meet the energy demand. ATP must therefore be made without the presence of oxygen. Let's look at the two subcategories of anaerobic metabolism that can create ATP.

ATP–CP Phosphagen System

This system provides fuel for up to 10 seconds at maximal intensity. ATP and CP are high-energy

TABLE 3.1 Expressions of Exercise Intensity

CLASSIFICATION OF INTENSITY	RPE	PERCENTAGE OF HRR	PERCENTAGE OF HRMAX
Very light	<10	<30%	<35%
Light	10-11	30%-49%	35%-59%
Somewhat hard	12-13	50%-74%	60%-79%
Hard	14-16	75%-84%	80%-89%
Very hard	>16	>85%	>90%

compounds stored in limited amounts (4-5 calories) in muscles and other cells. For the startup of intense activity, and especially for brief, very intense activity, this system provides the ATP for muscle contraction to occur. This system works in two phases:

- **ATP–CP phase 1: stored ATP (fuel for 1-2 seconds at maximal effort).** When the nervous system signals a muscle to contract the ATP is split

ATP (splits) → ADP + P + energy,

forming ADP and P (adenosine diphosphate and phosphate) with a concomitant release of energy to allow the muscle to contract:

Adenosine-P-P-P → ADP + P + E*.

E* = energy release.

- **ATP–CP phase 2: creatine phosphate (the phosphagen system).** CP is the backup for ATP. It is a high-energy chemical compound stored in the muscle cell in greater quantities than ATP. With the aid of an enzyme called *creatine kinase*, CP splits (releasing energy and a phosphate) to provide energy to re-form ATP from ADP. Creatine kinase is stimulated by the concentration of ADP in the cell. This provides a feedback mechanism for rapidly forming ATP from the high-energy phosphates, which allows the muscle to keep contracting until the ATP and CP levels decline to the point that the body must slow down and draw upon the lactic acid system to continue. This reaction is outlined here:

ADP + CP → ATP + creatine

⇑

creatine kinase

The breakdown of stored ATP and the resynthesis using CP are both anaerobic chemical reactions. In other words, the reaction occurs without oxygen being available to the cell.

The total amount of stored ATP and CP is limited to approximately 10 seconds of intense effort. Once the storage is depleted, the cells will no longer be able to provide ATP at the same high rate, and the body will have to slow down so that metabolism can match energy needs through glycolysis, the next fastest method to synthesize ATP.

Glycolytic System

This system provides fuel for up to 2 minutes at maximal intensity. The glycolytic energy pathway is a series of 10 enzymatically driven reactions that cause the breakdown of carbohydrate in the form of glycogen stored in the muscle cell or glucose found in the blood. These reactions take place in the cytoplasm of the cell. This method of metabolism creates energy in the form of two to three ATP molecules, depending on the source. From glucose, it produces two ATP molecules, and from glycogen, it produces three ATP molecules. The reason for the difference is due to one ATP being used in one of the reactions of glucose breakdown. A three-carbon compound called *pyruvate* is also formed. This breakdown occurs without oxygen and therefore is an incomplete chemical reaction. The glycolytic energy pathway results in the reduction of pyruvate to form a cellular by-product called *lactic acid* (LA).

The chemical reaction for the breakdown of glucose is

Glucose → 2ATP + 2LA + heat

As more glucose is metabolized, more lactic acid is produced. As the lactic acid gathers in the cell, it begins to lower the cellular pH (becoming more acidic) and begins to slow contraction speed and strength. This is felt as a burning sensation in the muscle after high-intensity exercise. Eventually the lactic acid can reach a high enough level to cause temporary muscle failure (meaning no contraction can occur). This is called *lactic acidosis.*

The production of ATP using the glycolytic pathway is limited because lactic acid accumulates, potentially resulting in the need to cease exercise if intensity is not reduced. The muscle cells can be trained to improve this energy pathway, resulting in the muscle cells producing less lactic acid at the same intensity so we can exercise harder for longer. This occurs because glycolytic enzymes increase by 10% to 25% when training this system through high-intensity exercise. Over time, cells also become more efficient at working with lactic acid in the cellular environment and may last longer at a higher intensity.

Glycolysis is the prime producer of ATP from 10 seconds to 2 minutes of intense exercise. Beyond 2 minutes of intense exercise, either the muscle will shut down, or, if the speed or intensity of contraction is reduced, the blood will be able to deliver adequate oxygen, thereby allowing aerobic metabolism to produce additional ATP.

Aerobic or Oxidative Energy System

When sufficient oxygen is available to the muscle cells for a given intensity of exercise, an abundance of ATP is produced in the cells. In this case, the supply of oxygen is delivered by the cardiorespiratory system to meet the demand for oxygen in the exercising muscles so that ATP is now being made in the presence of oxygen. There are two subcategories of aerobic metabolism that can create ATP: aerobic glycolysis and fatty acid oxidation.

Aerobic Glycolysis

This system provides fuel for more than 2 minutes of exercise at moderate intensity. Aerobic metabolism begins in the same way as the glycolytic pathway in that glycogen or glucose is broken down into pyruvate. However, because oxygen is present, instead of pyruvate being converted to lactic acid it then enters a series of reactions known as the *Krebs cycle* and the *electron transport chain*. Oxygen is made available to the muscle cells from nearby capillaries and the cell is able to take in that oxygen. The muscle cell can now begin to use the available oxygen to produce ATP aerobically through the oxidative system. Mitochondria, cellular structures with specialized enzymes to assist in aerobic metabolism, use either glucose or fat for fuel to create ATP.

With this continuous supply of oxygen, the muscle cell begins to break down glucose in the presence of oxygen to produce ATP. This chemical reaction is very efficient and produces large amounts of ATP (1 unit of glucose = 38 ATP). This is a complete breakdown of glucose and the waste products of the reaction are carbon dioxide (CO_2) and water (H_2O) as well as heat. These by-products are simply diffused into the bloodstream and taken away for disposal (carbon dioxide is exhaled and water is used elsewhere or lost through sweat).

The chemical reaction to break down glucose and glycogen for ATP is

$$\text{Glucose} + O_2 \rightarrow 38\text{ATP} + CO_2 + H_2O + \text{heat.}$$

This system of ATP production is limited only by the ability of the cardiorespiratory system to deliver oxygen. If oxygen is available, then glucose and glycogen are metabolized to make ATP. This system is especially useful for producing energy for long, continuous, moderate- to low-intensity exercise (see figure 3.1).

Fatty Acid Oxidation

This system provides fuel for over 2 minutes during low-intensity exercise. The muscle cell is also capable of using fatty acids to make ATP, and this metabolic pathway is called *fatty acid oxidation*. It occurs in the mitochondria of the muscle cells when a continuous supply of oxygen is present. This aerobic metabolism of fat produces a very large amount of ATP (1 unit of fatty acid = 100 ATP). Fatty acids are a high-energy fuel, but they are difficult to metabolize because a large amount of oxygen is required for this reaction to occur.

The chemical reaction for fatty acid oxidation is as follows:

$$\text{Fatty acid} + O_2 \rightarrow 100\text{ATP} + CO_2 + H_2O + \text{heat.}$$

This chemical reaction produces carbon dioxide and water as well as heat, and these by-products are easily disposed of elsewhere in the body. This energy system is virtually unlimited, but few people exercise for extreme durations; those who do use up a great deal of body fat.

At rest and at low intensities of exercise, muscle cells can use fatty acids as a fuel because the demand for energy is low and the supply of oxygen is adequate. However, because the intensity is low, the amount of fatty acids used is low. In addition, because energy demand is low and each unit of

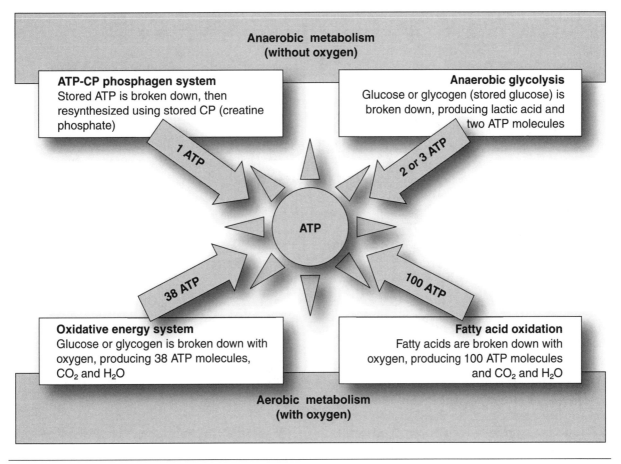

Figure 3.1 ATP production in a muscle cell.

fatty acids produces a large amount of energy, few units of fatty acids are used at rest.

From rest to a high level of intensity, the body tries to adjust its supply of energy to the required demand by automatically shifting the emphasis between the different energy systems. As exercise intensity increases, the cardiorespiratory system is limited in its ability to supply the required amount of oxygen quickly enough to allow fatty acid oxidation to occur. The metabolism of glucose and glycogen requires less oxygen, so glucose becomes the preferred fuel for the creation of ATP. Understanding exercise intensity becomes the key to understanding what method the muscle cell will choose to produce the necessary ATP for muscle contraction.

Interaction of the Energy Systems

The following sequence describes the transition from rest to exercise and back to recovery, illustrating how the three energy systems work together.

- **At rest:** Only small amounts of energy are needed, and they are supplied almost exclusively using aerobic metabolism of fatty acids.

- **At the beginning of exercise:** Depending on the difference between resting state and the level of exercise during the warm-up, the energy system used may vary. If the energy demand is only slightly higher than at rest, the aerobic system will continue to be used. If the energy demand is immediate and high, stored energy or ATP will be used (CP may also help to create more energy anaerobically until the aerobic system catches up or until the anaerobic glycolysis system kicks in after 20-30 seconds). This underscores the importance of a proper warm-up since commencing exercise that is too intense may result in the accumulation of lactic acid and impairment of the ability to continue exercise.

- **During steady-state exercise:** Once the supply of oxygen meets the demand, the muscle cell creates ATP using the breakdown of glucose through the oxidative system. This system works as long as needed, provided enough glucose is

Lactate Threshold

One concept that is important to understand regarding strenuous exercise is the **lactate threshold** (LT). The LT is the point at which the aerobic system cannot supply enough ATP for the needs of the body, forcing the anaerobic systems to increase their contribution of ATP. This occurs at approximately 85% to 90% of maximum heart or approximately 80% to 85% of $\dot{V}O_2$max in conditioned clients and 60% to 65% of maximal heart rate or 50% to 55% of $\dot{V}O_2$max in untrained clients, although it will vary 5% to 10% from client to client. When the LT is surpassed, anaerobic metabolism dominates and a significant accumulation of lactic acid begins as a by-product of high-intensity exercise. If exercise remains above the LT, this accumulation will lead to muscle fatigue and failure.

The point or intensity at which clients reach their lactate threshold depends on their fitness level and will change over time as they achieve greater fitness. Fitter clients have better oxygen delivery and extraction mechanisms and have a greater tolerance for lactic acid compared with deconditioned clients. The fitter you are, the harder you can exercise before surpassing the lactate threshold.

available. If the intensity is low enough, fat metabolism can occur as long as enough oxygen is available.

- **During strenuous exercise:** When energy demand is rapid and is expected for an extended period, the energy demand will require the anaerobic system to provide ATP. Once the ATP–CP phosphagen system is fatigued (approximately 10 seconds), the glycolytic system takes over the responsibility to produce ATP. The production and accumulation of lactic acid dictates the longevity of this system along with exercise intensity. Fatigue or failure may result if oxygen demand exceeds supply and high-intensity exercise continues beyond 2 minutes.

- **During recovery:** As the need for a higher supply of energy is reduced or eliminated, the body continues to take in more oxygen than it needs, thereby making it available to pay off the debt of oxygen that occurred at the beginning of exercise. The next section will explain how this excess oxygen is used.

Oxygen Deficit

As mentioned, when the need for a higher supply of energy is reduced or eliminated, the body continues to take in extra oxygen (more oxygen than would ordinarily be consumed at rest in the same amount of time). This oxygen is known as *excess post-exercise oxygen consumption* (EPOC). With mild aerobic exercise of relatively short duration, about half of the recovery oxygen occurs within

30 seconds. Complete recovery occurs within several minutes. There isn't a large oxygen deficit since steady state (enough oxygen to meet energy demands) is reached quickly in mild aerobic exercise, resulting in a faster recovery. With strenuous exercise, anaerobic metabolism increases along with increased levels of lactic acid, increased body temperature, and increased hormone levels. During exhaustive exercise, steady state is not reached and therefore a greater oxygen deficit is created. Depending on the intensity and duration of the exercise, it can take up to 24 hours to return to preexercise oxygen consumption due to the larger oxygen deficit. (See figure 3.2, which illustrates oxygen deficit and debt.)

EPOC is used for ATP and CP replenishment; resynthesis of a small portion of lactic acid to glycogen (most of the glycogen is restored from dietary carbohydrate); resolution in the disequilibrium in physiologic functions during steady-rate aerobic exercise (all physiologic systems that are activated with exercise increase their need for oxygen during recovery); reloading of oxygen to the blood returning to the lungs from active muscles; reloading of oxygen to the myoglobin in muscles; energy costs of ventilation above rest; energy requirements of a harder-working heart; tissue repair (redistribution of calcium, potassium, and sodium ions within muscle and other body compartments); and support for the elevated metabolism due to the thermogenic hormones released during exercise (epinephrine, norepinephrine, thyroxine, and glucocorticoids). In summary, EPOC is used for the recovery of both anaerobic and aerobic metabolism. The more

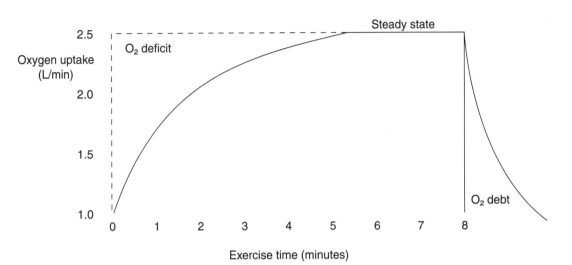

Figure 3.2 Oxygen deficit and oxygen debt.

anaerobic or intense the exercise is, the greater the oxygen deficit is and therefore the more EPOC is required to return the body to a preexercise state.

None of these systems works independently. All systems are working at the same time, but the predominance of one system over another depends upon the intensity of the activity. See table 3.2 for a comparison of the three systems with regard to the rate of energy production and the amount of ATP that can be made. The major limitations and primary use of each system are also included. The basic idea is if you need energy quickly (power, or energy per unit time), the ATP–CP system will be used predominately. If you need a lot of energy (capacity, or amount of ATP) but you do not need it quickly, such as for a long-distance hike, the oxidative system will be used predominately.

In discussing the interaction of the energy systems, the conditioning of clients for recreational and elite athletics becomes relevant. Table 3.3 shows the estimated contribution of each system for the performance of common sports.

The metabolic demands in table 3.3 reflect the relative contribution made by the three concur-

TABLE 3.2 Comparison of Energy Systems

SYSTEM	RATE AND AMOUNT OF ATP PRODUCTION	FUEL USED	CAPACITY OF SYSTEM	MAJOR LIMITATION	PRIMARY USE
ATP–CP (anaerobic)	Very rapid (1 ATP/unit of CP)	Stored ATP CP	Very limited	Small supply of ATP and CP.	Very high intensity, 1 to 10 s
Glycolytic (anaerobic)	Rapid (2-3 ATP/unit of glucose)	Blood glucose Muscle glycogen	Limited	Lactic acid by-product causes fatigue and failure.	High intensity, short duration, 10 s to 2-3 min
Oxidative	Slow (38 ATP/unit of glucose)	Blood glucose Muscle glycogen	Unlimited	Oxygen must be supplied constantly.	Mid to low intensity, 2+ min
Fatty acid oxidation (aerobic)	Slow (100 ATP/unit of fatty acid)	Fatty acids in bloodstream	Unlimited	Large amount of oxygen must be supplied constantly.	Low intensity, 2+ min

TABLE 3.3 Estimated Percentage Contribution of Each System in Common Sports

SPORT	ATP–CP SYSTEM	GLYCOLYTIC SYSTEM	OXIDATIVE SYSTEM
Basketball	High	Moderate-high	—
Volleyball	High	Moderate	—
Tennis	High	—	—
Golf	High	—	—
Baseball	High	—	—
Ice hockey	High	Moderate	Moderate
Standard marathon	—	—	High

Adapted, by permission, from National Strength and Conditioning Association, 2000, *Essentials of Strength Training and Conditioning*, 2nd ed. (Champaign, IL: Human Kinetics), p. 142.

rently operating metabolic systems for an average athlete. In other words, the dashes do not mean that the system is not working; they are an estimation of the predominance of the system during the main sport actions. These system contributions can change from moment to moment depending on the player position and game intensity. As a trainer, you still want to train all three systems; however, your emphasis on a particular system should reflect the estimated contribution of each system for the given sport or activity.

Developing the Energy Systems

It is beyond the scope of this chapter to discuss all methods of developing the energy systems, so we will focus on interval training as one method that may be used. It is imperative to develop a base of continuous training so that you are accustomed to exertion before undertaking an interval training program. Table 3.4 shows the program variables in designing interval training programs. The following sections provide questions and answers to aid in understanding the table.

Work-to-Rest Ratio

This ratio designates how much rest your client should have in relation to the amount of work that was completed during the work interval. With a work-to-rest ratio of 1:3, after completing an interval of 10 seconds, a client must rest 30 seconds before the next interval of work. The length of rest

TABLE 3.4 Program Variables in Interval Training Programs

ENERGY SYSTEM	WORK INTERVAL TIME	WORK–REST RATIO	WORK VOLUME	TYPE OF RELIEF	INTENSITY	SET AND REST TIMES
ATP–CP	10-20 s	1:3-1:6	2-8 min of accumulated work time	Rest relief (walking, stretching)	Maximal	1 set of intervals equals 60 s work (6 reps × 10 s intervals). Rest 5-10 min between sets.
Glycolytic	20 s-2 min	1:2-1:5	2-12 min of accumulated work time	Work relief (light exercise, jogging)	Maximal	1 set of intervals equals 3 min (6 reps × 30 s intervals). Rest 10-12 min between sets.
Oxidative	2+ min	1:0.5-1:1	20-60 min of accumulated work time	Rest relief	Upper edge of comfort zone or sport specific	Set should not exceed 60 min. Rest 10-15 min between sets.

will also depend on the fitness level of the client (more time is needed for a less conditioned client). This is why a range is given in the table.

Type of Relief

When training the ATP–CP system, you want to use rest relief. If work relief is used instead, the ATP that must be replenished is used to support the activity of the relief and therefore does not help to replenish intramuscular ATP and CP stores. If these stores are not repaid, the body will have to rely more on the lactic acid system for the next interval and the intensity will have to be lowered; thus, you are not developing the ATP–CP system. For the glycolytic intervals, work relief has been assigned because it will inhibit or partially block the complete restoration of the ATP–CP system, and as a consequence the lactic acid system rather than the ATP–CP system will dominate the subsequent work interval. Also, work relief aids the clearance of lactic acid, which encourages the improvement of this system and the ability to handle lactic acid. The oxidative system uses rest relief. The rationale for this is that with rest relief, the lactic acid developed during intense aerobic intervals will not be cleared effectively (work relief clears lactic acid better) and therefore for the next interval the glycolytic system cannot provide aid, giving a stronger training stimulus to the oxidative system.

Monitoring the Intensity of an Interval

One simple way to monitor intensity is through heart rate (HR) monitoring. For the ATP–CP and glycolytic systems, the intensity given in table 3.4 is maximal. Table 3.5 gives age-adjusted HRs (fitness level and activity specificity may alter these numbers) that you can use while monitoring interval conditioning.

Arranging Work and Rest Times

A set consists of a series of work and relief intervals such as 6 intervals of 10-second sprints followed by 30 seconds of rest. Repetitions are the number of work intervals within 1 set. As an example, let's say you would like to complete 2 minutes of work intervals for your 26-year-old client's ATP–CP system and you would like to use a 10-second interval time. This would amount to 12 intervals. For the ATP–CP system, 1 set of intervals is 60 seconds of work. You would have to complete 2 sets of 6 repetitions of 10-second work intervals with 30-second rest intervals if using a 1:3 work-to-rest ratio (work interval + rest interval = 1 repetition). The work interval should raise the client's HR to 180 beats per minute (bpm) or to what is appropriate for their fitness level. After each relief interval, the HR should be reduced to 140 bpm. After completing all reps for the set, the client would rest 5 to 10 minutes to get the HR down to 120 bpm. Then you would have the client complete another set of 6 repetitions of 10-second intervals with 30-second rest intervals. You can then build up the volume from there.

Important Considerations for Interval Conditioning

1. Fitness interval conditioning can be as simple as increasing the intensity up and down to challenge the client's anaerobic system in an informal way.

2. If you are training an athlete, the previous parameters may be useful, or you may have to complete a time-motion analysis of the client's sport demands.

TABLE 3.5 Age-Adjusted Heart Rates

AGE (YEARS)	WORK INTERVAL HR (BPM)	RELIEF INTERVAL HR (BPM)	RELIEF HR BETWEEN SETS (BPM)
Under 20	190	150	125
20-29	180	140	120
30-39	170	130	110
40-49	160	120	105
50-59	150	115	100
60-69	140	105	90

HR = heart rate; BPM = beats per minute

From E. Fox and D. Mathews, 1974, *Interval training* (Philadelphia, PA: W.B. Saunders), 60. By permission of Donald Mathews.

3. Exhaustion is not the goal of an interval conditioning program. It should be challenging and enjoyable.

4. Be sure the client has completed a warm-up of at least 5 to 10 minutes before interval conditioning and a cool-down of at least 5 minutes afterward. Ideally, the HR should feel like the preexercise levels after the cool-down.

5. Beginning exercisers should not participate in anaerobic intervals.

6. Anaerobic interval training should only be completed 2 to 3 times per week. Intersperse these sessions with easy cardiorespiratory training sessions.

7. Because this is just an introduction to energy system development, you may need to seek a sport conditioning course to learn more about this type of conditioning. There are many different activities that can be used for interval conditioning.

Developing all three energy systems will help with recreational sport performance and daily activities (running after a bus is anaerobic!), and it will provide all-around development of cardiorespiratory fitness. Just be sure that training progresses in a safe and logical manner.

Continuum of Energy Production

Every movement we make requires the production and use of energy. Our bodies are capable of movements of various intensities and durations, so understanding energy production is essential (see figure 3.3). It is important to know that the body does not use only one method to produce ATP. At any time, all of the energy systems are being used to produce energy, and the demand of the movement dictates which system will dominate in this production. This dynamic process is dictated by exercise intensity, exercise duration, and availability of oxygen.

Summary of Important Points

1. Energy is defined as the ability to do physical work. The body needs ATP in order to convert the chemical energy from food into muscle contraction for movement.

2. Metabolism includes all chemical reactions that allow large molecules to break down and other molecules to build up.

3. Energy is produced in the cells of the body using anaerobic metabolism (without oxygen) and aerobic metabolism (with oxygen).

4. Different time frames and intensities of exercise dictate which energy system produces the necessary energy for activity.

5. Interval conditioning is an effective method of developing the energy systems.

Case Studies

Roger

At this stage of Roger's fitness plan, he needs to focus on improving his aerobic fitness. The initial stage will encompass 4 to 6 weeks of aerobic exercise at an intensity of 40% to 60% of heart rate reserve (HRR) for 15 to 20 minutes (refer to chapter 4 for more information on HRR). This can then be followed by the improvement stage, which can last from the 6th week up to the 24th week of training, progressively working up to 60% to 85% of HRR for 20 to 40 minutes. The timing is variable; it depends on the progression of the client. Progress safely and watch for orthopedic tolerance. Once a good aerobic base is set, perhaps you can embark on development of energy systems. Since Roger is not training for any particular sport or event, you can create hard–easy intervals and use his rating of perceived exertion (RPE) as a guide for intensity to tax his glycolytic or ATP–CP system. The number of hard–easy cycles will depend on his fitness level and time availability. Be sure not to exhaust him, and also be sure to program easy and hard days. This will provide variety and train his energy systems.

Molly

Once Molly has established an aerobic base, it will be time to introduce interval training. Since she is playing volleyball and basketball, it would be advisable to conduct a time-motion analysis of her sport and style of play. How long does she work hard on court and how long are the active recovery breaks? You can then set the work-to-rest interval to match this for cardiorespiratory conditioning so she can develop the appropriate energy systems for her sports. The number of interval cycles will depend on her fitness level and time availability.

At Rest

Air is breathed in through the airways to the lung alveoli.
↓
A rich supply of oxygen surrounds the alveoli and permits the exchange of oxygen from the lungs to the capillaries. Carbon dioxide is exhaled.
↓
Hemoglobin in the red blood cell binds with the oxygen and carries it.
↓
The oxygenated blood is carried via the pulmonary vein to the left atrium of the heart.
↓
The left ventricle of the heart pumps the oxygenated blood through the aorta to all parts of the body, including the exercising muscles.
↓
The oxygenated blood is sent through the arteries, arterioles, and capillaries to the muscle.
↓
The oxygen diffuses through the capillaries to the muscle cells. Dissolved nutrients from food are also delivered.
↓
The muscle cell breaks down stored glycogen or glucose in the presence of the oxygen to produce ATP (if using aerobic metabolism).
↓
Carbon dioxide and water are the waste products and are carried away in the blood.
↓
Veins carry the deoxygenated blood back to the right atrium of the heart.
↓
The deoxygenated blood is pumped from the right ventricle to the lungs via the pulmonary artery. Carbon dioxide is exhaled and fresh oxygen is supplied to the blood. The cycle begins again.
↓
At rest, this cycle of oxygen transfer and energy creation takes about 20 seconds to occur.

At the Onset of Exercise

The respiratory rate and depth of breathing increase.
↓
The rate of gas exchange across the alveoli increases. More capillaries open to allow better gas exchange to occur in the lungs.
↓
The hemoglobin in the blood is saturated with oxygen.
↓
The left atrium of the heart fills to a greater capacity with oxygenated blood.
↓
More blood is pumped with each beat (stroke volume) and the heart rate increases, producing a greater output of blood (cardiac output) each minute.
↓
Blood is shunted toward areas of need (muscles) and away from areas of low activity.
↓
Blood pressure rises so that the blood is pumped out of the heart with more force (systolic pressure rises), but the pressure in the heart as it fills stays the same (diastolic pressure stays the same). The arterioles and capillaries dilate to carry more blood.
↓
At the muscle cell, the rate of gas exchange increases to deliver more oxygen.
↓
Exercising muscles force the veins to return the deoxygenated blood to the heart faster.
↓
The cardiovascular and respiratory systems cannot instantaneously increase the delivery of oxygen to the muscles to meet the ATP demands aerobically.
↓
At the start of exercise the anaerobic energy systems supply the ATP if the intensity of exercise is not low enough to allow the aerobic system to meet the energy needs.
↓
The volume of oxygen missing in the first few minutes of exercise is the oxygen deficit.
↓
When steady state is reached, oxygen supply meets demand and aerobic metabolism supplies the needed ATP.
↓
When exercising stops, there is still an elevated oxygen delivery. This extra oxygen is used to help the body recover from anaerobic and aerobic metabolism.
↓
The faster a person reaches steady-state exercise, the smaller the oxygen deficit.
↓
A less fit person takes longer to reach steady state and therefore creates a greater oxygen deficit and must produce more ATP using anaerobic methods.

Figure 3.3   An overview of energy production from rest to exercise.

Jennifer

After Jennifer has established an aerobic base, you can introduce interval training so that she can produce more work in less time. This will increase her fitness level and reduce her time commitment. You can informally create intervals to tax the ATP–CP and glycolytic systems since she is not training for a particular sport or event. Be sure not to exhaust her since she is a busy person. Her workouts need to give her energy for her busy days! Programming easy and hard days into her training schedule will allow for recovery and regeneration and will also add variety and fun to her program. Be creative with the intervals. This could mean doing step-ups on a step or BOSU balance trainer (if you have established proper acclimation of this modality) for the work portion and walking on the treadmill for the active recovery. Sometimes you do not have to use the same piece of equipment for both.

CHAPTER 4

Cardiorespiratory Concepts

Gregory S. Anderson, PhD
Brian Justin, MHK

CHAPTER OBJECTIVES

After completing this chapter, you will be able to

1. describe the anatomy of the heart;

2. explain the flow of blood from the heart to the body and back again;

3. discuss the mechanics of the cardiovascular system and its response to exercise;

4. explain the function and anatomy of the respiratory system;

5. discuss the mechanics of the respiratory system and its response to exercise;

6. identify the major benefits of cardiorespiratory training;

7. identify basic differences in developing cardiorespiratory training programs for beginner, intermediate, and advanced clients;

8. explain the major issues that affect the design of cardiorespiratory training based on the FITT formula;

9. discuss the concepts of cardiorespiratory recovery and relaxation as well as flexibility; and

10. determine appropriate exercises for cardiovascular recovery.

The cardiovascular and respiratory systems are essential to body motion. They work together to deliver oxygen and nutrients and remove wastes from body tissues. The respiratory system adds oxygen and removes carbon dioxide from the blood, while the circulatory system transports these substances and nutrients to and from body tissues.

Increased physical activity strengthens the heart, circulatory system, and lungs. As a personal trainer, you must understand how these systems assist in producing movement and how they adapt to training to make people feel healthier, move more easily, and live longer.

Cardiovascular System

The cardiovascular system is composed of the heart and a network of arteries and veins (blood vessels) that carry blood throughout the body. It is responsible for the circulation of blood throughout the body, transporting nutrients, oxygen, carbon dioxide, metabolic waste products, and key chemical messengers (hormones). The circulatory system is also involved in maintaining the core temperature of the body by transporting heat from the core to the skin where it can dissipate.

Cardiovascular Anatomy

The heart is a muscular pump that creates the pressure that is required to move blood through the circulatory system (figure 4.1). It has four chambers and functions as two pumps, one on the right side and one on the left. The right atrium and right ventricle form the right pump, collecting blood returning from the tissues and moving it through the lungs (referred to as *pulmonary circulation*); the left atrium and left ventricle combine to make the left pump that receives blood from the lungs and moves it through the tissues of the body and back to the right side of the heart (referred to as *systemic circulation*).

In the four-chamber system, the atria receive blood returning to the heart via veins and pass the blood into the ventricles, which are the mus-

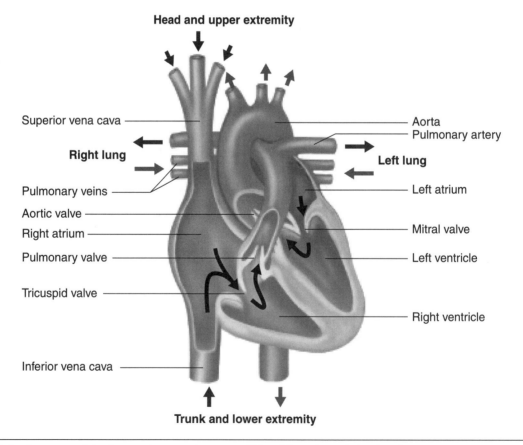

Figure 4.1   Structure of the human heart and course of blood flow through its chambers.

Reprinted, by permission, from T.R. Baechle and R.W. Earle (eds.), 2000, *Essentials of strength training and conditioning*, 2nd ed. (Champaign, IL: Human Kinetics), 116.

cular pumps that move the blood away from the heart via the arteries. Blood moves through the pulmonary circuit to the lungs and then through the systemic circuit to body tissues.

Circulation

Blood travels in arteries either to the lungs from the right side of the heart or to body tissues from the left side. It returns to the heart through veins, which bring blood back to the left atrium from the lungs or to the right atrium from body tissues. At the start of this loop, the oxygenated blood leaves the heart from the left ventricle through the aorta and travels from the arteries to microscopic vessels called *arterioles,* which then branch into even smaller vessels called *capillaries.* Capillaries are the smallest and most numerous of blood vessels. At the capillary level, the blood passes by cells, where oxygen and nutrients are dropped off and carbon dioxide and other waste products are picked up for transport. After this gas exchange, the deoxygenated blood carrying the extra carbon dioxide leaves the arterial system and begins making its way back to the heart by way of veins. Major veins from the upper and lower halves of the body empty directly into the right side of the heart. The blood passes from the right atria to the right ventricle, where it is pushed out through the lungs where the carbon dioxide will move out of the blood and oxygen will move in. In the lungs, the blood picks up oxygen and drops off carbon dioxide through diffusion. Oxygenated blood then returns to the left atria via pulmonary veins to start the circuit over again.

In a typical adult, 5 litres of blood circulate every minute at rest and up to six or seven times a minute during maximal exercise. It is the function of the left ventricle to force blood out of the heart through the aorta. Oxygen-rich (red) blood travels out of the aorta and is sent under pressure to all parts of the body (figure 4.2).

Blood Pressure

Blood pressure (BP) is the result of blood being pumped out of the ventricles, exerting force against the arterial walls. At rest, blood in the circulatory system is forced through the arteries at an average pressure of 120/80 millimetres of mercury (mmHg). The top number, or systolic pressure, is the pressure exerted on the walls of the arteries as the heart contracts, representing peak pressure in the system. The bottom number, or diastolic

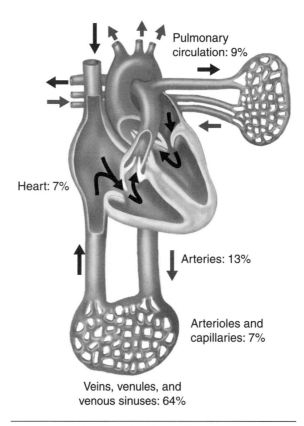

Figure 4.2 The arterial (right) and venous components of the circulatory system. The percent values indicate the distribution of blood volume throughout the circulatory system at rest.

Reprinted, by permission, from T.R. Baechle and R.W. Earle (eds.), 2000, *Essentials of strength training and conditioning,* 2nd ed. (Champaign, IL: Human Kinetics), 119.

pressure, is the pressure exerted on the walls of the arteries as the heart relaxes and fills again, representing the lowest pressure in the arteries. Even as a client becomes fitter, resting BP remains constant because exercise helps maintain the elasticity of vessels and keep the circulatory system healthy.

During exercise, the heart must pump harder to deliver the oxygen required by the working muscles, and stroke volume increases. As more blood is pumped into the aorta at once, the aorta is distended a greater amount, and thus it is normal for BP to increase during exercise. During moderate exercise, systolic pressure rises quickly to values above 200 mmHg and then levels off, whereas diastolic pressure remains relatively stable due to the opening of more capillary beds. During straining exercises such as weightlifting, BP may spike to much higher levels as the muscular contractions compress the arteries and produce a much greater resistance to the blood flow. During such nonrhythmic activities, the low-pressure veins are also compressed and blood flow back to the heart and brain may be reduced, resulting in dizziness or faintness. For people with hypertension, these types of activities may be dangerous.

Heart Rate

The heart pumps approximately 72 bpm at rest. Each time the heart pumps, it forces blood into the arteries to deliver oxygen and nutrients to the metabolically active tissues of the body. The wave of blood moving through the arties can be felt as a pulse at any of the major arteries that are close to the skin (i.e., radial artery, temporal artery, and carotid artery). The radial pulse is taken at the wrist along the outer edge of the lateral tendons and is the preferred location for manual heart rate (HR) measurement. HR monitors are excellent alternatives to taking HRs manually and are a basic requirement for working with clients in a personal training environment.

As the demand for oxygen increases with activity, the heart must pump faster to provide more oxygen. The link between metabolic demand and HR allows trainers to use HR as an indicator of exercise intensity.

Stroke Volume

Stroke volume (SV) is the amount of blood that the left ventricle ejects in one beat. Stroke volume at rest for a typical male averages around 70 millilitres. As a client becomes fitter, the ventricles become larger, allowing them to hold more blood and contract with more force. This causes stroke volume to increase; thus, a trained person will be able to deliver more blood per heartbeat than an untrained person of the same body size. Therefore, a fit heart does not have to work as hard at rest or during exercise.

Cardiac Output

Cardiac output (Q) is the amount of blood that the heart ejects in 1 minute. It is the product of HR and stroke volume (i.e., how many times the heart beats and how much blood it ejects per beat):

$$Q = SV \times HR.$$

Q = cardiac output, SV = stroke volume, HR = heart rate.

As demands for oxygen and nutrients increase during exercise, cardiac output increases by increasing both HR and stroke volume. Stroke volume

increases early in exercise and continues to rise through moderate exercise, after which it plateaus. HR increases with exercise intensity to maximal levels, where it plateaus before exhaustion.

While at rest, the body requires about 5 litres of blood to be circulated per minute; with improved fitness and increased stroke volume, resting HR decreases. A stronger heart creates a greater contraction, forcing more blood out with each beat. The trained heart is a more efficient pump and can pump out more blood per beat (larger stroke volume) than the untrained heart. For this reason, during rest the trained heart beats at a slower rate and gets more rest between beats, beating 28,000 fewer times in a day. This means that during exercise, the trained heart is capable of delivering greater amounts of oxygen to meet the demands of the exercise. To offer an example, we can compare the rest and exercise responses of both a trained and untrained person.

Rest

Untrained:
5,000 millilitres = 70 bpm × 71.4 millilitres

Trained:
5,000 millilitres = 50 bpm × 100 millilitres

Maximal Exercise

Untrained:
20,000 millilitres = 195 bpm × 102.6 millilitres

Trained:
35,000 millilitres = 195 bpm × 179.5 millilitres

Increasing cardiac output during exercise means the trained person is able to deliver more oxygen and nutrients to the working muscles. Further, during exercise the trained body learns to redistribute blood from less active tissues, such as digestive organs and kidneys, to the heart and skeletal muscles (table 4.1).

Respiratory System

The pulmonary or respiratory system is made up of the left and right lungs and air passageways. This system exchanges gas between the bloodstream and the environment. It provides a large interface between the air we breathe in and the blood circulating through our lungs, and it is at this interface where oxygen is brought into the bloodstream and carbon dioxide is removed from the blood. This exchange of gases occurs as a result

TABLE 4.1 **Distribution of Cardiac Output at Rest and During Strenuous Exercise**

BODY TISSUE	REST	STRENUOUS EXERCISE
Muscle	20%	84%
Liver	27%	2%
Kidneys	22%	1%
Brain	14%	4%
Skin	6%	2%
Heart	4%	4%
Other	7%	3%

of ventilation and diffusion. *Ventilation* refers to the mechanical process of moving air in and out of the lungs, whereas *diffusion* refers to the way gases are exchanged in the lungs.

Respiratory Anatomy

The respiratory system consists of the mouth, nose, nasal cavity, pharynx, larynx, trachea, bronchial tree, and lungs (figure 4.3). The mouth and nose inhale air from the atmosphere, which contains approximately 21% oxygen. The air travels through the trachea and enters the primary bronchi and their subdivisions, the secondary and tertiary bronchi. The ends of the tertiary bronchi branches contain bronchioles, which have tiny air sacs called *alveoli* at their ends. The alveolar sacs are microscopic, thin-walled elastic sacs where gas is exchanged. Air fills the alveoli, which are surrounded by capillaries where oxygen rapidly moves from the alveoli into the blood by a process called *diffusion*. At the same time, the alveoli receive carbon dioxide from the capillaries for removal through exhalation. This respiration process is a continuous cycle.

The average adult has a lung volume of 4 to 6 litres of mixed air, which contains nitrogen (89%), oxygen (21%), and a small amount of carbon dioxide (.4%). Within the lungs there are approximately 300 million alveoli, providing a very large surface area for diffusion to take place. With the alveolar surface spread out flat, this equates to approximately 60 to 80 square metres, or the size of a tennis court.

Ventilation

Air moves in and out of the lungs along pressure gradients created by diaphragm contraction and

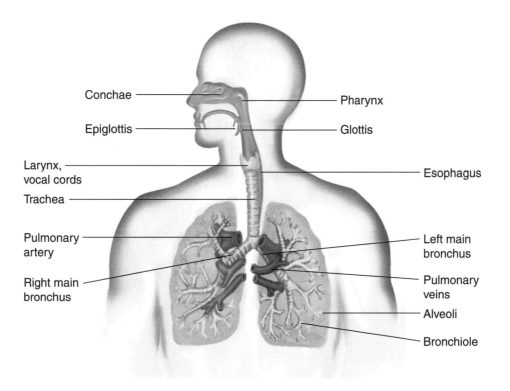

Figure 4.3 Anatomy of the lungs.

Reprinted, by permission, from T.R. Baechle and R.W. Earle (eds.), 2000, *Essentials of strength training and conditioning*, 2nd ed. (Champaign, IL: Human Kinetics), 120.

relaxation. Inspiration is the process of air moving into the lungs and occurs once lung pressure is below atmospheric pressure. This low pressure is created by the diaphragm contracting and pushing down into the abdomen while other inspiratory muscles lift the ribs upward and outward, increasing the volume of the thoracic cavity in which the lungs sit. This creates a partial vacuum and the lungs are sucked open, increasing their volume as a result of the enlarged chest cavity and reducing air pressure within the lungs. Because inspiration uses muscle contractions, it requires energy expenditure.

Expiration is the passive process of air moving out of the lungs, occurring when lung pressure exceeds atmospheric pressure. When the diaphragm and the other inspiratory muscles relax and the stretched lungs recoil, the chest cavity decreases in volume, lung air pressure increases above atmospheric pressure, and air is forced out of the lungs.

Exercise Response

At the onset of exercise, the cardiovascular system responds to a change in demand for oxygen. This response begins immediately, but there may be a delay in accommodating oxygen demands depending on the difference between the demands before exercise and during exercise. This is the rationale in support of a thorough warm-up.

The brain recognizes a need for more oxygen to the muscles. It signals the heart to increase HR and stroke volume, which increases cardiac output. The increase in blood volume increases the amount of blood (and therefore oxygen) that

is carried to the exercising muscles. Blood flow redistributes away from the abdominal area by **vasoconstriction** (narrowing of the arteries) and increases to the working muscles by **vasodilation** (widening of the arteries). There is also a change in BP to accommodate the increased demand for oxygen. As the demand for blood flow increases, systolic pressure elevates to force blood out of the heart faster and at a higher pressure. Diastolic pressure should stay the same or even slightly decrease due to vasodilation of vessels in the exercising muscles, which reduces the resistance and pressure of the blood.

At the onset of exercise, the rate of respiration also increases. This change in breathing rate and depth helps meet the demand for additional oxygen for energy production. During the first few minutes of exercise, pulmonary ventilation increases in a similar manner to exercise HR. At rest, ventilation is approximately 10 litres per minute. In the first minute of exercise, it can increase to approximately 45 litres per minute. After 2 minutes, when a person reaches steady-state exercise, it can increase to approximately 60 litres per minute. Pulmonary ventilation may increase to 220 litres of air per minute in well-conditioned endurance athletes in response to maximum metabolic demands. Figure 4.4 shows typical HR and ventilation responses for a fit person who is jogging on a treadmill.

Systems Integration

Aerobic fitness reflects the efficiency of the cardiovascular, respiratory, and muscular systems. It reflects the ability to perform continuous, repetitive

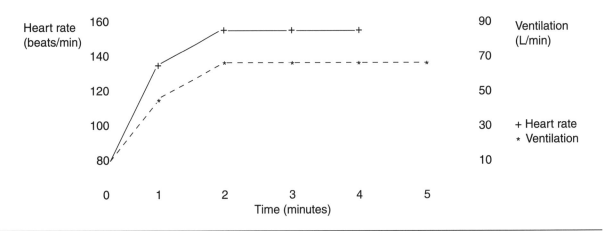

Figure 4.4 A concept diagram of HR and ventilation response.

movement using the large muscle groups of the body for an extended period of time without fatigue by generating energy for physical work through the aerobic energy pathways. This capacity is often reflected in terms such as *cardiorespiratory endurance, aerobic capacity,* and *maximal oxygen consumption.*

One measure of aerobic fitness level is aerobic capacity—the maximum amount of oxygen the body can extract and use in the process of energy production ($\dot{V}O_2$max). Your $\dot{V}O_2$max reflects the amount of energy that can be generated through the aerobic energy pathways and depends upon the ability to ventilate the lungs, the ease at which oxygen moves from the lungs to the blood, the capacity of the blood to carry the oxygen, the ability of the heart to pump the blood (cardiac output) and distribute it to the working musculature, and the ability of the muscles to extract and use the oxygen delivered. For this reason, $\dot{V}O_2$max reflects the ability to integrate the responses from various systems that are required to support increased activity. It can be measured in maximum volume of O_2 per minute in litres or relative to body mass (millilitres per kilogram minute). Normal values for an aerobically fit male and an unfit male weighing 70 kilograms are presented in table 4.2.

Factors that contribute to aerobic capacity can generally be divided into two categories: a central component involving the heart and its ability to distribute blood (and therefore oxygen), and a peripheral component involving the muscles and their ability to extract and use oxygen in the production of aerobic energy. This distinction is important because the components respond to different training regimes; what best develops the central component does not necessarily develop the peripheral component.

TABLE 4.2   Oxygen Uptake During Rest and Maximal Exercise

	RELATIVE $\dot{V}O_2$	ABSOLUTE $\dot{V}O_2$
Rest		
Fit (70 kg)	$3.5\ ml \cdot kg^{-1} \cdot min^{-1}$	0.25 L/min
Unfit (70 kg)	$3.5\ ml \cdot kg^{-1} \cdot min^{-1}$	0.25 L/min
Maximal exercise		
Fit (70 kg)	$60\ ml \cdot kg^{-1} \cdot min^{-1}$	4.2 L/min
Unfit (70 kg)	$35\ ml \cdot kg^{-1} \cdot min^{-1}$	2.5 L/min

Oxygen Uptake During Recovery

After exercise stops, oxygen consumption remains elevated above resting levels for awhile despite the fact that the oxygen demands placed on the body during exercise are no longer present. Referred to as *EPOC* (see chapter 3), this oxygen is used for recovery processes that bring the body back to homeostasis. The magnitude of the recovery period varies based on the intensity and duration of the exercise. Light activity causes little disturbance in the body and requires a recovery period that is usually short and relatively unnoticeable, whereas intense exercise can result in a recovery period lasting many hours, sometimes even days.

The rate of recovery is rapid for the first few minutes postexercise and then slows for the remainder of the recovery period. The fast portion of recovery helps replenish the ATP–CP stores and remove lactic acid, and the slower portion of recovery supports muscle tissue repair and adaptations that occur as a result of the exercise. EPOC has been shown to be smaller and occur at a faster rate for the same exercise following many weeks of aerobic training; thus training can affect recovery rate. Also, active recovery such as light aerobic exercise has been shown to be better than passive recovery, supporting the need for a cool-down period. Active recovery, where you keep moving instead of stopping, assists the heart and circulatory system in redistributing blood to all parts of the body. This prevents blood from pooling in the exercising muscles and helps cells reduce the oxygen debt created at the beginning of exercise when oxygen supply did not meet demand. Abruptly stopping activity (for example, suddenly ending a high-intensity run) places considerable stress on the cardiorespiratory system. Just as the warm-up gradually increases exercise intensity, active recovery, including a gradual decrease in the intensity of exercise, reduces the stress on the cardiorespiratory system, ensuring a safe and effective cardiovascular recovery.

The primary focus of cardiorespiratory recovery is to reduce exercise intensity. As a personal trainer, you can assist this recovery by

- reducing the intensity and impact of the exercise,
- reducing the range of motion of movements, and
- telling clients to consciously begin an active recovery.

Benefits of Cardiorespiratory Training

Many studies have shown the benefits of cardiorespiratory training, especially for helping reduce the risk of heart disease. Cardiorespiratory training also reduces resting HR, normalizes resting BP, and improves the ability to perform daily activities. Physiological improvements and their related benefits are listed in table 4.3.

These physiological benefits lead to an overall improvement in both oxygen delivery and oxygen extraction. The result is an increase in aerobic capacity or $\dot{V}O_2$max:

$$\dot{V}O_2\text{max} = \text{oxygen delivery} \times \text{oxygen extraction.}$$

TABLE 4.3 Benefits of Cardiorespiratory Training

IMPROVEMENTS	BENEFITS
Delivery of blood (central training effects)	
Increased stroke volume	Increased maximal cardiac output and delivery of oxygen and nutrients
Increased blood delivery	Greater amount of blood volume pumped per beat (due to stronger heart muscle)
Increased red blood cells	Increased amount of hemoglobin and hence oxygen-carrying capacity
Extraction of oxygen (peripheral training effects)	
Increased capillary density	Better distribution of oxygen and nutrients to the working muscles, as well as improved waste removal
Increased size and number of mitochondria	Improved aerobic production of ATP
Increased aerobic enzymes	Enhanced ability to utilize oxygen

Exercise Prescription

Client success in an exercise program depends on the personal trainer making correct decisions about exercise design. If a personal trainer does not interpret the client's expectations, experience, fitness level, and training goals correctly, the exercise plan will not be effective.

When designing exercise plans for clients, consider the FITT formula: frequency, intensity, time, and type. Health Canada and the Canadian Society for Exercise Physiology developed a guide called *Physical Activity Guide to Healthy Active Living* that offers specific recommendations for each of the four factors in the FITT formula. This guide for healthy adults, older adults, young people, and children can be found at www.phac-aspc.gc.ca/pau-uap/paguide/index.html.

The development of an individualized FITT design is influenced by many factors. Personal trainers must develop a strong knowledge base regarding each component of the FITT formula. The following sections examine the four components of the FITT formula as they pertain to the development of cardiorespiratory fitness.

Exercise Frequency

Frequency refers to the number of times the cardiorespiratory system is stressed each week. Frequency of activity depends upon the intensity and duration of the training periods. The *Physical Activity Guide to Healthy Active Living* recommends 4 to 7 training sessions a week for health improvement. Exercise frequency is influenced by the client's lifestyle. Ideally, all clients would have the time and motivation to exercise every day. The reality is that most people lead busy lives and have limited free time.

When planning exercise frequency, consider the following:

ISSUES	INFLUENCES
Number of sessions a client is able to commit to	Various factors affect this choice, including family, work, social, and financial commitments. The personal trainer works with the capabilities of the client to establish a reasonable expectation regarding frequency.
Client's current fitness level	If the client is not a regular exerciser, recommend a slow increase in activity level. If the client is already fit, the number of sessions can be more frequent.
Client's goals for cardiorespiratory conditioning	If the client is interested in weight reduction, recommend more frequent training to enhance results. Clients who seek improved health and fitness also need to exercise more frequently.

When counseling clients about exercise frequency, encourage them to modify their current activity patterns for improvement. Regular physical activity helps establish exercise as a habit and minimizes the risk of injury. Research shows that people can improve cardiorespiratory health in 2 exercise sessions a week. As exercise frequency increases, the results improve. A common recommendation is to exercise one day and rest the next. This approach leads to health benefits, fat reduction, and less risk of injury. Research indicates that dramatic improvements in aerobic fitness and cardiorespiratory health occur as training sessions increase from 2 to 4 per week. Improvements level off, with few extra cardiorespiratory effects occurring when moving from 4 to 7 sessions a week. Optimal aerobic training effects occur in 4 or 5 training sessions a week, with no need for training every day unless weight loss is the major objective.

Closely observe clients who wish to exercise every day to ensure that they do not overtrain. Frequent exercisers must pay close attention to exercise intensity in order to maintain a positive adaptation to exercise.

Exercise Intensity

Intensity refers to the rate of work being performed. The rate of work can be described as a speed (such as an 8-minute mile [1.5 kilometres]) or relative load placed on the body (% of maximum HR). Training intensity can have a significant impact on the success of the workout because it has considerable physiological and psychological effects on the client. For example, if the workout is too difficult, the client will be unable to complete the planned activity. From a physiological standpoint, the client's body is unable to supply the required energy, and from a psychological standpoint, the client might not enjoy the exercise session because it is too difficult. The result is a client who does not have fun and may want to avoid future workouts. When this occurs, you may have lost a client.

Since intensity is so closely linked to client success and enjoyment, it is critical that you understand the major ways to determine and evaluate exercise intensity. There are three primary methods of planning and detecting exercise intensity that are based on the physiological response of the body to exercise: oxygen uptake, HR monitoring, and perceived exertion. Most clients cannot monitor oxygen uptake during their exercise; this is only an option for elite athletes who have access to labora-

tory testing and training. Physiological (HR) and psychological (perceived exertion) responses to exercise are intensity specific and act as adequate markers for the prescription of exercise intensity during cardiorespiratory training sessions.

The most common method of evaluating intensity during cardiorespiratory exercise is exercise HR. HR increases linearly with oxygen uptake (or exercise intensity) throughout the majority of the exercise range. Clients understand what their HR is and can be trained to use an HR monitor or take their HR manually, so it is a natural indicator to use for prescribing exercise intensity. The two primary ways of using HR for prescribing exercise intensity include a percentage of either HR maximum or reserve. Both rely on knowing the client's maximum HR, or HRmax.

Most clients will not know their HRmax, and it can be dangerous to determine in many clients. However, a general indicator of HRmax can be determined by using the following equation:

$$HRmax = 220 - age.$$

Due to changes in the nervous system, the capacity of the heart decreases with age. The previous equation determines a theoretical HRmax and provides a good guess as to what a client's HRmax may be. However, these values can be incorrect, and you should observe clients carefully when first prescribing exercise intensity in order to determine its appropriateness. For example, in theory a 20-year-old should have an HRmax of 200 bpm; however, maximum HRs as low as 180 and as high as 220 are common. Using this equation will overpredict the intensity for people with a lower HRmax and underpredict the intensity of people with a higher HRmax.

Percentage of Maximum Heart Rate

Using HRmax to determine exercise intensity is simply an estimate of how hard the client should exercise. In general, research shows that an appropriate range of recommended exercise intensity falls between 55% and 90% of HRmax, and this is known as the **target heart rate training zone**. This range encourages clients to exercise hard enough for cardiorespiratory gains, but not so hard that the aerobic energy system is unable to provide enough energy, making the exercise anaerobic. Where a client belongs in this intensity range is based on exercise experience, exercise goals, and current fitness level. This is not the most accurate method of setting exercise intensity, but it is easily understood by most clients.

Target HR Zone Calculations: Percentage of HRmax

Target HR = (220 – age) × percent

Case Study

40-year-old female with a resting HR of 75

Lower target HR = (220 – 40) × .55

= 180 × .55

= 99 bpm

Upper target HR = (220 – 40) × .9

= 180 × .9

= 162 bpm

If the client is a beginner or has low fitness levels, we would use exercise values near the lower end of the target HR zone (55%-64% of HRmax). For an intermediate fitness client, we would use values in the middle (65%-74% of HRmax), and for an advanced fitness client, we would use values in the upper range (75%-90% HRmax).

Table 4.4 shows recommended HRs for various ages.

TABLE 4.4 **Heart Rate Chart**

AGE	PERCENT HRMAX	HR (BPM)
20	55	110
	60	120
	70	140
	80	160
	90	180
30	55	105
	60	114
	70	133
	80	152
	90	171
40	55	99
	60	108
	70	126
	80	144
	90	162
50	55	94
	60	102
	70	119
	80	136
	90	153
60	55	88
	60	96
	70	112
	80	128
	90	144

If clients do not have a HR monitor, they can take an exercise pulse at the radial or carotid pulse sites. Ask them to count the number of beats in 15 seconds and multiply that number by 4 to determine bpm. However, be aware that this method can be inaccurate by as much as 10 to 15 bpm.

To determine how hard clients should exercise, consider their current fitness level. The fitter the client, the more stress the body is capable of handling. The more stress the body can handle, the more intense the workout should be. Fit clients need to train at higher intensities to continue to develop their cardiorespiratory system.

When planning exercise intensity, consider the following:

ISSUES	INFLUENCES
Client's exercise experience	Clients with minimal exercise experience should begin training at the lower end of the intensity spectrum (55%-64%).
Client's current fitness level	Fitter clients should work in the moderate (65%-74%) to high (75%-90%) range of the target zone.
Client's goals for cardio-respiratory conditioning	Improving cardiorespiratory health requires clients to exercise in their target zone. Fat loss requires increased total caloric expenditure.

Heart Rate Reserve

A second method of determining exercise intensity using HR is heart rate reserve (HRR). This calculation takes resting HR into account and calculates the number of beats you can increase your HR during the exercise (HRmax – resting HR). It also takes into consideration fitness level because when clients become fitter, resting HR decreases. Using the HRR calculation is most appropriate for clients who know their resting and maximum HRs, have exercise experience, know their current cardiorespiratory fitness level, and have been working out with a trainer.

Target HRs should fall within 50% and 85% of HRR when using the Karvonen formula described next.

Target HR Zone Calculations: HRR Method

Target HR = [(HRmax – resting HR)
× percentage] + resting HR

Case Study

40-year-old female with a resting HR of 75 bpm

Lower target HR = $\{[(220 - 40) - 75] \times .5\} + 75$
$= [(180 - 75) \times .5] + 75$
$= (105 \times .5) + 75$
$= 52.5 + 75$
$= 128$ bpm

Upper target HR = $\{[(220 - 40) - 75] \times .85\} + 75$
$= [(180 - 75) \times .85] + 75$
$= (105 \times .85) + 75$
$= 89.2 + 68$
$= 157$ bpm

When both maximum and resting HRs are known, HRR may be a good option, but when calculating HRmax, the same error is added as when using percentage of HRmax, and this method will not produce better results than the simpler method. Further, cardiorespiratory fitness must be known and percentage values for lower target HR adjusted accordingly; otherwise, as clients gain fitness, their lower target HR would actually decrease, which is incorrect. Using our previous example, let's explore this concept after the person has considerable training experience and resting HR is now 62 bpm:

Lower target HR = $\{[(220 - 40) - 62] \times .5\} + 62$
$= [(180 - 62) \times .5] + 62$
$= (118 \times .5) + 62$
$= 59 + 62$
$= 121$ bpm

In this situation, as the person became fitter, the estimated lower target HR decreased. Thus it is imperative to increase the percentage of HRR as clients become fitter in order to be accurate. For example, if the woman is now well above average fitness and we use a percentage value of .75 for her lower target HR, we would get a lower target HR of 151 bpm. The HRR method must be interpreted with caution unless all the variables are known to be true and the trainer has experience in determining the lower target HR multiplication (percentage) factor based on measured aerobic capacity.

Rating of Perceived Exertion

Many personal trainers use HR monitors with clients. An HR monitor gives the client immediate, accurate, and continual feedback about exercise intensity. Clients can combine HR monitoring with rating of perceived exertion (RPE) to establish an understanding of how their bodies respond to exercise.

Encourage your clients to communicate with you about intensity throughout the exercise session. They can do this by rating their exertion using a numeric system and descriptive statements. Dr. Gunnar Borg developed a scale for rating perception of physical effort (figures 4.5 and 4.6). You can use this standardized scale to help clients express their level of fatigue during the workout. A person's RPE has been shown to be reliably related to work intensity as well as both HR and oxygen consumption during cardiorespiratory activities.

Comparing the Methods

The relationships among RPE, percentage of HRmax, and percentage of HRR are relatively stable across the population and are detailed in table 3.1.

Research has demonstrated that a person's RPE during exercise is closely related to exercise HR—for example, from measures of perceived exertion, young people's HR can be approximated by multiplying their RPE by 10.

Exercise Time

Exercise time is often also referred to as *duration* and reflects the length of time a training stimulus is applied without rest. For example, if you warm up for 10 minutes, jog for 25 minutes, and cool down for 5 minutes, the duration is 25 minutes since this is the amount of time that the body is stressed enough to stimulate an adaptation or improvement in fitness.

Exercise time is linked to intensity because the harder the exercise, the shorter the duration. You must establish a proper combination of intensity and duration to produce fitness gains for clients based on their needs and goals.

Research shows that health improves with approximately 20 to 30 minutes of exercise in the target HR zone. The *Physical Activity Guide to Healthy Active Living* recommends a range of exercise duration depending on the effort of the activity. In general, there is an inverse relationship between intensity and duration for health benefits to occur—the easier the exercise, the longer it should last.

To determine appropriate exercise duration, consider each client's current level of fitness,

6	No exertion at all
7	
8	Extremely light
9	Very light
10	
11	Light
12	
13	Somewhat hard
14	
15	Hard (heavy)
16	
17	Very hard
18	
19	Extremely hard
20	Maximal exertion

Borg RPE scale
© Gunnar Borg, 1970, 1985, 1994, 1998

Figure 4.5 Borg scale.

G. Borg, 1998, *Borg's Perceived Exertion and Pain Scales* (Champaign, IL: Human Kinetics), 47.

0	Nothing at all	"No P"
0.3		
0.5	Extremely weak	Just noticeable
1	Very weak	
1.5		
2	Weak	Light
2.5		
3	Moderate	
4		
5	Strong	Heavy
6		
7	Very strong	
8		
9		
10	Extremely strong	"Max P"
11		
✦		
●	Absolute maximum	Highest possible

Borg CR10 scale
© Gunnar Borg, 1981, 1982, 1998

Figure 4.6 Modified Borg scale.

G. Borg, 1998, *Borg's Perceived Exertion and Pain Scales* (Champaign, IL: Human Kinetics), 50.

goals, and needs. Duration can increase as the client becomes fitter in order to impose overload for positive adaptation. Be aware that as exercise duration increases, the risk of injury also increases. Careful consideration is required when determining proper exercise time.

When planning exercise time, consider the following:

ISSUES	INFLUENCES
Client's exercise experience	An inactive client should start with 10 to 15 minutes of activity, then gradually increase exercise time in small increments (5 minutes) every week.
Client's current fitness level	Beginner clients can start with some activity, adding duration as they adapt to increased workload.
Client's goals for cardio-respiratory conditioning	Fitter clients exercise between 30 and 60 minutes as desired. Improving cardiorespiratory efficiency requires more than 20 minutes of elevated HR. Weight reduction requires longer exercise time to maximize caloric expenditure.

Exercise Type

Exercise type refers to the type of activity performed, or mode. An obvious starting point is to choose an activity that the client enjoys or has performed previously with some success. Incorporating fun into each workout improves your clients' chances for success. Many people choose not to exercise because they do not find it enjoyable. Your goal is to find fun in all activities for clients.

All activities have specific difficulty levels. To maximize client success, you must match the right activities with the right client. Training modes and equipment should be based on the client's current fitness level, past fitness experience, goals, and needs. Many clients prefer activities that are continuous in nature, such as walking, swimming, running, stepping, cycling, and skating. Clients can perform many continuous cardiorespiratory activities outdoors or indoors on machines such as treadmills, stair climbers, and cross-trainers. This type of training allows clients to gradually build to steady-state exercise and stay there before cooling down.

Different types of equipment and exercises have different levels of difficulty. Factors that affect exercise difficulty include skill, coordination, and caloric expenditure. Activities such as tennis, squash, basketball, in-line skating, skiing, aerobics, step aerobics, and swimming require skill and coordination.

The caloric expenditure required to perform an activity is another consideration. The two major factors that affect caloric expenditure are amount of muscle mass used and type of movement. As a general rule, more muscle mass and more movement (especially in the vertical plane) require more effort. The greater the effort, the more calories are burned. Closely examine the exercises you recommend to clients to determine which exercise type is best for maximizing their results.

When planning exercise type, consider the following:

ISSUES	INFLUENCES
Client's exercise experience	Inexperienced clients should begin on equipment that requires minimal skill, coordination, and caloric expenditure.
Client's current fitness level	New exercisers should choose exercises that limit movement in the vertical plane and involve less muscle mass. Fitter clients can be challenged with equipment and activities that involve complex movements in horizontal and vertical planes.
Client's goals for cardiorespiratory conditioning	Clients working to improve cardiorespiratory conditioning can experiment with many types of exercise equipment. When weight reduction is the goal, clients should maximize caloric expenditure.

Putting It All Together

Research has determined the optimal combinations of exercise frequency, intensity, time, and type.

- Frequency: Training at 60% of $\dot{V}O_2$max 4 days a week. Research indicates that substantial gains are made when frequency of training increases up to 4 days a week, after which improvements plateau (see figure 4.7).

- Duration: Training at 60% of $\dot{V}O_2$max 30 minutes per session. Research indicates that substantial gains are made when duration increases up to 30 minutes, after which improvements plateau (see figure 4.8).

- Intensity: Training for 30 minutes 3 or 4 times a week. Research indicates that there are substantial gains when increasing the intensity of the training sessions up to 80% of $\dot{V}O_2$max, after which improvements plateau (see figure 4.9).

Table 4.5 provides general guidelines for program development. Each client will respond differently, and keeping communication channels open with clients will be essential to your success, allowing for program modifications before problems arise.

Summary of Important Points

1. The decisions you make in developing thorough cardiorespiratory training programs for clients are crucial.

2. The cellular benefits of cardiorespiratory conditioning include increased number of aerobic enzymes, increased number and size of mitochondria, improved blood delivery, and increased capillary density.

3. Energy or ATP is produced through anaerobic and aerobic metabolism. When oxygen

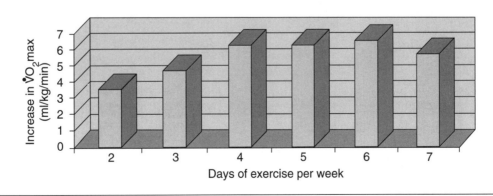

Figure 4.7   Frequency chart.

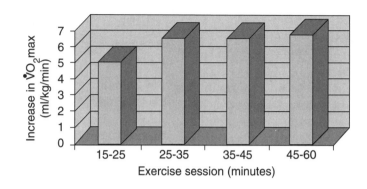

Figure 4.8   Duration chart.

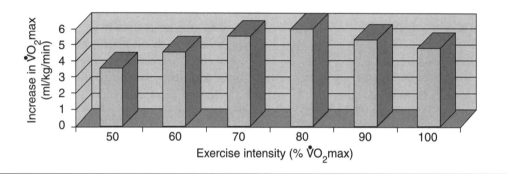

Figure 4.9   Intensity chart.

TABLE 4.5   **Cardiorespiratory Training Guidelines**

DESCRIPTION	BEGINNER (VERY LOW TO LOW FITNESS)	INTERMEDIATE (AVERAGE FITNESS)	ADVANCED (ABOVE-AVERAGE FITNESS)
Program focus	Improved health profile Increased energy Daily activities made easier Weight reduction	Weight reduction Program variety	Increase $\dot{V}O_2$max Weight maintenance Sport training Competition
Frequency	1-3 times/week	3-5 times/week	4-6 times/week
Intensity	55%-64% HRmax RPE 9-12	65%-74% HRmax RPE 12-15	75%-90% HRmax RPE 13-16
Time	15-30 min	20-45 min	40-60 min
Type	Walking Stationary cycling Swimming Water aerobics Basic fitness classes	Stair climbing Treadmill Fitness classes Cycling classes Cross-training	Complex movements Sports Cross-training Interval training

supply can't meet demand, the client reaches an anaerobic threshold and can no longer produce energy aerobically.

4. Follow the FITT formula for program design (frequency, intensity, time, and type).

5. Exercise frequency should range from 2 to 7 sessions per week.

6. Exercise intensity should range from 55% to 90% of HRmax.

7. Exercise time should range from 10 to 60 minutes.

8. Exercise type should match the client's needs.

9. Cardiorespiratory training design should

10. Recovery is the final phase of cardiorespiratory exercise. Its primary purpose is to assist the body in recovering from exercise and gradually return to a preexercise state.

11. The cardiorespiratory system is a transport system for oxygen. It picks up oxygen in the lungs and takes it to cells in the body.

12. Resting HR for the average person is 72 bpm; resting BP is 120/80 mmHg.

13. Aerobic capacity is measured by the amount of oxygen that can be delivered to the muscle cell compared with the amount of oxygen used by the muscle cell to make energy for muscle contraction ($\dot{V}O_2$max).

14. At the onset of exercise, the cardiovascular system responds to the increased demand for oxygen by increasing HR, stroke volume, and cardiac output.

15. The respiratory system provides oxygen to the body and gets rid of carbon dioxide.

16. At the onset of exercise, the respiratory system provides additional oxygen to the working muscles by rapidly increasing the rate of ventilation (similar to the increase in HR).

Case Studies

Roger

Roger's resting HR is 81 bpm and his resting BP is 137/92 mmHg. His $\dot{V}O_2$max is 32 millilitres per kilogram per minute. Although Roger's aerobic capacity is fair, he is borderline hypertensive. At this stage of his fitness plan, he needs to focus on improving his aerobic fitness through walking, cycling, or swimming. The initial stage will encompass 4 to 6 weeks of aerobic exercise at an RPE of 9 to 12, or 55% to 60% of maximum HR (HRmax), for 15 to 20 minutes, 2 to 3 times a week. This can then be followed by the improvement stage, which may last from the 6th week until the 24th week of training progressively, working up to an RPE of 12 to 13, or 65% of HRmax, for 20 to 40 minutes a minimum of 3 days per week. During this phase, progress time and not intensity. Once he is comfortable with this, encourage him to add a fourth day of aerobic activity on his own since frequency of activity is important for helping regulate his BP.

Molly

Molly's resting HR is 75 bpm and her resting BP is 115/78 mmHg, well within normal ranges. Her $\dot{V}O_2$max is 35 millilitres per kilogram per minute, which is average. Because Molly wants to lose weight, volume of activity will be important. She should be encouraged to perform aerobic activity (such as using a treadmill or taking fitness classes) 3 to 4 times a week for 20 to 40 minutes. She should exercise at an RPE of 12 to 15, or 65% to 70% of her HRmax. In the beginning, she should be encouraged to increase time rather than intensity.

Jennifer

Jennifer's resting HR is 80 bpm and her resting BP is 120/80 mmHg. Her resting HR is high for her age, although her blood pressure is well within normal ranges. Jennifer's $\dot{V}O_2$max is 29.5 millilitres per kilogram per minute, which is average. She should be encouraged to perform aerobic activity (such as using a treadmill or taking fitness classes) 3 times a week for 20 minutes for the first 4 weeks at an RPE of 12 to 13, or 65% of her HRmax. Over the next 4 weeks, she should be encouraged to increase the intensity to an RPE of 14 to 15, or 70% of HRmax. Once she has achieved this goal, she can work toward 30 to 40 minutes.

CHAPTER 5

Skeletal Anatomy and Flexibility Concepts

Carmen Bott, MSc

CHAPTER OBJECTIVES

After completing this chapter, you will be able to

1. list the primary functions of bones,
2. identify the classifications of bones,
3. locate and name major bones in the body,
4. define anatomical position,
5. locate important structures in the body using proper anatomical terms,
6. identify classifications of joints and types of synovial joints,
7. describe joint movement using correct terminology,
8. identify movements that occur in the major joints,
9. define flexibility and its relationship to fitness,
10. identify joint mechanics and explain how stretching promotes flexibility,
11. describe the changes that occur after regular stretching,
12. identify the purpose of flexibility training,
13. determine appropriate durations for flexibility training,
14. perform various techniques that promote flexibility, and
15. identify basic guidelines for flexibility training.

Skeletal System Overview

The average human adult skeleton has 206 bones joined to ligaments and tendons to form a protective, supportive framework for the attached muscles and the soft tissues that underlie it (figure 5.1). There are only minor differences between male and female skeletons: men's bones tend to be larger and heavier than corresponding women's bones and the pelvic cavity is wider in women to accommodate childbirth. The skeleton plays an important part in movement by providing a series of independently movable levers that the muscles can pull to move different parts of the body. It also supports and protects the internal organs. Babies are born with 270 soft bones—about 64 more than an adult—and many of these fuse together by the age of 20 or 25 into the 206 hard, permanent bones.

The skeleton is not just a movable frame. Without bones, we would not be capable of standing upright, let alone moving. The skeleton serves four essential functions:

1. Protects the vital organs and soft tissue.
2. Serves as the factory where red blood cells are produced.
3. Serves as a reservoir for minerals (calcium and phosphate).
4. Provides attachments for muscles to produce movement.

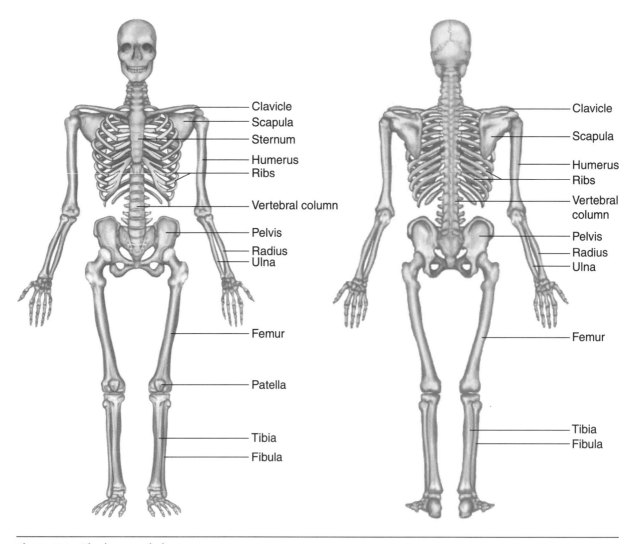

Figure 5.1 The human skeleton.

Reprinted, by permission, from T.R. Baechle and R.W. Earle (eds.), 2000, *Essentials of strength training and conditioning,* 2nd ed. (Champaign, IL: Human Kinetics), 27.

Classifications of Bones

As discussed, the human skeleton has more than 200 bones, and most of them are involved in movement. Bones are 50% fluid and 50% solid. Minerals make them rigid and protein makes them strong. Bones are classified according to shape: long, short, flat, and irregular (table 5.1).

Parts of the Skeleton

The skeleton has two main parts: the axial skeleton and the appendicular skeleton. The axial skeleton consists of the skull, spine, ribs, and sternum (breastbone) and includes 80 bones. The appendicular skeleton includes two limb girdles (the shoulders and pelvis) and their attached limb bones. This part of the skeletal system contains 126 bones, 64 in the shoulders and upper limbs and 62 in the pelvis and lower limbs.

What Is the Anatomical Position?

The anatomical position is a position where a person stands with arms at the sides, palms facing forward. This is the point of reference when describing body parts or movements. From this position, parts of the body can be described in relation to one another and movement can be described using selected terms, as described next.

Anterior and Posterior

Anterior describes the front of the body; *posterior* describes the back of the body.

Medial and Lateral

When standing in an anatomical position, we refer to body parts that are closest to the midline of the body as *medial*; parts that are away from the midline of the body are *lateral*.

Superior and Inferior

When one body part is above another, it is *superior*; when one body part is below another, it is *inferior*.

Supine and Prone

When the body lies faceup, it is *supine*; when the body lies facedown, it is *prone*.

Dorsal and Plantar

The top of the foot is referred to as the *dorsal* surface; the bottom of the foot is called the *plantar* surface.

Proximal and Distal

The end of a bone or muscle that is closest to the body is called the *proximal* end; the end that is farthest from the body is called the *distal* end.

Joint Movement Terminology

To describe movement at a joint, we use specific terminology to identify the direction in which the movement occurs. This terminology is listed next.

Flexion, Extension, and Hyperextension

Straightening a joint is called *extension* (i.e., the joint angle increases). Bending a joint is called *flexion* (i.e., the joint angle decreases). When a

TABLE 5.1 **Classifications of Bones**

CLASSIFICATION	EXAMPLES	FUNCTION
Long bones	Femur Humerus	Serve as levers for movement.
Short bones	Tarsals (ankle) Carpals (wrist)	Give strength to joints, but with limited mobility.
Flat bones	Ribs Scapulae	Provide a broad site for muscle attachment; protect internal organs.
Irregular bones	Ischium Pubis Vertebrae	Protect internal organs; support the body.

movement occurs beyond the normal joint range of motion (ROM), it is called *hyperextension*.

Abduction (Protraction) and Adduction (Retraction)

Abduction occurs when a bone moves away from the midline of the body. Bringing the bone toward the midline of the body is called *adduction* of the joint.

Circumduction

Circumduction is a circular movement that combines flexion, abduction, extension, and adduction. This type of movement occurs at ball-and-socket joints.

Medial and Lateral Rotation

To rotate a joint, you turn the moving bone about its axis or centre. Rotation toward the midline of the body is called *medial* or *internal rotation*. Rotation away from the midline of the body is called *lateral* or *external rotation*.

Supination and Pronation

The forearms and lower body are capable of producing two movements. External movement, or movement away from the midline of the body, is called *supination*. Internal movement, or movement toward the midline of the body, is called *pronation*.

Inversion and Eversion

These movements occur at the ankle joint. Turning the medial, or inner, side of the foot off the ground is called *inversion*. Turning the outer side off the ground is called *eversion*.

Elevation and Depression

Typically, *elevation* is produced by shrugging the shoulders upward (scapular elevation), whereas *depression* is produced by lowering the shoulders below anatomical position (scapular depression).

Joints

The place where bones meet is called a *joint*. We classify joints based on the amount of movement that occurs at this joining point between bones (figure 5.2). There are three classifications of joints: fibrous, cartilaginous, and synovial.

Joint	Movements
Shoulder girdle (scapula, clavicle)	Elevation–depression
	Abduction or protraction–adduction or retraction
	Upward rotation–downward rotation
Shoulder joint	Flexion–extension
	Abduction–adduction
	Medial–lateral rotation
	Transverse flexion–extension (flexion or extension along a transverse plane)
	Circumduction
Elbow joint	Flexion–extension
Radioulnar joint	Pronation–supination
Wrist joint	Flexion–extension
	Radial flexion–ulnar flexion
Vertebral column Spine	Flexion–extension
	Lateral flexion
	Rotation
Lumbosacral joint	Flexion–extension (anterior pelvic tilt–posterior pelvic tilt)
Hip joint	Flexion–extension
	Abduction–adduction
	Medial–lateral rotation
	Circumduction
Knee joint	Flexion–extension
	Rotation at 90° flexion
Ankle joint	Plantar flexion–dorsiflexion
	Eversion–inversion

Figure 5.2   Joint movement summary.

Fibrous Joints

Fibrous joints connect bones without allowing any movement. The bones of the skull and pelvis are held together by fibrous joints. The union of the spinous processes and vertebrae are also fibrous joints.

Cartilaginous Joints

Cartilaginous joints are joints in which the bones are attached by cartilage. These joints allow for only a little movement, such as in the spine or ribs.

Synovial Joints

Synovial joints allow for much more movement than cartilaginous joints. These freely movable joints have cartilage along the surface of the bones that join together to reduce friction and absorb shock. They are also enclosed by an articular capsule that holds the synovial fluid (a lubricating fluid produced by the synovial membrane) inside the joint cavity. There are six types of synovial joints providing various amounts of movement. The three major types of synovial joints are described in table 5.2.

TABLE 5.2   **Types of Synovial Joints**

TYPE	MOVEMENT	EXAMPLES
Hinge	Allows movement in one direction.	Elbow Knee
Condyloid	Allows movement in two directions.	Wrist Ankle
Ball and socket	Allows movement in three directions and the largest ROM.	Shoulder Hip

Connective Tissue

Ligaments and tendons are forms of fibrous connective tissue. A ligament is a short band of tough, fibrous connective tissue composed mainly of long, stringy collagen molecules. Ligaments connect bones to other bones in joints. A tendon is a tough band of fibrous connective tissue attached on one end to a muscle and on the other to a bone.

Flexibility

Flexibility is needed to perform everyday activities with relative ease. To get out of bed, lift children, or sweep the floor, we need flexibility. Flexibility tends to deteriorate with age, often due to a sedentary lifestyle. Without adequate flexibility, daily activities become more difficult to perform. Over time, we create body movements and posture habits that can lead to reduced mobility of joints and compromised body positions. Staying active and stretching regularly help prevent this loss of mobility, which ensures independence as we age. Being flexible significantly reduces the chance of experiencing occasional and chronic back pain.

What Is Flexibility?

Flexibility is a measure of the range of motion around a joint (e.g., knee) or series of joints (e.g., lower back). Flexibility is most limited by the joint's physical structure, including the bone, connective tissue, and muscle. Both men and women can improve flexibility with training.

Purpose of Flexibility Training

It is important to include flexibility training as part of your clients' regular fitness routines. Improved flexibility may enhance performance in aerobic training and muscular conditioning as well as in sport. There is scientific evidence that the incidence of injury decreases when people include flexibility training in their routines due to the enhanced ability to move unimpeded through a wider ROM. The only exception to this would be when there is an excessive or unstable ROM, which may increase the likelihood of injury. When used appropriately, flexibility training allows clients to become more in tune with their body. It is a form of active relaxation that can improve both mental and physical recovery.

Once the workout is complete, clients can focus on relaxation and rejuvenation of mind and body. After pushing the body to work hard, it is time to encourage recovery. This is an excellent time for flexibility training because the muscles are warm and pliable, allowing them to stretch farther.

Following are some of the major benefits of flexibility training:

- Reduces stress in the exercising muscles and releases tension developed during the workout.

- Assists with posture by balancing the tension placed across the joint by the muscles that cross it. Proper posture minimizes stress and maximizes the strength of all joint movements.

- Reduces the risk of injury during exercise and daily activities because muscles are more pliable.

- Improves performance of everyday activities as well as performance in exercise and sport.

As with all other components of the workout, flexibility training should be based on the FITT formula (see chapter 4). The following sections examine each component of the FITT formula more closely as it relates to flexibility.

Frequency of Flexibility Training

Stretching should be included after every workout to encourage improvement and maintain overall flexibility. Canada's *Physical Activity Guide to Healthy Active Living* recommends flexibility training 4 to 7 days a week.

Intensity of Flexibility Training

Stretching should never be painful. The focus should be on bringing the muscle to a point of slight tension. Encourage clients to continue their breathing pattern throughout the stretch.

Duration of Flexibility Training

The length of the flexibility component depends on the needs and motivation of the client. In most cases, flexibility training should last at least 5 to 10 minutes. Stretching is one area of the workout that tends to get cut short when time is running out. Don't assume that clients will perform their own recovery and flexibility once their session with you has ended. Being organized with workout design ensures that there is always time for stretching.

Flexibility Techniques

To increase or restore muscle ROM, it is necessary to overload the muscle with flexibility training. To improve joint ROM, it is necessary to lengthen the muscle and surrounding connective tissue in safe and effective ways.

Two main methods of flexibility training (static and dynamic) can be used, but all types of flexibility training will be more effective after a thorough warm-up, when the body temperature is elevated.

Static Stretching

This method of flexibility training involves taking a specific joint or set of joints through a ROM to a comfortable end point (at least 20 seconds), resting for approximately 20 seconds, and then repeating the stretch two to three times.

The goal of static stretching is to overcome the stretch reflex (the automatic tightening of a muscle when stretched, which relaxes after approximately

20 seconds) to coax a joint into a wider ROM. This is done by holding the stretch gently and not overstretching the muscle.

- **Example:** Sit on the floor with your legs in front of you and bend forward at the hips with your spine in a neutral position until you feel a slight tension in the hamstring group. This stretch requires relaxation of the hamstrings and will increase ROM at the hip joint. Keep in mind that if you also flex the spine, you will be including the ROM of the vertebral joints, which may decrease the effect on the hamstrings.

- **Advantages:** Static stretching can be used by virtually anyone; it is easily taught and usually very safe. Once learned, it can be performed in almost any environment without external assistance or equipment.

- **Disadvantages:** Static stretching will improve flexibility at a specific body position and only to a small degree outside of that position, limiting its effectiveness for athletes or those wanting to increase flexibility in multiple ROMs. It is best suited to noncompetitive clients or as a complement to other methods of flexibility training.

Dynamic Stretching

This method of flexibility training uses increasingly dynamic movements through the full ROM of a joint. Dynamic stretching develops active ROM through the process of reciprocal inhibition, where the agonist muscle is contracting while the antagonist or opposite muscle is carried through the lengthening process.

When performed correctly, dynamic stretching warms up the joints, maintains current flexibility, and reduces muscle tension. The exercise begins at a slow pace and gradually increases in speed and intensity. This method of stretching is best performed before exercise or activity that is movement based, like tennis or hiking.

- **Example:** While standing on one foot, flex the hip joint of the nonsupporting leg (knee extended, like a pendulum). This motion contracts the hip flexors (agonists) and requires inhibition or relaxation of the hamstring group (antagonists).

- **Advantages:** Dynamic ROM is extremely useful for athletes and those who are warming up for an activity that requires a wide ROM, especially when speed is involved. Dynamic and static stretches combined can prepare the joints for explosive movements more than either type alone.

- **Disadvantages:** Dynamic ROM should be used gradually and only by those who have been shown an appropriate series of movements. If inappropriate movements are used, small trauma may be experienced over time in the joints or connective tissue from movements that are too fast or through a ROM that is too extreme.

Stretching

Common stretches for each major muscle group are found in Appendix B. Can-Fit-Pro recommends performing dynamic stretches prior to an exercise session in a warm-up, and static stretches after an exercise session in a cool-down. While other types of stretching exist, they are typically for therapeutic purposes and often outside of a personal trainer's scope of practice.

Guidelines for Flexibility Training

- Don't overdo it; work within your limits.
- Breathe comfortably. Exhale as the muscle lengthens to assist in relaxation.
- Perform flexibility exercises for each muscle group for total-body improvements.
- Work with warm muscles because they lengthen more easily and with less discomfort. The best time to do flexibility training is after the cardiorespiratory workout.
- Modify. You can alter the difficulty of a stretch by paying attention to
  - single-joint versus multijoint movements (complexity),
  - position of the stretch (whether it involves balance),
  - available ROM (individual limits),
  - length of the lever (longer is more difficult),
  - degree of exercise difficulty,
  - chosen stretching technique, and
  - effect of gravity (as an assistance or resistance).

Choose activities that serve two functions: relaxation and flexibility. This does not mean that the entire time has to be spent stretching. There are many methods of flexibility training that promote relaxation, such as yoga, meditation, Pilates, tai chi, visualization, and breathing. Try these alternatives to assist clients in relaxing and encourage them to de-stress from their busy lives.

Summary of Important Points

1. Bones protect the internal organs and provide the body with structure and the ability to move.

2. Bones are divided into four classifications: long, short, flat, and irregular.

3. The anatomical position is when the body is erect with arms at sides and palms facing forward.

4. The axial skeleton consists of the head, trunk, and vertebrae. The appendicular skeleton consists of the appendages and the pelvis.

5. Joints are classified by the amount of movement they possess. There are three types of joints that differ due to the amount of movement they can create.

6. The three most common types of synovial joints referred to in fitness are the hinge, condyloid, and ball-and-socket joints.

7. Ligaments connect bone to bone and tendons connect muscle to bone.

8. Various terms are used to describe joint movement.

9. To understand the big picture of human movement, it is important to identify the possible movements that can occur at each joint and the muscles that produce these movements.

10. Flexibility training serves two primary purposes: relaxation and rejuvenation of the mind, body, and spirit, and development of flexibility.

11. The flexibility component should be performed 4 to 7 days a week.

12. Stretching should never be painful.

13. The flexibility component should last at least 5 to 10 minutes (longer for clients with special needs).

14. Flexibility training may also include the following techniques to promote relaxation:

yoga, meditation, Pilates, tai chi, visualization, and breathing.

15. It is important to follow the guidelines for flexibility training to achieve the best results for clients of all abilities.

16. Flexibility enhances performance in sport, aerobic conditioning, muscular conditioning, and daily activities.

17. There are two methods of training flexibility: static stretching and dynamic stretching.

Case Studies

Roger

Roger spends the majority of his day sitting at a desk. This pattern can lead to shortened muscles and poor posture. Roger should be encouraged to follow a flexibility routine daily, even on the days he does not visit the gym. He should also be guided in breathing deeply to allow for muscle relaxation and making sure he stretches when his body is warm (i.e., at the end of his workout). A flexibility exercise should be prescribed for each major muscle group, paying special attention to his hamstrings, pectoralis major and pectoralis minor, and hip flexors since these muscles undergo more shortening with prolonged sitting. Each stretch should be held gently for 1 minute, and areas that need more stretching should be repeated more than once.

Molly

Molly is quite young and may not realize the importance of flexibility training. In particular, it's likely that specific areas of her body are tighter than others due to her school and studying schedule. Specifically, a greater emphasis may need to be placed on the muscle groups in the back (latissimus dorsi and trapezius) and hip flexors, although she will benefit from a total-body flexibility routine at the end of each workout. It is important to spend time educating her on how restoring muscles to their resting length after exercise is important so that she can participate in the sports she loves on a daily basis. Molly might also enjoy trying a yoga class to work on this parameter in a more social environment.

Jennifer

For Jennifer, flexibility training must provide an opportunity to relax. She should be coached on breathing deeply and slowly moving into each stretch, thus heightening her body awareness. With so many things going on in her life, Jennifer should be encouraged to stretch as often as possible. Yoga and tai chi would be great additions to Jennifer's fitness routine, and these can also be followed in the comfort of her own home once she learns some simple techniques or follows video instructions. Rejuvenation of the mind, body, and spirit during flexibility training is important for Jennifer.

CHAPTER 6

Muscular Concepts

Carmen Bott, MSc

CHAPTER OBJECTIVES

After completing this chapter, you will be able to

1. identify the major muscles,

2. identify the origins and insertions of the major muscles,

3. list and locate major muscle pairs,

4. describe the structure of skeletal muscle,

5. describe the sliding filament theory of muscular contraction,

6. define types of muscle fibres and list their characteristics,

7. differentiate among types of muscle contractions, and

8. name the muscles that produce all possible movements in the major joints.

Muscles are attached to bone by tendons, and they exert force by converting chemical energy into tension and contraction. They move and make us capable of a variety of actions by simply contracting and becoming shorter; they pull but they cannot push. They are made up of millions of tiny protein filaments that work together to produce motion in the body. Each of more than 600 muscles is served by nerves that link the muscle to the spinal cord and brain. Bodily needs demand that muscles accomplish different chores, so we are equipped with three types of muscles: cardiac, smooth, and skeletal. Cardiac muscle, found only in the heart, powers the action that pumps blood throughout the body. Smooth muscle surrounds or is part of the internal organs. Skeletal muscle, which is the focus of this chapter, carries out voluntary movements and is what may ache after strenuous exercise. Skeletal muscle is the most abundant tissue in the body, making up about 23% of a woman's body weight and about 40% of a man's body weight.

Muscle Structure

Skeletal muscles consist of bunches of elongated, rod-shaped cells called **muscle fibres.** Each fibre is packed full of thinner fibres called *myofibrils,* a smaller structural component that runs the length of the muscle. Each myofibril is composed of a long series of *sarcomeres.* A sarcomere is the basic unit of muscle contraction and comprises two types of protein: a thin filament called *actin* and a thick filament called *myosin.* These protein filaments slide along each other when a muscle contracts.

Figure 6.1 illustrates the levels of organization within a skeletal muscle.

Muscle Contraction

In a relaxed muscle, thick and thin myofilaments overlap each other a bit. When a muscle cell is stimulated by a nerve impulse, these myofilaments slide past each other until they completely overlap. Thick filaments (myosin) pull on the thin filaments (actin) in order to pull the ends of the sarcomere closer together. The cell shortens, and as other cells shorten at the same time, so does the entire muscle (this is known as the All-or-None law of muscle contraction). This happens without the contractile proteins changing in size or shape. For the muscle to contract or shorten, the muscle cells convert energy (ATP) into mechanical work (contraction). Relaxation occurs when the myosin and actin return to their unbound state. The mechanism of shortening is called the *sliding filament theory.* Figure 6.2 demonstrates the movement of the actin over the myosin during contraction.

Types of Muscle Contractions

When muscles produce movement, they contract and relax. The resulting movements are based on the response of the muscle, as described in table 6.1.

Basic Organization of the Nervous System

The ability to perform coordinated and skilled movement requires coordination between the muscular system and the nervous system. The nervous system is divided into two parts: the central nervous system (CNS) and the peripheral nervous system (PNS). The CNS is composed of the brain and spinal cord and is enclosed by the skull and spinal column. It is the control centre of the nervous system because it receives information from the PNS and develops an appropriate response. The PNS is made up of

Table 6.1   Three Types of Muscle Contractions

TYPE OF CONTRACTION	DESCRIPTION	EXAMPLES
Isotonic—concentric	Movement occurs when the muscle contracts with enough force to shorten.	Lifting phase of a biceps curl
Isotonic—eccentric	The muscle generates tension, but as it exerts force, it lengthens (e.g., like a braking mechanism).	Lowering phase of a biceps curl
Isometric	In this static contraction, the muscle exerts force to counteract an opposing force; no change in muscle length occurs.	Holding the arm at a fixed angle of 90° with resistance in one's hand

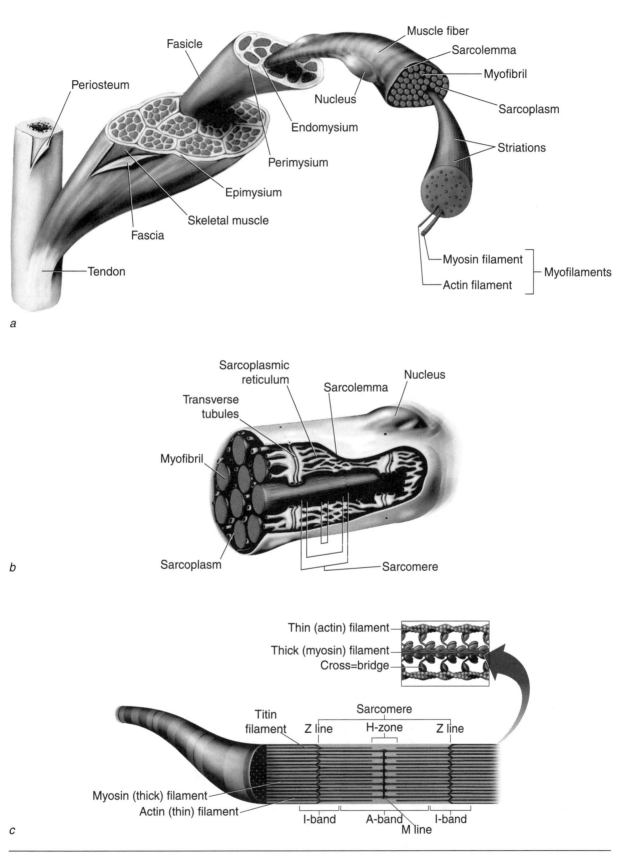

Figure 6.1 Levels of organization within a skeletal muscle: *(a)* skeletal muscle, *(b)* muscle fibre, and *(c)* sarcomere.

Reprinted, by permission, from W.C. Whiting and S. Rugg, 2006, *Dynatomy* (Champaign, IL: Human Kinetics), pp. 69-70.

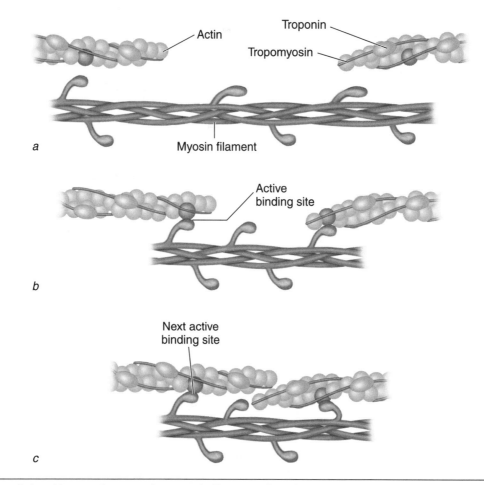

Figure 6.2 Sliding filament theory with a muscle fiber *(a)* relaxed, *(b)* contracting, and *(c)* fully contracted.

Reprinted, by permission, from J.H. Wilmore and D.L. Costill, 2004, *Physiology of sport and exercise,* 3rd ed. (Champaign, IL: Human Kinetics), p. 42.

nerves that connect the extremities to the brain (CNS). It continuously delivers information about all body parts to the brain for processing.

Each muscle has several nerve fibres that lie within the body of the muscle. Some nerves activate only a few muscle fibres, whereas other nerves may activate hundreds of fibres. The nerve and fibres that it commands are called a *motor unit* (figure 6.3). When the nerve is stimulated, all of the associated muscle fibres will create tension (the All-or-None law). Motor units consisting of many muscle fibres produce strong contractions, and motor units with only a few muscle fibres result in weaker contractions.

Nerve signals are transported in the body by neurons, or nerve cells. There are two kinds of neurons: sensory and motor. Sensory neurons carry information and sensations from the body and environment to the CNS. Motor neurons carry information from the CNS back to the muscles to create a response or movement.

Proprioceptors are specialized sensory receptors found in joints, muscles, and tendons. They are sensitive to pressure and tension and are responsible for sending messages to the CNS in order to maintain muscle tone and perform coordinated movements. *Muscle spindles* are proprioceptors that consist of several modified muscle fibres enclosed in a blanket of connective tissue. These spindles provide information concerning muscle fibre length and the rate of change in its length. Spindles tell the muscle how much it needs to contract to overcome a given stretch.

Golgi tendon organs (GTO) are proprioceptors located in tendons. GTOs are activated when the tendon attached to an active muscle is stretched. They function similarly to the muscle spindles in that they also measure changes in the muscle. However, whereas the muscle spindle is active even while the muscle is at rest, the GTO only becomes activated when the muscle contracts. Further, GTOs are not concerned with changes in muscle

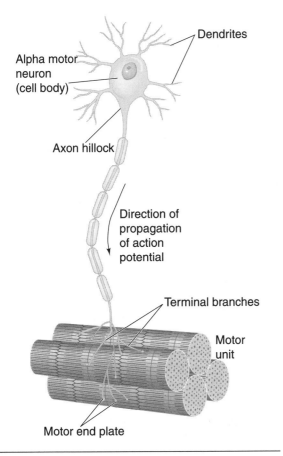

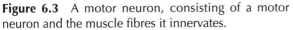

Figure 6.3 A motor neuron, consisting of a motor neuron and the muscle fibres it innervates.

Reprinted, by permission, from J.H. Wilmore and D.L. Costill, 2004, *Physiology of sport and exercise*, 3rd ed. (Champaign, IL: Human Kinetics), p. 40.

length, but rather with the increased tension of the muscle as a result of a change in its length. GTOs are high-threshold, slowly adapting receptors and apparently serve, at least in part, to prevent excessive stresses at joints. If the strain on the muscle and tendon becomes excessive, the GTO sends an impulse to the CNS, causing the muscle to relax and thereby preventing injury.

Force of Muscle Contraction and Fibre Types

Although all fibres within a motor unit function in a similar manner, there are differences among motor units related to the types of muscle fibre being recruited. Skeletal muscle can be classified according to its fibre type. In basic terms, fibres can be distinguished as either slow twitch or fast twitch (see figure 6.4). All muscles have a combination of these fibre types, and the percentage of fibre types in each muscle varies according to the function of the muscle, training, and genetics. Slow-twitch fibres are best suited for endurance work because they have a greater ability to use oxygen. Exercise that requires short, intense bursts of activity uses fast-twitch fibres. During exercise, the nervous system generally recruits slow-twitch fibres first. As muscle contractions become more intense, fast-twitch fibres are added.

Factors Related to Strength

Strength is not as simple as the idea that bigger muscles are stronger muscles. Several factors play a role in a muscle or muscle group's ability to generate force (strength):

- Neural control—Muscle force is generally greater when
  - more motor units are involved in a contraction,
  - the motor units are bigger in size, and
  - the rate at which the motor units fire is faster.

  Note: Most of the gains made in the first few weeks of a strength program can be attributed to neural adaptation as the brain learns how to tell the muscles to generate more force.

Fast twitch	**Slow twitch**
Produce most ATP or energy within the cell.	Contain lots of mitochondria and capillaries for oxygen delivery.
Contract quickly and produce a great deal of force, but fatigue quickly.	Contract slowly and produce a smaller amount of force than fast-twitch fibres, but are resistant to fatigue.
Work anaerobically.	Work aerobically.

Figure 6.4 The major differences between fibre types.

- Muscle size—The force a muscle can generate is related to its size.
- Muscle length—A muscle can generate its greatest force when it is at its resting length because the actin and myosin filaments lie next to each other and all potential cross-bridges are exposed.
- Speed of contraction—For concentric muscle actions, maximal force can be achieved with slower contractions, whereas eccentric contractions produce more force with faster movements.

Muscle Anatomy

We have examined the different muscle fibre types, how a muscle produces a contraction, and how the nervous system plays a role in coordinated movement. Now we can move back to the macroscopic level and take a closer look at how muscles and muscle groups work together to produce movement. In order to understand how to produce and perfect human movement, we study the science of anatomy in action, also known as *kinesiology*.

Movement occurs when muscles, bones, and joints work together to set the body or a body part in motion. Muscles pull on bones to create movement at a joint.

Interactions of Skeletal Muscles and Group Actions

Muscles that assume the major responsibility for producing a specific movement are called prime movers, or *agonists*. The biceps brachii is the prime mover of elbow flexion, for example.

Muscles that oppose, or reverse, a particular movement by a prime mover are called *antagonists*. When a prime mover is active, the antagonist muscle is relaxed, yielding to the movement of the prime mover. Antagonists can also help to regulate the action of the prime mover by partially contracting to provide some resistance or to slow or stop the action. During elbow flexion, the triceps brachii is the antagonist.

Most movements also involve muscles called *synergists*, which reduce undesirable or unnecessary movements that might result as the prime mover contracts. For example, when a muscle crosses two or more joints, its contraction causes movement at all of the joints unless the synergists act as muscle stabilizers. Muscles that help to maintain posture are also synergists.

Figure 6.5 illustrates the concepts of agonist, antagonist and synergist muscle groups.

Depending on the movement, muscles can act as prime movers, antagonists, or synergists at any one time.

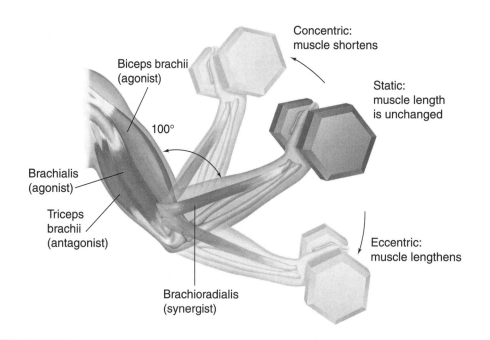

Figure 6.5 The actions of agonistic, antagonistic, and synergistic muscles during elbow flexion.

Reprinted, by permission, from J.H. Wilmore and D.L. Costill, 2004, *Physiology of sport and exercise*, 3rd ed. (Champaign, IL: Human Kinetics), p. 53.

Muscle Origin and Insertion

Skeletal muscles produce movement by exerting force on tendons, which then pull on bones. Most muscles cross a joint and attach to the articulating bone that forms a joint. The attachment of the muscle tendon to the stationary bone is called the *origin* of the muscle. The attachment of the muscle tendon to the moving bone is called the *insertion* of the muscle. In limbs, the origin is usually proximal and the insertion is usually distal. When a muscle contracts, it pulls its insertion toward its origin. The fleshy portion between the origin and insertion is called the *muscle belly.*

Major Muscles

The major muscles of the body are described based on anatomical location. For simplicity and ease of learning, the origin and insertion points for these muscles are labeled as approximate anatomical positions only.

Shoulder Girdle

Muscles of the Shoulder Girdle

The shoulder girdle is an articulation between the scapula and the clavicle. It is considered a group of floating bones because the bones are secured only by muscles. The floating nature of this joint makes the area very unstable, but it allows for a large ROM. Figure 6.6 shows the posterior and anterior views of the upper body. Note that on the right-hand side of the posterior diagram, the superficial muscle (trapezius) has been removed to show the deep muscles that lie below it (levator scapulae and rhomboids).

Movements of the Shoulder Girdle

As mentioned, the shoulder girdle region is considered a floating joint because it is stabilized by muscles. To generate maximum force and optimal contraction of upper-body muscles, the shoulder girdle must be stable (not moving) before contraction. The best way to cue clients to stabilize the shoulder girdle is to ask them to lift the shoulder blades (elevation), pull the shoulder blades back (retraction), and pull them down (depression) (see table 6.2). This is called the *set position.* When the shoulder girdle is in the set position, it is stable. Cue the set position before all upper-body movements to enhance muscle contraction.

Shoulder

Muscles of the Shoulder

The shoulder joint is an articulation between the humerus bone (upper arm) and the scapula and clavicle. It is a synovial ball-and-socket

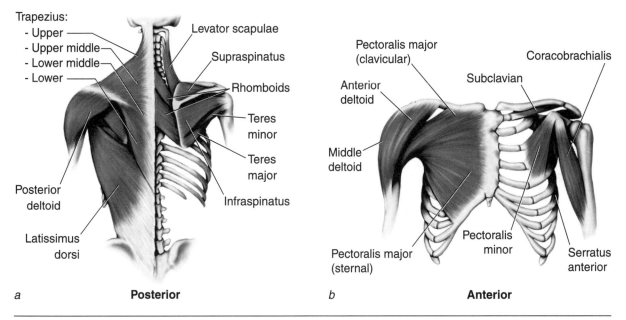

Figure 6.6 Muscles of the shoulder girdle: *(a)* posterior and *(b)* anterior views.
Reprinted, by permission, from R.S. Behnke, 2006, *Kinetic anatomy,* 2nd ed. (Champaign, IL: Human Kinetics), p. 47.

TABLE 6.2   **Movements of the Shoulder Girdle**

MUSCLE	ORIGIN	INSERTION	FUNCTION
Trapezius • 1 and 2 upper fibres • 3 middle fibres • 4 lower fibres	Base of skull Vertebrae C1-T12	Clavicle Scapula (upper medial and medial surface)	1 and 2: Elevation 3: Adduction or retraction 4: Depression and upward rotation and stability of scapula
Levator scapulae	Vertebrae C1-C4	Scapula (upper medial surface)	Elevation of scapula
Rhomboids • Major • Minor	Vertebrae C7-T5	Scapula (medial surface)	Adduction or retraction of scapula
Pectoralis minor	Ribs 3-5	Scapula (coracoid process)	Depression and abduction or protraction of scapula
Serratus anterior	Ribs 1-8	Scapula (lateral surface)	Abduction or protraction and upward rotation of scapula

joint that has a large ROM in all three planes of movement. Although it has great ROM, it also has a great amount of instability. The muscles of the rotator cuff are essential for joint integrity in this area.

The rotator cuff muscles are also known as the SITS (i.e., supraspinatus, infraspinatus, teres minor, subscapularis) muscles (figure 6.7). They stabilize the shoulder joint and allow for rotation of the humerus in the scapula.

Movements of the Shoulder

The muscles of the rotator cuff provide stability for the shoulder joint (i.e., they keep the ball in the socket). Three muscles lie as a group on the posterior surface (supraspinatus, infraspinatus, and teres minor) of the scapula, and one muscle lies on the anterior surface of the scapula (subscapularis). The muscles of the rotator cuff assist in rotation of the joint and give the joint stability to produce power (see table 6.3 and figures 6.8 and 6.9).

TABLE 6.3   **Movements of the Shoulder**

MUSCLE	ORIGIN	INSERTION	FUNCTION
Pectoralis major • Clavicular (upper) • Sternal (lower)	Clavicle, sternum, upper 6 ribs	Upper humerus	Flexion, adduction, medial rotation, horizontal adduction, flexion
Deltoid • Anterior • Medial • Posterior	Clavicle, scapula (spine of scapula)	Upper humerus	Abduction, external rotation; assists in flexion, extension, adduction
Coracobrachialis	Scapula (coracoid process)	Middle of humerus	Flexion, adduction
Teres major	Scapula (lateral surface)	Upper humerus	Adduction, extension, medial rotation
Latissimus dorsi	Vertebrae T6-S5	Upper humerus	Extension, adduction, medial rotation
Rotator cuff • Supraspinatus (posterior) • Infraspinatus (posterior) • Teres minor (posterior) • Subscapularis (anterior)	Scapula	Upper humerus	Rotation and stabilization of shoulder joint

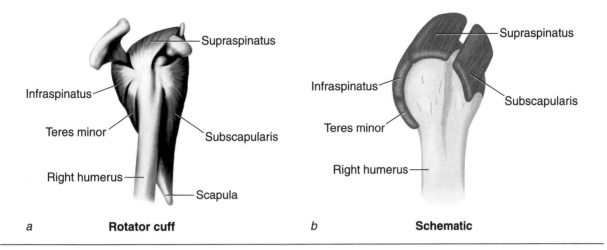

a **Rotator cuff** b **Schematic**

Figure 6.7 Lateral view of the muscles of the rotator cuff.

Reprinted, by permission, from R.S. Behnke, 2006, *Kinetic anatomy,* 2nd ed. (Champaign, IL: Human Kinetics), 52.

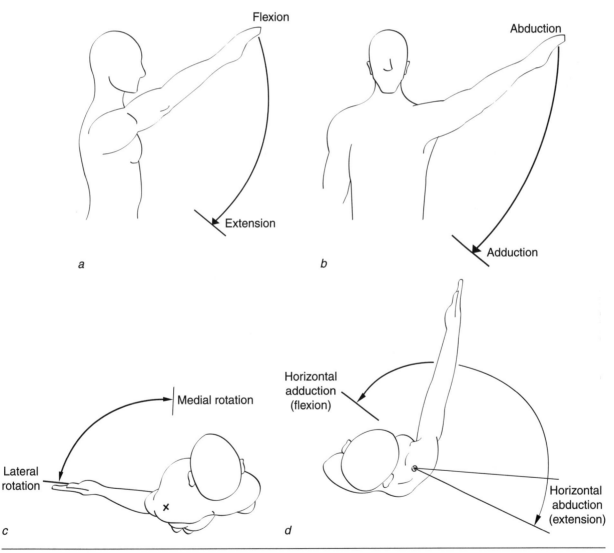

Figure 6.8 Glenohumeral (shoulder) movements: *(a)* flexion and extension, *(b)* abduction and adduction, *(c)* internal (medial) and external (lateral) rotation, and (d) horizontal abduction and adduction.

Reprinted, by permission, from W.H. Whiting and S. Rugg, 2006, *Dynatomy* (Champaign, IL: Human Kinetics), p. 59.

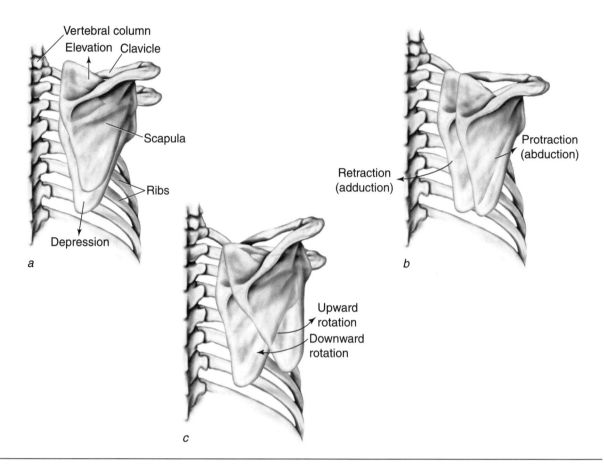

Figure 6.9   Movements of the scapula: *(a)* elevation and depression, *(b)* retraction and protraction, and *(c)* upward and downward rotation.

Reprinted, by permission, from W.H. Whiting and S. Rugg, 2006, *Dynatomy*, (Champaign, IL: Human Kinetics), p. 59.

The Forearm

For simplicity, we will discuss two distinct joints in this section. The first joint is the elbow and the second is the articulation between the radius and ulna bones called the *radioulnar joint.*

Elbow

Muscles and Movements of the Elbow

The elbow joint is an articulation between the humerus bone (upper arm) and the radius and ulna bones (forearm). Movement in this joint is very limited because of the bone structure. However, there is movement between the radius and the ulna at the radioulnar joint. From an anatomical position, the palms turn forward so that the anterior view shows the inside surface of the lower arm (figure 6.10a). The posterior view shows the back of the arm (figure 6.10b). Movements of the elbow are described in table 6.4 and illustrated in figure 6.11.

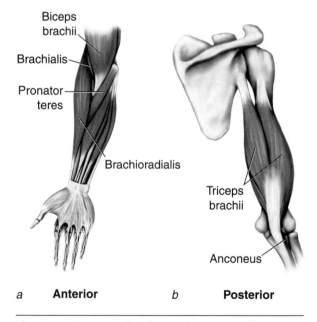

Figure 6.10   Superficial muscles of the elbow and forearm: *(a)* anterior and *(b)* posterior views.

Reprinted, by permission, from R.S. Behnke, 2006, *Kinetic anatomy*, 2nd ed. (Champaign, IL: Human Kinetics), 66.

TABLE 6.4 **Movements of the Elbow**

MUSCLE	ORIGIN	INSERTION	FUNCTION
Biceps brachii • Long head • Short head	Scapula	Radius	Elbow flexion, supination of forearm
Brachialis	Humerus	Ulna	Flexion
Pronator teres	Humerus	Radius	Pronation (weak flexion)
Brachioradialis	Humerus	Radius	Flexion
Triceps brachii	Upper humerus, scapula	Ulna	Extension of elbow
Anconeus	Humerus	Ulna	Extension of elbow

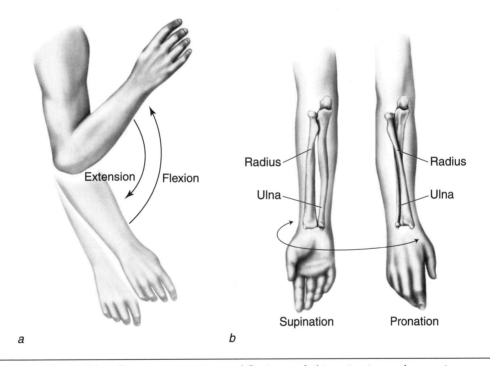

Figure 6.11 Movements of the elbow: *(a)* extension and flexion and *(b)* supination and pronation.

Reprinted, by permission, from W.H. Whiting and S. Rugg, 2006, *Dynatomy* (Champaign, IL: Human Kinetics), p. 61.

Wrist

Muscles and Movements of the Wrist

The wrist joint is an articulation between the radius and ulna bones and the bones of the upper hand (scaphoid, lunate, and triquetrum). There are also joints between the carpals (bones) in the hand, as well as between the metacarpals (fingers). This large number of bones allows us to create fine movements with our hands, fingers, and thumbs. From an anatomical position, the palms turn forward so that the anterior view shows the inside of the wrist and palm. The posterior view shows the back of the hand. The anterior view illustrates the muscles that flex (bend) the wrist (figure 6.12); the posterior view shows the muscles that extend (straighten) the wrist. Movements of the wrist are described in table 6.5 and in figure 6.13.

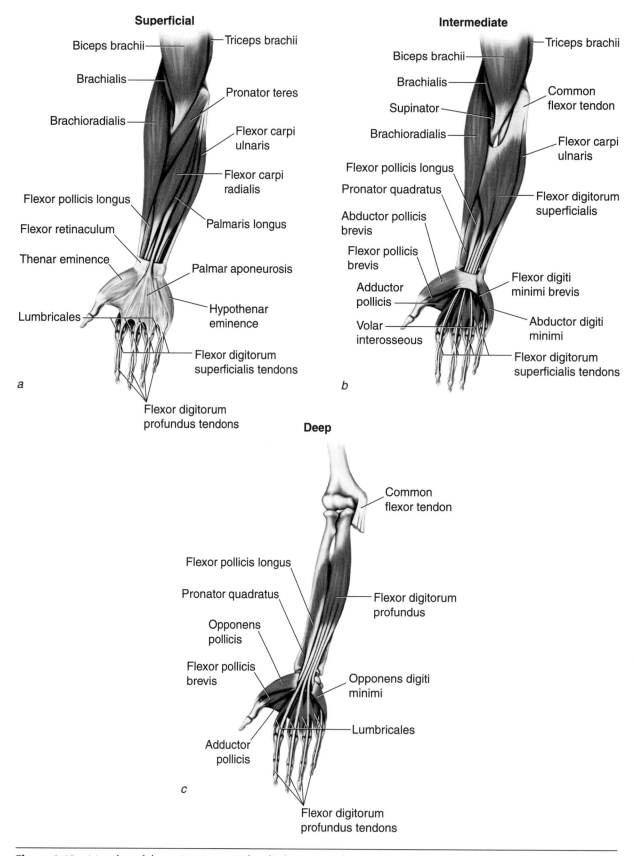

Figure 6.12 Muscles of the wrist: *(a)* superficial, *(b)* intermediate, and *(c)* deep layers.

Reprinted, by permission, from R.S. Behnke, 2006, *Kinetic anatomy,* 2nd ed. (Champaign, IL: Human Kinetics), 81.

TABLE 6.5   **Movements of the Wrist**

MUSCLE	ORIGIN	INSERTION	FUNCTION
Flexors of the wrist • Flexor carpi radialis • Flexor carpi ulnaris • Palmaris longus • Flexor digitorum superficialis • Flexor retinaculum	Medial surface of lower humerus	Carpals, metacarpals, fingers	Wrist flexion • Radial flexion • Ulnar flexion
Extensors of the wrist • Extensor carpi radialis longus • Extensor carpi radialis brevis • Extensor digitorum • Extensor carpi ulnaris • Adductor pollicis longus • Extensor indicis • Extensor pollicis brevis • Extensor retinaculum • Interossei	Lateral surface of humerus	Carpals, metacarpals, fingers	Wrist extension • Radial flexion • Ulnar flexion

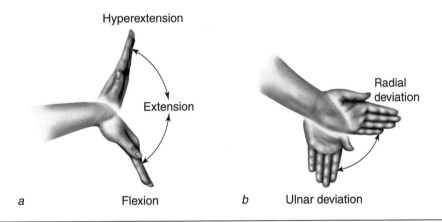

Figure 6.13   Movements of the wrist: *(a)* flexion, extension and hyperextension; and *(b)* radial and ulnar deviation.

Reprinted, by permission, from W.H. Whiting and S. Rugg, 2006, *Dynatomy* (Champaign, IL: Human Kinetics), p. 61.

Torso

Muscles of the Torso

Movement of the torso occurs at two primary joint locations. Spinal movement occurs at the intervertebral joints (the joints between the vertebrae of the spine). There is also an articulation between the fifth lumbar vertebra and the sacrum of the pelvis that produces movement of the pelvis (pelvic tilt). The core or torso area is best illustrated by viewing the anterior (front) of the body and the posterior (back) of the torso (figure 6.14).

Movements of the Torso

In this region, there are two distinct joint areas: movement that occurs at the spine and movement that occurs at the pelvis (table 6.6 and figure 6.15). Movement of the spine occurs between intervertebral discs that comprise the entire spinal column. Movement also occurs in the lumbosacral joint, where there is an articulation between the lumbar vertebrae and the sacrum of the pelvis. As discussed, this joint allows the pelvis to tilt.

Research shows that core stability increases the ability to produce power from the appendages

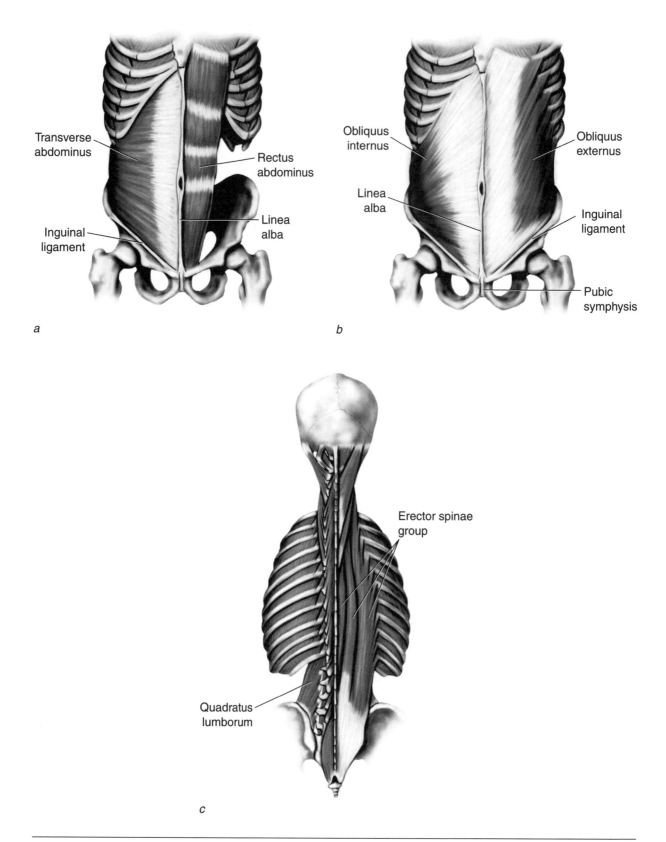

Figure 6.14 Muscles of the torso: *(a)* transverse and rectus abdominus, *(b)* obliquus internus and externus, and *(c)* erector spinae.

Reprinted, by permission, from R.S. Behnke, 2006, *Kinetic anatomy,* 2nd ed. (Champaign, IL: Human Kinetics), 132, 136.

TABLE 6.6 **Movements of the Torso**

MUSCLE	ORIGIN	INSERTION	FUNCTION
Rectus abdominis	Pubis	Ribs 5-7, sternum	Spinal flexion, posterior pelvic tilt
Internal oblique	Pelvis	Lower ribs	Spinal rotation, lateral flexion, posterior pelvic tilt
External oblique	Lower 8 ribs	Pelvis	Spinal rotation, lateral flexion, posterior pelvic tilt
Transverse abdominis (deep muscle not shown)	Lateral torso	Linea alba, pelvis	Internal stability
Erector spinae	Lower thoracic vertebrae, lumbar spine	Cervical and thoracic vertebrae, ribs, base of skull	Spinal extension
Quadratus lumborum	Pelvis (iliac crest)	Rib 12, lumbar vertebrae	Lateral flexion

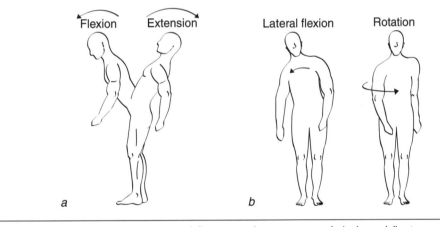

Figure 6.15 Movements of the torso: *(a)* spinal flexion and extension and *(b)* lateral flexion.

Reprinted, by permission, from W.H. Whiting and S. Rugg, 2006, *Dynatomy*, (Champaign, IL: Human Kinetics), p. 64.

(arms and legs). A stable core provides the arms and legs with a solid anchor to produce force and movement. Clients with strong core muscles can experience better body control, balance, and coordination. The torso also provides an anchor for force production.

Hip

Muscles of the Hip

The articulation of the femur bone with the base of the pelvis forms the hip joint. Several ligaments help support this synovial ball-and-socket joint. The hip joint has great ROM and a large amount of muscle surrounding it. Like the shoulder joint, there are a number of deep muscles that allow for hip stability and rotation. Figure 6.16 illustrates the anterior and the posterior of the hip area.

Movements of the Hip

The hip joint is an articulation between the femur bone and the base of the pelvis. This synovial ball-and-socket joint provides good ROM. Note that there is also medial and lateral movement at the hip. The hip joint gains stability from deep ligaments and deep muscles that create rotation and hold the ball in the socket (figure 6.17 and table 6.7).

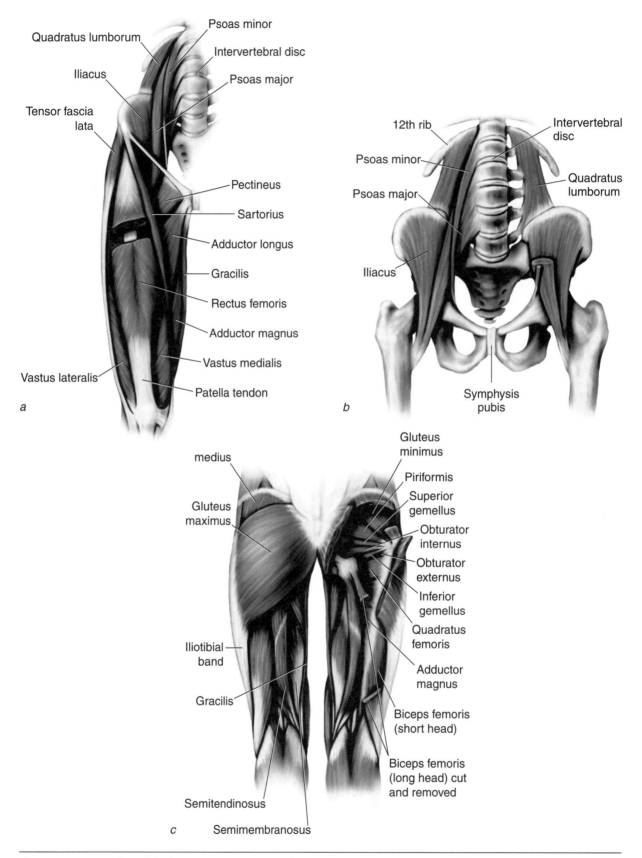

Figure 6.16 Muscles of the hip: *(a)* anterior view; *(b)* psoas major, psoas minor, and iliacus; and *(c)* posterior view.

Reprinted, by permission, from R.S. Behnke, 2006, *Kinetic anatomy,* 2nd ed. (Champaign, IL: Human Kinetics), 178, 180.

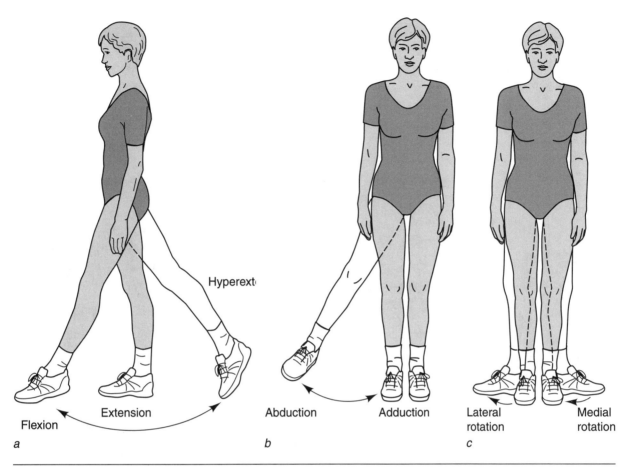

Figure 6.17 Movements of the hip: *(a)* flexion, extension and hyperextension; *(b)* abduction and adduction, and *(c)* lateral and medial rotation.

Reprinted, by permission, from E.T. Howley and B.D. Franks, 2007, *Fitness professionals handbook,* 5th ed. (Champaign, IL: Human Kinetics), p. 426.

Table 6.7 **Movements of the Hip**

MUSCLE	ORIGIN	INSERTION	FUNCTION
Psoas major	Thoracic (bottom few) and lumbar vertebrae	Femur	Hip flexion
Iliacus	Pelvis (iliac crest)	Femur	Hip flexion
Adductor group • Adductor longus • Adductor magnus • Adductor brevis • Gracilis • Pectineus	Base of pelvis	Length of femur (medial edge)	Adduction
Tensor fasciae latae	Pelvis (iliac crest), IT band (lies in the middle of the muscle)	Lateral femur, head of fibula	Hip flexion, abduction, medial rotation
Rectus femoris	Pelvis (iliac spine)	Patella and patellar ligament (to the tibia)	Hip flexion
Sartorius	Pelvis (iliac spine)	Tibia (medial edge)	Hip flexion, lateral rotation

(continued)

TABLE 6.7   *(continued)*

MUSCLE	ORIGIN	INSERTION	FUNCTION
Gluteus medius	Pelvis (iliac spine)	Upper femur	Hip extension, abduction
Gluteus maximus	Pelvis (sacrum and iliac crest)	Upper femur	Hip extension
Hamstrings • Biceps femoris • Semitendinosus • Semimembranosus	Base of pelvis	Upper tibia, fibula	Hip extension

Knee

Muscles of the Knee

The knee joint is the articulation between the femur bone of the thigh and the tibia and fibula bones of the lower leg. The joint itself is not very stable (i.e., the bones do not fit together very well); therefore, the knee requires additional support from a collection of ligaments. The medial and lateral collateral ligaments provide lateral stability for the knee in order to prevent excessive side-to-side motion. The anterior and posterior cruciate ligaments cross inside the knee joint, providing internal stability and preventing displacement of the tibia and femur. The knee joint provides limited ROM, but it is important for weight bearing and for many major lower-body movements. Figure 6.18 shows muscles in the anterior and the posterior of the lower leg.

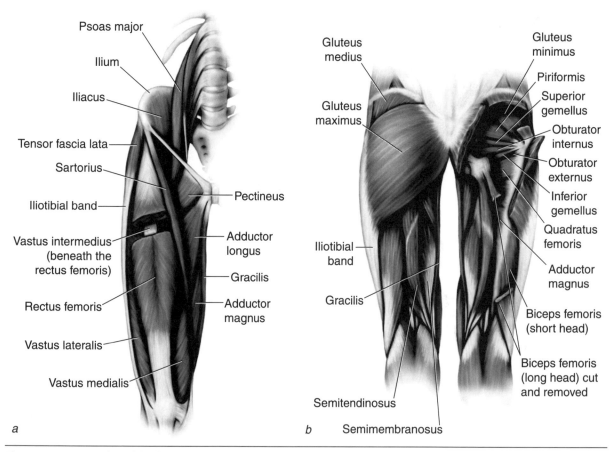

Figure 6.18   Muscles of the knee: *(a)* anterior and *(b)* posterior views.

Reprinted, by permission, from R.S. Behnke, 2006, *Kinetic anatomy,* 2nd ed. (Champaign, IL: Human Kinetics), 198, 201.

Movements of the Knee

As mentioned, the knee is an important joint for weight bearing and mobility, but it is also very unstable due to its construction. Ligaments in the knee area hold the bones together to increase joint stability. The medial and lateral collateral ligaments provide lateral stability, and the anterior and posterior cruciate ligaments provide stability to the front and back of the joint (figure 6.19 and table 6.8).

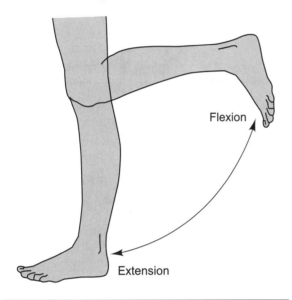

Figure 6.19 Movements of the knee.

Reprinted, by permission, from E.T. Howley and B.D. Franks, 2007, *Fitness professionals handbook*, 5th ed. (Champaign, IL: Human Kinetics), p. 426.

Ankle

Muscles of the Ankle

The ankle joint is a synovial joint formed by the articulation of the tibia bone and the foot (talus bone). Due to weight bearing and gravity, the ankle joints endure a great deal of stress. They gain stability from a number of ligaments that prevent excessive forward, backward, and sideways motion. In order to identify the muscles important to this joint, we will examine the ankle and foot from an anterior view, a lateral view, and a posterior view in figure 6.20.

Movements of the Ankle

The ankle joint is an articulation between the tibia and fibula and the talus. This synovial condyloid joint provides the ability to move the foot upward and downward (table 6.9 and figure 6.21).

Major Muscle Pairs

Many muscles work in opposition to each other, with one muscle producing movement in one direction and its partner or pair producing movement in the opposite direction. Common muscle pairs are shown in figure 6.22.

Summary of Important Points

1. The origin of a muscle is usually closer to the midline of the body (proximal), and the insertion is usually away from the midline of the body (distal).

TABLE 6.8 **Movements of the Knee**

MUSCLE	ORIGIN	INSERTION	FUNCTION
Quadriceps • Rectus femoris • Vastus lateralis • Vastus medialis • Vastus intermedius	Pelvis (rectus femoris only), upper femur (all others)	Patella and patellar tendon (to tibia)	Knee extension
Hamstrings • Biceps femoris • Semitendinosus • Semimembranosus	Base of pelvis	Upper tibia, fibula	Knee flexion
Plantaris	Lower femur	Heel	Knee flexion
Popliteus	Lower femur	Medial tibia	Knee flexion
Gastrocnemius	Base of femur	Heel (Achilles tendon)	Knee flexion

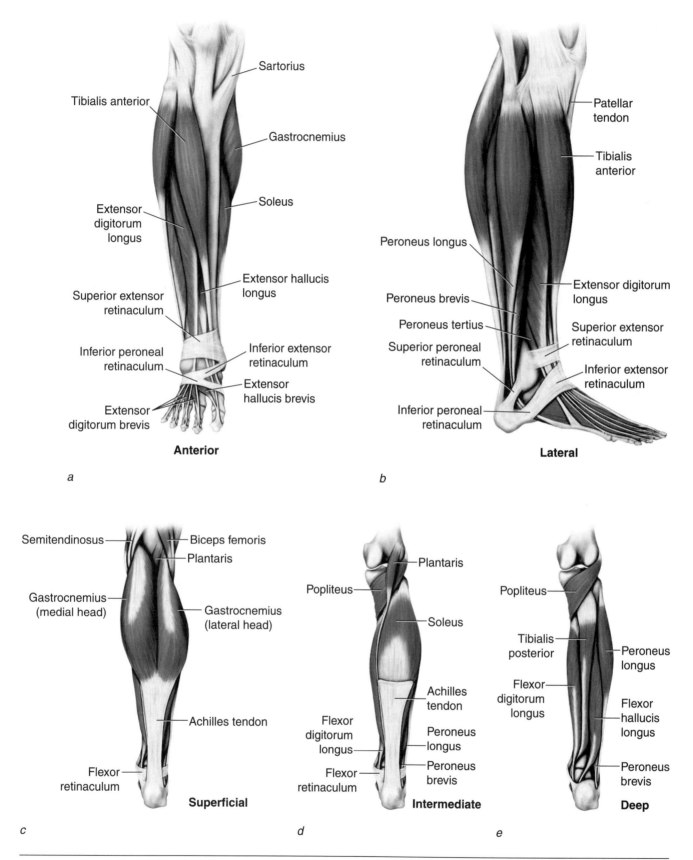

Figure 6.20 Muscles of the ankle: *(a)* anterior, *(b)* lateral, *(c)* superficial, *(d)* intermediate, and *(e)* deep posterior views

Reprinted, by permission, from R.S. Behnke, 2006, *Kinetic anatomy,* 2nd ed. (Champaign, IL: Human Kinetics), 216, 217.

TABLE 6.9 Movements of the Ankle

MUSCLE	ORIGIN	INSERTION	FUNCTION
Tibialis anterior	Top 2/3 of tibia	Metatarsal	Dorsiflexion, inversion
Extensor digitorum longus	Anterior tibia, fibula	Top of 2nd-5th toes	Dorsiflexion, eversion
Extensor hallucis longus	Anterior fibula	Big toe	Dorsiflexion, inversion
Peroneus tertius	Anterior fibula	Metatarsal	Dorsiflexion. eversion
Gastrocnemius	Base of femur	Heel (Achilles tendon)	Plantar flexion
Soleus	Top of tibia, fibula	Heel (Achilles tendon)	Plantar flexion
Tibialis posterior	Posterior tibia, fibula	Bones in foot, 2nd-4th toes	Plantar flexion, inversion
Flexor digitorum longus	Posterior tibia	Bottom of 2nd-5th toes	Plantar flexion, inversion
Flexor hallucis longus	Lower posterior tibia	Bottom of big toe	Plantar flexion, eversion
Peroneus • Longus • Brevis	Lateral fibula	Side of foot and 5th toe	Plantar flexion, eversion

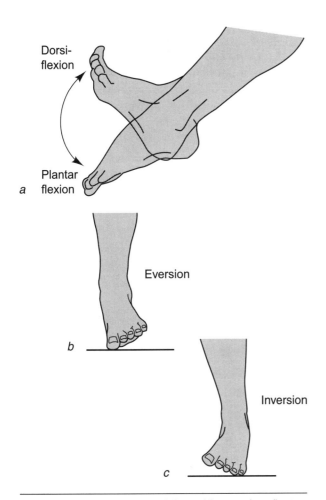

Figure 6.21 Movements of the ankle: *(a)* dorsiflexion and plantar flexion, *(b)* intertarsal eversion, and *(c)* intertarsal inversion.

Reprinted, by permission, from E.T. Howley and B.D. Franks, 2007, *Fitness professionals handbook,* 5th ed. (Champaign, IL: Human Kinetics), p. 426.

Rectus abdominis	Erector spinae
Biceps	Triceps
Quadriceps	Hamstrings
Anterior tibialis	Gastrocnemius and soleus

Figure 6.22 Muscle pairs.

2. Skeletal muscle comprises many muscle fibres that are made up of myofibrils. Myofibrils contain protein filaments called *actin* and *myosin.*

3. The sliding filament theory explains how a muscle contracts.

4. There are two primary muscle fibre types: fast twitch for hard, short exercise and slow twitch for moderate, long exercise.

5. The three types of muscle contractions are isotonic (where the muscle shortens and lengthens), isometric (where force is produced with no change in muscle length), and isometric (where the muscle exerts force to counteract an opposing force with no change in muscle length)

6. Several factors determine the force of a muscle contraction, including the neural stimuli for contraction, size and length of the muscle, joint angle, and speed of the contraction.

Adaptations to Resistance Training

Muscle is a very adaptable tissue. With proper training, muscles grow stronger and larger, which enables us to perform everyday activities more easily. Conversely, they can also become smaller and weaker if they are not used on a regular basis. Therefore, resistance training should be part of everyone's exercise program.

Benefits of Resistance Training

When we impose demands on our muscles and perform physical work that is greater than usual, they get stronger. This increase in strength is due to increased

- muscle fibre size,
- muscle contractile strength,
- coordination among muscle groups,
- tendon and ligament contractile strength, and
- bone strength.

Positive changes in the muscular system have a large influence on our everyday lives. Personal trainers need to identify reasons why clients should be involved in regular resistance training.

What Is Muscular Strength?

Muscular strength is the maximum amount of force that a muscle or muscle group can generate.

What Is Muscular Power?

Muscular power is the explosive aspect of strength. It is the product of strength and speed of movement: power = (force × distance) / time.

What Is Muscular Endurance?

Muscular endurance is the ability of a muscle to repeatedly exert force over a period of time.

Muscular strength and endurance are related; an increase in strength can lead to improvements in endurance. A reasonable amount of strength and endurance may help clients be more efficient in daily tasks and reduce the chances of having low back pain. Power is a key component for most athletic performances.

Resistance Training Program

Frequency of Resistance Training

Adequate rest is required between resistance training workouts to create a muscle-building process. Generally, about 48 hours between workouts is needed to avoid overtraining, injury, and poor results. Figure 6.23 lists the scenarios that have an impact on the frequency of resistance training.

Muscle building and recovery is very individualized. The *Physical Activity Guide to Healthy Active Living* recommends 2 to 4 strength workouts per week. For most clients, more rest is better than not enough rest, especially when beginning a new training program.

Intensity of Resistance Training

Intensity in resistance training is based on repetitions, sets, and loads.

Figure 6.24 lists the scenarios that have an impact on exercise intensity.

When determining repetition range, be aware of the inverse relationship between number of repetitions and load or amount of resistance. Choose a number of repetitions the client can complete

Ways Resistance Training Can Benefit Clients

- Reduces the incidence of joint and muscle overuse injury.
- Complements the maintenance of a healthy body weight.
- Makes everyday activities easier.
- Improves core strength and posture.

- Helps prevent osteoporosis.
- Improves strength for cardiovascular exercise.
- Improves sport performance.
- Reduces loss of muscle mass due to inactivity and aging.

Scenario	Solution
Client's goals	Clients who are working toward muscular endurance can train every other day (24 hours recovery). Clients who train for muscle strength, hypertrophy (growth) or power require a minimum of 48 hours recovery for positive results.
Intensity of the workout	Clients who train at a moderate intensity require less recovery between workouts compared with those who train at a high intensity.

Figure 6.23   Scenarios that affect the frequency of resistance training.

Scenario	Solution
Client's experience	Resistance training design is based on the client's experience. A new weightlifter should train at a reduced intensity and focus on developing technique before increasing intensity.
Client's goals	Clients have different goals with respect to resistance training. Common goals include muscle growth (hypertrophy), muscle definition, and overall improved strength or endurance. Intensity varies based on these goals.

Figure 6.24   Scenarios that affect exercise intensity.

with proper technique and safety, keeping in mind their goals: strength or power, hypertrophy or endurance. This concept can be illustrated with an intensity continuum (see figure 6.25).

The decision to perform more than 1 set of an exercise is based on clients' goals and amount of time they have to spend training.

The following are purposes of multiple sets:

- Help the client learn the correct technique—practice makes perfect.

- Increase fatigue of the muscle fibres, which encourages greater muscle growth during the recovery stage. (Many clients do not lift

a heavy enough weight to promote muscle failure in a single set. To encourage growth, use multiple sets of each exercise. The amount of time clients have to complete the workout may affect the number of sets they perform.)

Workout intensity significantly affects the results of resistance training. In the first 6 to 8 weeks of a resistance training program, beginners experience significant results. This is due to improvements in motor unit (mentioned in chapter 5) recruitment of previously underused muscle fibres. Seeing changes so quickly helps to motivate beginners;

Reps		1	3	5	7	9	11	13	15	17
%1RM	100	90		80			70			
Results		Power			Strength				Endurance	
Adaptation		Neural			Hypertrophy				Metabolic	

Figure 6.25   Intensity continuum.

however, the rate of change in muscle recruitment slows significantly after the first 8 weeks.

The force output of a muscle can vary widely. The more fibres are recruited during exercise, the more force will be produced. If an activity requires near-maximal performance, more muscle fibres are recruited (see figure 6.26).

Duration of Resistance Training

Time is the third component of the FITT formula. How long should a resistance training session last? This depends on clients' personal goals, experience, and how long they are resting between sets and exercises. Figure 6.27 lists the scenarios that have an impact on exercise time.

To help make workouts more time efficient, you can modify routines for clients using split programs, which are explained later in this chapter.

Type of Resistance Training

Consider the type of muscle contraction (isometric or isotonic), the type of equipment (constant versus variable resistance), and the most appropriate exercises for the client. This area allows for a considerable amount of variety and imagination.

Resistance training programs use isometric, isotonic (with and without variable resistance), and isokinetic protocols.

Isometric Training

Isometric training involves static muscle contraction in which the length of the muscle does not change

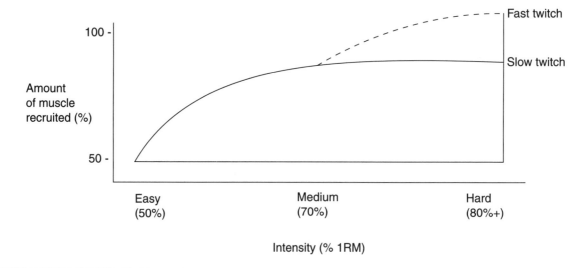

Figure 6.26   Muscle fibre recruitment.

Scenario	Solution
Client's experience	When beginning a resistance training routine, new clients may have a low fitness level or lack confidence. Begin resistance training for a short duration (20-30 minutes) until the client develops proper technique, form, and confidence.
Client's goals	As the client's goals become more serious and focused on developing muscle mass, time in the weight room must increase. To properly fatigue and develop muscles, clients should complete multiple sets at a high intensity. The harder the workload is, the longer the rest between sets should be. More sets and more rest result in a longer workout time.

Figure 6.27   Scenarios that affect exercise time.

when force is applied against a fixed resistance. Isometric training has certain limitations. One major criticism of isometric training is that it does not require the limbs to move. As a result, strength gains occur only at the joint angle at which the exercise takes place rather than through a full ROM.

Isotonic Training

Isotonic training involves concentric and eccentric muscle contractions. In a concentric contraction, the muscle shortens as the weight moves against the force of gravity. In an eccentric contraction, the muscle lengthens as the weight moves with gravity.

Isotonic training includes either constant or variable resistance. An arm curl with a dumbbell is an example of an isotonic exercise that uses constant resistance because the weight stays constant through the entire ROM. The lifter experiences changes in exercise intensity due to changes in the length of the lever arm at various stages of the lift. Variable, or accommodating, resistance equipment requires the lifter to exert maximum effort throughout the entire ROM. Theoretically, this equipment provides more resistance at the joint angles where the lifter is stronger and less resistance at weaker positions; in other words, it accommodates the lifter's leverage or strength. This mechanical change is achieved through cams, which change the direction of the force (e.g., Nautilus equipment), and leverage, which varies the length of the moment arm of the resistance (e.g., Universal equipment).

Isokinetic Training

Isokinetic training is done on specialized equipment that controls the speed of movement through the ROM. This equipment offers accommodating resistance (i.e., the resistance matches the strength of the muscle and accommodates changes in mechanical advantage). Figure 6.28 lists scenarios that have an impact on exercise type.

Resistance Training Guidelines

Clients of all ages and fitness levels can benefit from resistance training. The demand for more information and instruction on resistance training has increased the demand for personal trainers. Clients understand that they should perform resistance training, but they are often unsure about what exercises they should do and how to perform them safely.

One of your roles as a personal trainer is to introduce clients to resistance training and alleviate their intimidation about being in a weight room. Personal trainers must have experience and a solid knowledge base in resistance training, including proper choice of exercises, mechanically correct technique, and training results. The best way to learn how to train others is to train yourself first.

Errors in program design can be costly. An improper resistance training program can lead to

1. injury,
2. dissatisfaction or lack of enjoyment,
3. lack of results, and
4. loss of clients.

This section offers a basic introduction to guidelines, technique, and exercise choice for resistance training. The exercises presented here are not intended as a complete list of resistance

Scenario	Solution
Client's experience	An inexperienced client can have major safety and confidence problems when getting started. Beginners should use weight machines that put them in a fixed position and allow for muscle isolation. As clients become more experienced, they can begin to use equipment that provides less structure and control, such as free weights and pulleys.
Client's goals	Clients who work toward general muscular endurance could benefit from resistance machines. Clients who want functional strength and muscle growth should use a combination of equipment, including free weights, pulleys, and machines. Exercise type is limited only by the trainer's enthusiasm to teach new techniques and add program variety.

Figure 6.28   Scenarios that affect exercise type.

training exercises. The focus is on developing knowledge and feeling comfortable with standard resistance exercises. These are exercises that most clients would begin with before attempting more advanced training methods. Table 6.10 summarizes basic resistance training guidelines.

Summary of Important Points

1. Resistance training is an essential component of a balanced and effective training program.

2. Regular resistance training increases muscle fibre size, contractile strength, bone strength, and ligament strength.

3. Clients experience many positive health benefits from resistance training, including improved body composition, reduced injury, better posture, improved daily activities, improved sport performance, and better body awareness.

4. To develop a sound resistance training program, it is important to consider principles such as exercise selection, muscle balance, exercise order, rest, breathing, speed, technique, and loading.

5. The FITT formula for resistance training is based on a client's goals and experience. In general, the more weight you lift, the harder the workout and the more muscle mass you build.

6. There are many ways to vary a client's exercise routine using new exercises and programs. Variety is essential to success and adherence.

Proper Exercise Choice and Technique

Appendix A contains over 100 exercises that are the basis for most resistance training programs. This is not a complete list of possible exercises; instead, it

TABLE 6.10   **Resistance Training Guidelines**

DESCRIPTION	BEGINNER (MINIMAL EXPERIENCE)	INTERMEDIATE (REGULAR EXERCISER)	ADVANCED (SERIOUS LIFTER)
Program focus	Learning proper technique Learning correct exercises Developing core strength Gaining muscular endurance	Refining proper technique Learning new exercises Developing core strength Gaining muscular strength Exercise variety	Exercise variety Increasing muscular size Maximizing core strength Maximizing training time
Workouts/week	2-3	3-4	4-6
Intensity %1RM	Less than 70% 1RM	70%-80% 1RM	80%-100% 1RM
Result	Muscular endurance	Muscular strength and hypertrophy	Maximum strength and power
Reps	12-15, no muscle failure	8-12	1-8, reaching failure
Sets	1-3	1-4	1-6
Rest between sets	30 s-1 min	30 s-2 min	2+ min
Equipment choice	Weight training machines Body weight exercises Stability ball	Weight training machines Pulleys Free weights Body-weight exercises Stability ball	Weight training machines Pulleys Free weights Body-weight exercises Stability ball Medicine ball
Routine choice	Total body Balanced workout	Total body Split program 2 muscle groups per workout	Split programs Advanced designs (e.g., circuits, splits, pyramids) Many possible modifications

is intended as an introduction to show you how to teach and spot basic resistance training exercises. Once you master teaching these exercises, you can choose more advanced movements, equipment, and routines.

Case Studies

Roger

Roger has been working behind a desk for a long time. Some of the expected characteristics of office workers are weak low back (quadratus lumborum) and abdominal (rectus abdominis) muscles. He most likely also has tight hip flexors due to the constant sitting. If he is doing a lot of typing at his desk, he may also have tightness in his shoulders (trapezius).

Roger has decided to work with a personal trainer twice per week. A guided strength program will help Roger attain his goal of gaining more muscle mass and losing 5-7 kilograms (10-15 pounds) of body fat. Roger's physical testing results of 11 push-ups and 7 curl-ups indicate that he is a beginner, so choosing exercises that are appropriate for his ability and level is important. Joint function and mobility are also critical to counteract the stiffness he may feel from his desk job; therefore, exercises that involve large ranges of motion with careful control should be prescribed. Whole-body movements such as squats, lunges, rows, and presses will help Roger restore joint integrity and mobility. Exercises for the middle and lower trapezius, rhomboids, and erector spinae muscle groups must be incorporated to improve Roger's posture, which could be affected by the many hours he spends sitting at his job. Excellent technique must also be a focus before he begins lifting weights more intensely.

Multiple sets (2-3) are encouraged to help him learn proper form and increase fatigue of the involved muscle fibres. A resistance training session that lasts 20 to 30 minutes is a great start, and he can add more volume as he adapts to the training. That way he also has time to devote to cardiorespiratory exercise. Since at least 48 hours are needed between training sessions for the same muscle groups, Roger could allow a day or two between sessions with his trainer.

Molly

As a former athlete, Molly likely has stronger muscles in her lower body (i.e., quadriceps, hamstrings, gastrocnemius). The sports she has played have built strength and power in her lower body and most likely her torso (rectus abdominis and quadratus lumborum). These muscle groups will likely react the quickest to strength training and will most likely be able to handle a disproportionately higher level of resistance.

Molly has a unique background in that she has a long history of physical activity through participation in sport, which will likely give her a keen sense of body awareness and training intensity. According to Molly's physical testing results, her fitness levels have declined considerably since her high school sporting days. Her ability to do 5 push-ups and 12 curl-ups places her in a beginner category. Since Molly is seeing her trainer once per week and changing her body composition is a goal, it is crucial that her training program focus on energy expenditure during the workout. One way to achieve this is to follow a cardio–strength circuit. The circuit should involve continuous exercises in the following format: One cardio exercise for 2 minutes, a push–pull superset such as push-ups and standing rows (8 to 12 reps each), and a core exercise (8-12 reps). Another example of a push–pull superset is a squat (push) and a chin-up (pull), which also alternates the lower and upper body.

She should perform this circuit for 20 to 30 minutes to start, adding exercises as she improves her fitness level. The goal of this program is to keep Molly moving from one exercise to the next. Since she is young, healthy, and likely energetic, this type of exercise prescription will cover a great deal of ground in a short amount of time.

Jennifer

Even though we do not have much information on what Jennifer does for a living, we can see from her assessment that she ranks in the lower third in both of her strength tests. She would benefit from improving her strength and muscular endurance in her rectus abdominis, pectoralis major, deltoids, and latissimus dorsi. With young children at home, she would also benefit from an overall strength increase in her upper body since she no doubt picks up her kids on a regular basis.

Jennifer's programming and adherence will be largely based on feasibility, keeping in mind that she is also a beginner. It is important that Jennifer learns exercises she can do at home so she doesn't feel pressured to get to the gym or to skip the exercise if she doesn't have time. Many exercises she learns from her personal trainer can be performed at home. For example, Jennifer can follow a body-weight exercise and core stability routine involving stability-ball squats, planks, crunches, back extensions, and various forms of push-ups. It is recommended that Jennifer first focus on learning safety on the ball and proper technique, perhaps starting with 4 or 5 exercises, repeating each 1 to 3 times with correct form. The stability ball will also target Jennifer's core, which should be a focus of any beginner's resistance training program. After she has mastered the technique, you can add new exercises in your one-on-one meetings that she can incorporate in her at-home workouts.

CHAPTER 7

Injury Recognition Concepts

Terry Kane, BPHE, BSc

CHAPTER OBJECTIVES

After completing this chapter, you will be able to

1. distinguish two types of pain a client could experience,

2. define *scope of practice* and the implication to how you handle clients with undiagnosed pain,

3. define and describe the two types of musculoskeletal injuries a client could experience,

4. describe and differentiate an acute musculoskeletal injury from an overuse musculoskeletal injury,

5. define and differentiate the *signs* of an injury and the *symptoms* of an injury,

6. define the goals and action steps you should take, as a personal trainer, in the immediate management of an acute injury,

7. define the goals and action steps you should take, as a personal trainer, in the immediate management of a chronic injury,

8. identify what to do in the event a client presents to you for your recommendations with undiagnosed pain,

9. identify what to do in the event a client presents to you for your recommendations if they are currently in treatment for an injury,

10. identify the importance and rationale behind securing written authorization from a licensed health care professional before resuming exercising an injured client,

11. identify and differentiate the two categories of risk factors for common musculoskeletal injuries,

12. identify what steps you can take to prevent an acute injury, and

13. identify the steps you can take to prevent an overuse injury.

As a personal trainer, at some point in your career one of your clients will complain to you of pain before, during, or following a training session. This chapter is intended to educate you on how to manage this situation in the most appropriate manner. The information contained in this chapter will not only empower you with strategies to advise your clients on what to do, it will also help you use this information to prevent injuries. For more detailed information review the sources listed in the references.

Pain

Not unlike a fire alarm, pain is a message originating somewhere in the body that indicates a lack of normal tissue function or homeostasis. For all intents and purposes, pain is how the body tells us that something is wrong and needs investigation and possible treatment.

There are two types of pain, which are categorized by their origin. Both can result in permanent disability or even death if ignored or mismanaged.

1. **Mechanical pain** is the result of damage to the musculoskeletal system in which pain is created by a mechanical action or motion (e.g., falling from a ladder to the floor).
2. **Systemic pain** is the result of a disease, infection, or medical condition (e.g., rheumatoid arthritis, heart disease).

Despite your experience and knowledge, diagnosing a client's pain is beyond the scope of practice of a personal trainer. Given the potential for permanent disability and possibly death from either a delayed diagnosis or mistreatment, any client who reports undiagnosed pain to you should be referred to a physician, and further exercise should be postponed until medical clearance has been given by a licensed health care professional (i.e., physician, physical therapist) to resume it.

What Is Scope of Practice?

Scope of practice refers to the actions for which a person has been educated and considered competent, usually following successful completion of an examination by a recognized professional or academic organization. In the case of diagnosing the source of pain, this remains the sole domain of physicians.

Scenario 1

A 50-year-old male client begins a weight training program involving push-ups and bench presses. When he wakes up the following morning, he experiences severe chest pain while standing in the shower. His wife wants to take him to the hospital, but instead he calls you to find out if it could just be a muscle strain. What would you tell him and why? For a possible solution, see page 91.

Given the number of systemic conditions that can cause pain, the specificity of treatment for each condition, and the limited space available in this text, the remainder of this chapter will restrict itself to mechanical musculoskeletal pain.

Types of Musculoskeletal Injury

There are two categories of musculoskeletal injury, defined by their mechanism of injury and onset of symptoms.

1. An **acute injury** results from the application of a single force or load, creating tissue damage and leading to immediate pain and dysfunction.
2. An **overuse injury** results from repetitive loading, leading to the gradual onset of pain and dysfunction over days or weeks.

Even though both of these categories of injury are mechanical in origin, their symptoms and treatment differ depending on the injured tissue and severity of injury.

In order to help you educate and direct your injured clients, the following sections will describe a number of details specific to each category of musculoskeletal injury.

Acute Injuries

Acute injuries result from the application of a single force that exceeds the threshold of tensile strength of the loaded tissue, creating tissue damage and generating immediate pain. It's impossible to determine the tensile strength from one tissue to another and from one person to another. Rather than assuming that everyone has the same capacity to exercise and giving them the same exercise program, the default in personal training is to err on the side of caution and individualize exercise programs to prevent injuries. A client's age, family medical history, past medical history, and previous injuries can raise or lower the threshold of tissue strength and consequently change the risk of acute injury. As a result, personal trainers are encouraged to ask their clients to complete a PAR-Q form and it is vital to conduct an initial interview and physical assessment of clients before designing an exercise program.

Scenario 2

A 50-year-old sedentary stockbroker with a history of back surgery for a disk injury 10 years ago finds his 19-year-old son's fitness program on the coffee table at home. His son's program includes squats, lunges, medicine-ball exercises, plyometrics, and spin classes. He calls you and asks if it's safe to do his son's program. What do you tell him and why? For a possible solution, see page 94.

Signs and Symptoms of Acute Injuries

Clients will typically describe their injury based on how the injury feels (symptoms) and the resulting impact of the injury (signs).

What Are Symptoms of an Acute Injury?

Symptoms of an acute injury can include one or more of the following: immediate pain, stiffness, and muscle spasm.

What Are Signs of an Acute Injury?

Signs of an acute injury can include one or more of the following: immediate swelling at the injury site, bruising, redness and increased warmth at the injury site, tenderness to touch, loss of normal function at the injury site, loss of muscle strength, and loss of motion.

Immediate Management of Acute Injury

The two goals in the immediate management of an acute injury are minimizing the tissue damage and minimizing the inflammatory response associated with the injury. The time required to recover from an acute injury is largely dependent on how well these goals are achieved in the 72-hour window of time following injury. If excessive inflammation is allowed to establish itself at the site of injury, it can compound the impact of the injury, add additional treatment time to reduce it, and delay a return to full activity.

Based on these two goals and the importance of this initial 72-hour window, the following actions are encouraged in the event of an acute injury.

1. **Professional medical opinion**—Despite your experience and knowledge of injuries, any musculoskeletal injury can result in a neurovascular injury (i.e., nerve, artery, or vein injury) that could lead to permanent disability and even death. Any client with acute undiagnosed pain should be referred to a physician for a diagnosis as soon as possible.

2. **Rest**—Discontinue any activity known to aggravate the condition and restrict motion through the injured tissue. This facilitates the formation of a primitive scar at the site of injury. Length of rest varies depending on the injured tissue and severity of injury.

3. **Ice**—Applying ice reduces the immediate inflammatory response, swelling, and pain. The frequency and length of icing depend on how superficial the injured tissue is to

TABLE 7.1 **Examples of Acute Injuries**

TISSUE	INJURY	DIAGNOSIS	MECHANISM OF INJURY
Bone	Fracture	Fracture of distal radius	Tripping and falling on an outstretched arm
Ligament	Sprain	Sprained anterior talofibular ligament in ankle	Rolling an ankle by falling off a piece of balance equipment
Muscle	Strain	Strained hamstring	Rapid contraction during a plyometric exercise
Tendon	Rupture	Ruptured Achilles tendon	Sudden lunge or plyometric exercise

the surface, the patient's sensitivity to cold temperatures and whether they have any medical condition for which icing would be considered contra-indicated, such as lack of sensation to temperature or peripheral vascular disease. As a rule, ice should not be applied for longer than 20 minutes at a time and should not be reapplied until the tissue has regained full sensation (i.e., it's no longer numb to the touch).

4. **Compression**—Compression of the injured tissues prevents swelling. Any time the injured tissue is below the level of the heart (i.e., leg injury) it should have some form of external compression stocking or wrap on it. If a client changes their posture, such as lying down, resulting in the injured tissue being elevated above the heart, compression is no longer necessary. If the client lowers the injured tissue below the heart, then some form of compression would be helpful in minimizing the swelling.

5. **Elevation**—Elevating the injured tissue above the heart helps to minimize swelling and therefore is encouraged if at all possible.

Thus, the most effective strategy for managing an acute injury is to (1) see a physician as soon as possible, (2) unload and rest the injured tissue immediately, (3) lie down to elevate and ice the injured tissue, and (4) apply a compression bandage, wrap or sleeve any time the injured tissue is below the level of the heart.

Your Recommendations as a Personal Trainer: Acute Injury

1. If your client has *not been examined by a physician*, this should be your first recommendation.

2. If your client has seen a physician, it is important to know the diagnosis and whether the physician has endorsed continued exercise under your guidance. For your own liability protection and that of your facility, you should discontinue exercising with any injured client until you receive written endorsement from a licensed health care professional.

3. If your client is currently undergoing treatment for an acute injury, you should ask the client to contact the treating health care professional to determine if exercising with you is indicated or

contraindicated at that time. Due to privacy laws in Canada and the United States, health care professionals cannot discuss a patient's injury with you without written permission to do so; an authorization form signed by the physician and their patient (your client). The most effective route to get feedback on your client's injury and exercise program is to give clients a copy of their exercise program and to have your client ask their health care professional whether they are ready to resume training with you. **In order to reduce the risk of complicating any injury, you should postpone any exercise program until you have written permission from a licensed health care professional.**

4. Unless otherwise instructed by a licensed health care professional, you should recommend that your client continue icing the injury until the site of injury is no longer stiff and does not appear swollen, bruised, red, or warm to the touch. While some clients may prefer applying heat to an injury, physiologically, heat increases blood flow to the injured tissue, can increase swelling and delay a return to full activity.

Scenario 3

Your client sustains a dislocated shoulder that is diagnosed by a physician. The client is referred to physiotherapy for rehabilitation, but she thinks the physiotherapist is being too conservative for not letting her resume her arm and chest exercises. The client calls you and says she wants to start exercising with you again. What do you tell her? For a possible solution, see page 94.

Prevention of Acute Injuries

In terms of injury prevention, two categories of risk factors warrant consideration: intrinsic factors and extrinsic factors.

1. **Intrinsic risk factors** are those that affect the tensile strength of a tissue during exercise and increase the risk of injury. These factors are personal to the client, such as muscle weakness, muscle inflexibility, muscle imbalances, joint laxity, discrepancy in leg length, psychological state of mind, and cognitive function. Other intrinsic risk factors that can increase the risk of injury

include a history of previous injury at the injury site, degenerative changes such as arthritis, history of surgery at the site, and the use of medications that can alter the perception of pain or reduce a client's ability to accurately monitor the intensity of exercise (e.g., beta blockers)

2. Extrinsic risk factors are external to the client's physical and psychological status and include environmental factors such as temperature and humidity, exercise equipment, and fitness apparel and the running shoes worn by clients.

As a personal trainer, it's your responsibility to prevent acute injuries by following these steps:

- Profile your client for the presence of any intrinsic risk factors.
- Use the client profile (PAR-Q, interview, and assessment findings) to select the safest and most appropriate exercises for your client.
- Use the profile to determine a safe and appropriate dose (frequency, intensity, volume) of exercise.
- Ensure that your client is instructed on proper technique in all exercises, including warming up and cooling down.
- Ensure that your client can independently demonstrate proper execution of all exercises, including safe operation of any associated exercise equipment (e.g., turning a treadmill on and off).

- Ensure the safety of the exercise environment by maintaining all exercise equipment in proper working order (e.g., make sure all safety features are fully operational).

Overuse Injuries

Overuse injuries result from repetitive tissue loading over time in which no single load is sufficient to cause significant tissue damage and immediate pain. If the motion or exercise is repeated without adequate time to recover, there will be an accumulation of tissue damage and inflammation and ultimately discomfort and pain.

Not unlike in an acute injury, the presence of intrinsic risk factors such as muscle tightness, muscle weakness, history of prior injury or altered biomechanics can increase the risk of an overuse injury (see table 7.2). Extrinsic risk factors such as the size and fit of running shoes can also increase the risk of overuse injury if they don't fit properly. A common example of an overuse injury is carpal tunnel syndrome, which is the result of repetitive computer keyboard work day after day and insufficient recovery time.

What Are the Symptoms of an Overuse Injury?

Symptoms of an overuse injury include one or more of the following: low-grade discomfort at the site of the injury, discomfort in activities of daily living

TABLE 7.2   **Examples of Overuse Injuries**

TISSUE	INJURY	DIAGNOSIS	MECHANISM OF INJURY
Bone	Fracture	Tibial stress fracture	Long-distance running
	Periostitis	Epicondylitis (tennis elbow)	Overuse of forearm Faulty mechanics in tennis
Tendon	Inflammation	Achilles tendinitis	Running on uneven terrain or in poor shoes
	Inflammation	Shoulder impingement	Overuse in overhead movements
Fascia	Inflammation	Plantar fasciitis	Repetitive trauma to foot with poor biomechanical support
	Inflammation	IT band friction	Friction of IT band at lateral femoral epicondyle
Cartilage	Inflammation	Osteoarthritis	Repetitive weight-bearing or impact activity on degenerative joint
	Inflammation	Patellofemoral pain	Repetitive load on a bent knee Biomechanical malalignment
Bursa	Inflammation	Greater trochanteric bursitis	Repetitive load
Skin	Inflammation	Blisters	Friction between layers of skin

other than exercise (such as descending stairs or sleeping), sensation of stiffness at the site of the injury, and a progression in the intensity of pain with continued exercise or activity.

Signs of an overuse injury include one or more of the following: an alteration of normal biomechanics to avoid pain (e.g., limping downstairs to avoid patello-femoral pain), swelling, loss of pain-free motion with normal activities, and tenderness to touch.

Immediate Management of Overuse Injuries

The low level of pain and gradual onset associated with overuse injuries often mislead clients into believing that their pain

- is insignificant,
- will go away by itself, and
- does not require medical attention.

During the initial 72-hour window following onset of pain or discomfort, clients are encouraged to rest and ice the injured tissues as outlined earlier in the section on acute injury.

The distinguishing feature of an overuse injury is the persistence of pain beyond 72 hours, typically located within 2.5 centimetres of a joint or a tendon attachment (e.g., pain at the elbow where the tendons of the forearm muscles attach). Under these circumstances, a physician should investigate the pain before the client returns to any exercise or sport known to trigger the pain. As a default, medical attention should be sought in the event of any undiagnosed slow-onset pain if it persists longer than 3 days and is noticeable in other activities of daily living (e.g., walking, sitting, dressing, washing, sleeping).

Once clients have written permission from a health-care professional to return to exercise it is important that they are educated to the fact that despite the absence of pain, they may be vulnerable to reinjury for 3 to 6 months (depending on the injury). This isn't to suggest that your clients can't exercise during this period, but that they should

- modify their training program,
- explore changes to their exercise technique or equipment, and
- monitor their symptoms with any progression in training volume.

Continuing to exercise or perform any activity that reproduces pain will make the injury worse and can result in permanent disability.

Prevention of Overuse Injuries

Prevention strategies for overuse injuries focus on three concepts. In short, you should educate the client, choose the proper dose of exercise, and progress the exercise program wisely.

Client Education   For all intents and purposes, overuse injuries are preventable through good communication and education with your clients. As mentioned, what often causes a low-grade ache to turn into an overuse injury is continued participation and aggravation of the original tissue damage. The concept of stopping exercise is particularly difficult for clients who believe in the old saying, "No pain, no gain." Unfortunately, clients who believe in this saying commonly don't report their pain and continue aggravating their injury until it's too late and they require medical treatment and time off in order to heal. One of the most important steps in preventing an overuse injury is educating clients from the outset that there is *no gain with pain*. You also need to create an environment where clients feel comfortable telling you that they are sore without fear of ridicule or embarrassment.

Before implying a client may be to blame for an overuse injury, you need to ask yourself two questions:

1. Did you educate your clients about the importance of not exercising with pain?
2. Did you create an environment where your clients felt they could acknowledge their pain to you?

Dose and Volume of Exercise   One of the most important physiological qualities we possess is the ability of the body to repair itself from damage and to adapt at any age. Whether your client is 20 years old or 80 years old, there is a wealth of scientific evidence supporting the capacity to undergo physiological adaptations to exercise. The capacity and degree of potential change are not only age related but based on a client's family medical history and past medical history.

The primary cause of overuse injuries is an imbalance between the physiological tissue damage created by an exercise or motion and the degree of tissue repair that's achieved before repeating the exercise. Not unlike prescribing a medication, the key to preventing overuse injuries is ensuring the exercise is not only appropriate for the client and their health profile but also the dose of exercise is appropriate, specifically in terms of frequency, intensity, and volume. Note that frequency refers to the number of times per week a client can safely exercise without causing injury and depends largely on the intensity and volume of exercise in a given workout. The more intense and greater the volume of exercise in a given workout, the more time is often required for tissues to recover and repair before repeating the workout. Volume refers not only to the duration or repetitions of a given exercise but also the number of exercises for a given muscle group in a given workout (e.g., squats, leg presses, and knee extensions all work the quadriceps and load the patellofemoral joint).

Before clients reattempt a given workout routine or exercise, they should be entirely free of pain in the given muscle and surrounding joints. If clients are still experiencing pain or discomfort before a workout, it indicates that they need more time to repair and recover before exercising the painful muscle group or joint.

Given the potential to create injury, encouraging clients to work through pain is negligent and unprofessional. Therefore, the key to preventing overuse injuries is recognizing the importance of selecting the most appropriate exercises for your client's profile and the safest dose of exercise.

Progressing a Training Program   When it comes to progressing an exercise program, it is crucial to appreciate the physiological capacity of your clients to adapt to exercise. To avoid an imbalance, the rate of progression should not exceed the client's rate of adaptability for their age and health profile. For example, if a client has the capacity to adapt at 10% per week and you increase their exercise program by 20%, at some point in time the imbalance will result in tissue damage, inflammation, and pain. In order to reduce the risk of overuse injury in a new client, for whom you may be unfamiliar, an argurment could be made to error on the side of safety and limit any progression in a given exercise program to 10% per week.

Responsibilities

In addition to the responsibilities outlined in the acute injury section of this chapter, as a personal trainer it is your responsibility to prevent an overuse injury by following these steps:

- Educate your clients on the consequences of exercising through pain.
- Educate your clients that exercising a painful muscle or joint will likely only make their pain worse and potentially force them to discontinue that exercise.
- Create an environment where clients are under no fear or pressure to exercise with pain.
- Ask your clients before every training session if they are pain free. If not, their program must be modified for that workout in order to avoid aggravating their injury and creating more pain.
- Profile your client (PAR-Q, interview and assessment) for the presence of any intrinsic risk factors, particularly excessive muscle tightness or any biomechanical abnormality that may arise through highly repetitive exercises or motions.
- Ensure that any equipment used by your client fits well and is in good operational condition.
- Use the client profile to select the most appropriate exercises.
- Use the client profile to determine the dose (frequency, intensity, volume) of exercise.
- Using your profile, educate your client on a safe and appropriate rate of exercise progression.
- Forms 7.1 and 7.2 can be used to document injuries that your clients may have.

Solutions to Scenarios

Scenario 1

"Although there is a chance your chest pain could be just a muscle ache, the reality is that I can't tell you and it could well be something more serious such as a heart attack. I'd suggest that you call 9-1-1 and explain the situation to them. They'll be able to tell you exactly what to do. Do you understand?" Following the conversation, you need to document in writing the time of the call and your instructions.

Why?

Diagnosing pain is beyond the personal trainer's scope of practice. Given the information from

Personal Training Injury Report

Client Name: _____

Street Address: _____

Contact Telephone Number:

Daytime _____

Evening _____

Date of Report: (M/D/Y) _____

Onset Date of Symptoms: (M/D/Y) _____

Body Region List injured body regions below

_____

_____

_____

Symptoms as reported to trainer

Check box(es)

☐ Pain
☐ Loss of Range of Motion
☐ Muscle spasm
☐ Other: Describe

_____

Trainer's recommendations to the client

☐ Seek medical attention and secure written permission / authorization from a physician or physical therapist before resuming, supervised or unsupervised, physical exercise of the injured body region(s) listed in this report

☐ Other: Describe

_____

Signatures

Client Name (Print) _____

Client Name (Signature) _____

Trainer's Name (Print) _____

Trainer's Name (Signature) _____

Date _____

Form 7.1 Sample report used to document a client's injury.

From Can-Fit-Pro, 2008, *Foundations of Professional Personal Training* (Champaign, IL: Human Kinetics).

Return to Personal Training Report

Client Name:	_____
Street Address:	_____
Contact Telephone Number:	Daytime _____
	Evening _____
Date of this report:	(M/D/Y) _____
This form relates to the injury reported dated	(M/D/Y) _____

Return to Personal Training Criteria

Has the client seen a physician or physical therapist for all of the complaints listed in this report?   Yes / No

Has the client provided written authorization from a physician or physical therapist to resume personal training and exercising all of the injured body region(s) listed in this report? (If so, please staple authorization to this report)   Yes / No

Did the written authorization identify restrictions to either type of exercise or dose of exercise the client should not participate in? (If so, please describe any and all restrictions, in writing, on separate sheet and staple to this report)   Yes / No

Trainer's Notes _____

_____

_____

_____

Signatures

Client Name (Print)	_____
Client Name (Signature)	_____
Trainer's Name (Print)	_____
Trainer's Name (Signature)	_____
Date	_____

Form 7.2   Sample report to document a client's return to training.

From Can-Fit-Pro, 2008, *Foundations of Professional Personal Training* (Champaign, IL: Human Kinetics).

the client, this could be a medical emergency, and your role is to act accordingly by engaging an emergency medical response as taught in CPR training.

Scenario 2

"Your son's program was tailored to his medical profile as well as his goals and objectives—not yours. Although there may be some exercises you can do, the reality is that there are some that may reinjure your back or create another injury. Under the circumstances, I can't endorse you following your son's program, but I would be more than willing to get together with you and tailor a program that is safe and appropriate for you, your medical history, and your goals." Following the conversation, you need to document in writing the time of the call and your instructions.

Why?

The most important principle in exercise program design isn't to achieve a client's goals at any cost, but rather to work within the client's medical profile and to ensure the client's health and safety en route to improved fitness. Although the exercise program may be safe for the son, it may not be for the father; hence the recommendation to meet and design a separate program for the father.

Scenario 3

"I understand that you're frustrated and want to work out, but there are reasons why your physiotherapist doesn't think it's safe and I think you need to discuss this with her directly. As much as I want to help you out, the reality is that I need written permission from your physiotherapist or physician to start exercising your shoulder again, so talk to them and see what they say before doing anything that you may regret later."

Why?

First, if a licensed health care professional has said that the client should not exercise her shoulder, it is an absolute contraindication for you to exercise the injured tissue with the client. Second, many professional insurance policies for personal trainers contain a clause that releases them from covering you and your actions if clients are still in medical treatment for a condition and you do not have written permission to train them. You need to check your insurance policy.

Summary of Important Points

1. It is not uncommon for clients to complain of pain with exercise training.

2. As a personal trainer, your responsibility is not to ignore pain nor to diagnose or recommend treatment, but rather to stay within your scope of practice and act in the best interest of the client at all times.

3. In the event a client reports undiagnosed complaints of pain, you should refer the client to a physician.

4. In the event a client is undergoing treatment for an injury or has recently been discharged from treatment for an injury, you should secure written authorization from the treating health care professional before resuming training the injured joint or muscle.

5. As a personal trainer, you can play a significant role in helping your clients manage their injuries through

   - taking appropriate steps to manage an injury immediately,
   - referring clients to a physician, and
   - educating your clients effectively.

6. As a personal trainer, you can play a significant role in preventing musculoskeletal injuries through

   - screening clients for potential risk factors,
   - creating a safe and appropriate exercise program design, and
   - ensuring a safe and effective training environment.

Case Studies

Roger

Even though Roger answered *no* to all questions on his PAR-Q, the fact that he has joined a gym to exercise suggests that he has been prompted to take action by something important to him. This may be knowledge of his family's medical history (e.g., his older brother recently suffered a heart attack) or early signs or symptoms of disease (e.g., chest pain, osteoarthritis). A review of his medical history, his family's medical history, and his past and current use of medications would help to reveal any musculoskeletal or systemic vulnerabilities that may show up during exercise (e.g., pain, reinjury). In addition, given Roger's lack of exercise over the years, it is possible that he may subscribe to the no pain, no gain philosophy of training, which could easily result in either an acute or overuse injury. In order to prevent injury, it would be beneficial to not only perform a preexercise screening assessment but also to take the time to educate him on realistic goals and timelines, proper exercise program design, proper exercise technique, and how to operate exercise equipment safely.

Molly

Based on Molly's sport career and her educational background, it is easy to assume that she knows everything there is to know about exercise, but the fact that she has engaged your services suggests she is lacking something (i.e., motivation, compliance) or she has a goal she is eager to achieve quickly (i.e., return to sport, weight loss). Training clients who work or are studying in health sciences can be difficult because of the assumption that the client has the same knowledge of exercise as yourself; however, again, the fact that someone like Molly has sought your services suggests otherwise and shows acceptance that she needs your help to achieve her goals. Understanding Molly's motivation may be important in preventing an overuse injury, especially if her fitness goals and timelines are unrealistic. You have the opportunity to help prevent an injury by educating Molly on realistic goals and timelines, proper exercise program design, proper exercise technique, and how to operate exercise equipment safely.

Jennifer

Given her profile, Jennifer appears to be at a low risk for injury, especially since she's working with a personal trainer and only working out once or twice a week. The greater risk for Jennifer is performing unsupervised exercises on equipment at home that you may not be familiar with. In this circumstance, not only should you perform a preexercise screening assessment and educate Jennifer on exercise program design, you should also book at least one training session in her home to make sure she executes proper technique and operation of her own equipment. In addition to your gym-based program, you should draft a home program so she understands the intensity and volume of exercise you believe is safe. In the event she plans to work out independently at home or at work, getting Jennifer to create a training diary can help you make sure you do not progress her program too quickly and cause an overuse injury.

PART II

Screening and Assessment

CHAPTER 8

Preexercise Screening

Gregory S. Anderson, PhD

Brian Justin, MHK

CHAPTER OBJECTIVES

After completing this chapter, you will be able to

1. explain the reason for using health screening with all clients,

2. discuss the necessity for having all clients complete and sign a PAR-Q form,

3. develop and implement a health screening questionnaire, and

4. identify the scope of a personal trainer's capabilities with reference to medical conditions.

It is the legal and ethical obligation of every trainer and facility to ensure that clients entering a facility are reasonably safe. This obligation is part of your duty of care to the client, and any breach of the duty to exercise due care may result in negligence. Negligence may leave trainers or the facility (or both) liable for damages should a client get injured due to inadequate screening and assessment, defective equipment, faulty supervision, incompetent instruction, or trainers working outside their scope of practice. Therefore, in order to provide a safe and effective training environment, every fitness facility and personal trainer should screen clients for health problems before allowing to use a facility or before developing a fitness program.

Preexercise screening is a crucial first step in the personal training process. It is essential to understand your clients' health before you counsel them, plan an exercise program, or even decide whether you are capable of becoming their personal trainer.

A client's personal health history is a serious and private matter, and all information must be kept confidential. If you encounter a client who has significant medical concerns or risks outside your expertise, it's your responsibility to suggest that the client search for a more qualified personal trainer or medical professional.

Preexercise Screening

Preexercise screening is part of fitness professionals' duty of care and therefore is part of their legal responsibility. This screening is designed to identify clients who have medical conditions that leave them at risk of injury or death when performing moderate to vigorous physical activity. Preexercise screenings allow you to do the following:

1. Be professional and fulfill legal responsibilities (duty of care).
2. Identify a possible need to refer the client to additional health professionals.
3. Understand the client better and establish good communication.
4. Identify areas of strength or weakness based on previous injury.
5. Develop a precise, individualized exercise program.
6. Determine safe and effective exercises.

Preexercise screening must be able to identify people who have any of the following:

- Known disease
- Signs and symptoms of a disease that is as of yet undiagnosed
- Increased cardiac risk
- Risks inherent in activity due to their age

Screening for each of these factors provides the minimal evaluation required before allowing people to train in a facility or taking them on as clients for personal training.

Known Disease

People with known disease must have medical clearance for exercise. Their medical practitioner should provide guidelines as to the most appropriate activities and intensities, as well as which exercises to avoid.

Signs and Symptoms

Signs and symptoms of a disease process may be well established prior to diagnosis by a medical practitioner and act as early warning signals. Signs and symptoms of cardiovascular, metabolic, or respiratory disease that should prompt medical referral include

- pain and discomfort in the chest, lower jaw, or left shoulder;
- ankle swelling;
- feelings of rapid, throbbing HR;
- severe pain in leg muscles when walking;
- unusual fatigue and general feelings of lethargy;
- difficulty breathing when standing or at night;
- shortness of breath at rest or during light activity; and
- feelings of dizziness or fainting.

Increased Cardiac Risk

Trainers should be well aware of cardiovascular risk factors and be adept at screening clients for these risk factors:

- Age (men older than 45 years and women older than 55 years)

- Family history of heart disease (a father or grandfather having a heart attack or dying suddenly before the age of 55 years, or a mother or grandmother having a heart attack or dying suddenly before the age of 65 years)

- Smoking

- High BP, or hypertension (systolic pressure greater than 139 or diastolic pressure greater than 89)

- High cholesterol levels (total cholesterol over 200 milligrams per decilitre)

- Diabetes

- Sedentary lifestyle (less than 60 min of light effort performed daily, less than 30 min of moderate-intensity activity 4 times a week, or less than 20 minutes of vigorous activity 4 times a week)

Age Risk

Men over the age of 45 and women over the age of 55 are encouraged to have a medical exam before initiating an exercise program. Although medical exams may not be required of active individuals who have no other cardiac risks and want to participate in light to moderate exercise programs, they should be mandatory if the potential clients were previously sedentary, are initiating a new exercise regimen, or combine an age risk with any other risk factor.

Physical Activity Readiness Questionnaire

To begin the client screening process, have the client complete and sign a Physical Activity Readiness Questionnaire (PAR-Q). Developed by the Canadian Society for Exercise Physiology (CSEP) and Health Canada, this form is used as an initial health screening tool and is administered before clients begin a physical activity program. The PAR-Q includes seven questions designed to identify people who require medical clearance before participating in a new exercise program, and it helps cover two prescreening topics: known disease and signs and symptoms. Clients' responses to the PAR-Q give you an idea of their known health problems and medical conditions that might be affected by exercise. However, it is only a general prescreening tool, appropriate for people between 15 and 69 years of age.

If clients answer "yes" to one or more questions on the PAR-Q, they should seek medical advice before becoming more physically active. We recommend that you do not work with clients who have existing health risks until you have gained adequate experience working with healthy adults, and the clients have been cleared for unrestricted physical activity by their medical practitioner.

It is your legal responsibility to have a signed PAR-Q for all clients that you train. Since health is a dynamic process that can change in a short period of time, it is recommended that clients complete the PAR-Q on an annual basis. A copy of the PAR-Q is included (see figure 8.1) as a resource, and can be downloaded for free at www.csep.ca/forms.asp.

Health History Questionnaire

To gather more specific information concerning a client's health, it is a good idea to develop a second health screening questionnaire to supplement the PAR-Q. This second tool might include the following areas:

1. Client details (e.g., name, address, phone numbers, emergency contact)
2. Current medical conditions (e.g., diabetes, asthma, arthritis)
3. Medication use and allergies
4. Current or past injuries
5. Treatment from health care professionals
6. Cardiac risks (e.g., high BP, high cholesterol)
7. Family health history
8. Past and present exercise history
9. Past and present nutritional information
10. Past and present work history

Many personal trainers use a standardized form for all clients or develop their own questionnaire that works best for their interests and needs. See figure 8.2 for a copy of a health history questionnaire.

Other Resources

Several forms and questionnaires are available that are useful to the personal trainer. These questionnaires monitor such things as physical activity, cardiovascular risk, and lifestyle. You may also

PAR-Q & YOU

(A Questionnaire for People Aged 15 to 69)

Regular physical activity is fun and healthy, and increasingly more people are starting to become more active every day. Being more active is very safe for most people. However, some people should check with their doctor before they start becoming much more physically active.

If you are planning to become much more physically active than you are now, start by answering the seven questions in the box below. If you are between the ages of 15 and 69, the PAR-Q will tell you if you should check with your doctor before you start. If you are over 69 years of age, and you are not used to being very active, check with your doctor.

Common sense is your best guide when you answer these questions. Please read the questions carefully and answer each one honestly: check YES or NO.

YES	NO		
☐	☐	1.	Has your doctor ever said that you have a heart condition <u>and</u> that you should only do physical activity recommended by a doctor?
☐	☐	2.	Do you feel pain in your chest when you do physical activity?
☐	☐	3.	In the past month, have you had chest pain when you were not doing physical activity?
☐	☐	4.	Do you lose your balance because of dizziness or do you ever lose consciousness?
☐	☐	5.	Do you have a bone or joint problem (for example, back, knee or hip) that could be made worse by a change in your physical activity?
☐	☐	6.	Is your doctor currently prescribing drugs (for example, water pills) for your blood pressure or heart condition?
☐	☐	7.	Do you know of <u>any other reason</u> why you should not do physical activity?

If you answered

YES to one or more questions

Talk with your doctor by phone or in person BEFORE you start becoming much more physically active or BEFORE you have a fitness appraisal. Tell your doctor about the PAR-Q and which questions you answered YES.

- You may be able to do any activity you want — as long as you start slowly and build up gradually. Or, you may need to restrict your activities to those which are safe for you. Talk with your doctor about the kinds of activities you wish to participate in and follow his/her advice.
- Find out which community programs are safe and helpful for you.

NO to all questions

If you answered NO honestly to <u>all</u> PAR-Q questions, you can be reasonably sure that you can:

- start becoming much more physically active — begin slowly and build up gradually. This is the safest and easiest way to go.
- take part in a fitness appraisal — this is an excellent way to determine your basic fitness so that you can plan the best way for you to live actively. It is also highly recommended that you have your blood pressure evaluated. If your reading is over 144/94, talk with your doctor before you start becoming much more physically active.

DELAY BECOMING MUCH MORE ACTIVE:

- if you are not feeling well because of a temporary illness such as a cold or a fever — wait until you feel better; or
- if you are or may be pregnant — talk to your doctor before you start becoming more active.

PLEASE NOTE: If your health changes so that you then answer YES to any of the above questions, tell your fitness or health professional. Ask whether you should change your physical activity plan.

<u>Informed Use of the PAR-Q</u>: The Canadian Society for Exercise Physiology, Health Canada, and their agents assume no liability for persons who undertake physical activity, and if in doubt after completing this questionnaire, consult your doctor prior to physical activity.

No changes permitted. You are encouraged to photocopy the PAR-Q but only if you use the entire form.

NOTE: If the PAR-Q is being given to a person before he or she participates in a physical activity program or a fitness appraisal, this section may be used for legal or administrative purposes.

"I have read, understood and completed this questionnaire. Any questions I had were answered to my full satisfaction."

NAME _____

SIGNATURE _____ DATE _____

SIGNATURE OF PARENT _____ WITNESS _____
or GUARDIAN (for participants under the age of majority)

Note: This physical activity clearance is valid for a maximum of 12 months from the date it is completed and becomes invalid if your condition changes so that you would answer YES to any of the seven questions.

© Canadian Society for Exercise Physiology   Supported by: 🍁 Health Canada Santé Canada

continued on other side...

Figure 8.1 PAR-Q & You

PAR-Q & YOU

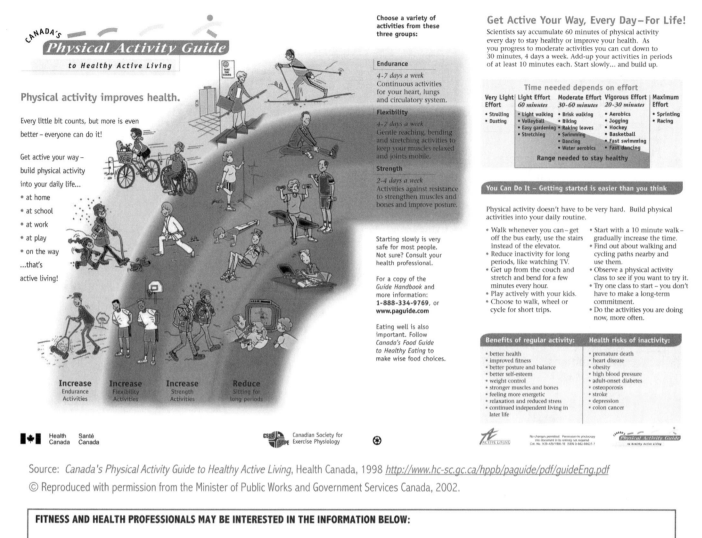

Source: *Canada's Physical Activity Guide to Healthy Active Living*, Health Canada, 1998 http://www.hc-sc.gc.ca/hppb/paguide/pdf/guideEng.pdf

© Reproduced with permission from the Minister of Public Works and Government Services Canada, 2002.

FITNESS AND HEALTH PROFESSIONALS MAY BE INTERESTED IN THE INFORMATION BELOW:

The following companion forms are available for doctors' use by contacting the Canadian Society for Exercise Physiology (address below):

The **Physical Activity Readiness Medical Examination (PARmed-X)** – to be used by doctors with people who answer YES to one or more questions on the PAR-Q.

The **Physical Activity Readiness Medical Examination for Pregnancy (PARmed-X for Pregnancy)** – to be used by doctors with pregnant patients who wish to become more active.

References:

Arraix, G.A., Wigle, D.T., Mao, Y. (1992). Risk Assessment of Physical Activity and Physical Fitness in the Canada Health Survey
Follow-Up Study. **J. Clin. Epidemiol.** 45:4 419-428.

Mottola, M., Wolfe, L.A. (1994). Active Living and Pregnancy, In: A. Quinney, L. Gauvin, T. Wall (eds.), **Toward Active Living: Proceedings of the International Conference on Physical Activity, Fitness and Health**. Champaign, IL: Human Kinetics.

PAR-Q Validation Report, British Columbia Ministry of Health, 1978.

Thomas, S., Reading, J., Shephard, R.J. (1992). Revision of the Physical Activity Readiness Questionnaire (PAR-Q). **Can. J. Spt. Sci.** 17:4 338-345.

To order multiple printed copies of the PAR-Q, please contact the:

Canadian Society for Exercise Physiology
202-185 Somerset Street West
Ottawa, ON K2P 0J2
Tel. 1-877-651-3755 • FAX (613) 234-3565
Online: www.csep.ca

The original PAR-Q was developed by the British Columbia Ministry of Health. It has been revised by an Expert Advisory Committee of the Canadian Society for Exercise Physiology chaired by Dr. N. Gledhill (2002).

Disponible en français sous le titre «Questionnaire sur l'aptitude à l'activité physique - Q-AAP (revisé 2002)».

Supported by: Health Santé
Canada Canada

Figure 8.1 *(continued)*

Sample Client information

Name: _____

Address: _____

Home Phone: _____ Work Phone: _____

Date of Birth: _____ Occupation: _____

Height (cm): _____ Weight (kg): _____ BMI: _____ [BMI = wt (kg)/ht (m)^2]

Blood pressure: Systolic _____ mmHg   Diastolic _____ mmHg   Pulse: _____ bpm

Please mark each statement that is true.

_____ You are a man over the age of 45 years.

_____ You are a woman over the age of 55 years.

_____ You are physically inactive (active less than 30 minutes 3 times a week).

_____ You are overweight (9 kg or more, or BMI over 30).

_____ You presently smoke or have quit within the past 6 months.

_____ You have high blood pressure or take blood pressure medication.

    _____ Systolic blood pressure over 140mmHg

    _____ Diastolic blood pressure over 90 mmHg

_____ You have been told you have high cholesterol.

_____ Your father or brother had a heart attack or heart surgery before the age of 55.

_____ Your mother or sister had a heart attack or heart surgery before the age of 65.

Exercise habits

_____ Intensive occupational and recreational exertion

_____ Moderate occupational and recreational exertion

_____ Sedentary work and intense recreational exertion

_____ Sedentary work and moderate recreational exertion

_____ Sedentary work and light recreational exertion

_____ Complete lack of occupational or recreational exertion

Any reason why you can't exercise regularly? _____

_____

What exercises do you enjoy or have enjoyed in the past?

1. _____

2. _____

3. _____

Existing medical conditions

Please check the appropriate conditions.

_____ Anemia   _____ Epilepsy   _____ Pregnancy

_____ Arthritis   _____ Heart condition   _____ Thyroid problems

_____ Asthma   _____ Hernia   _____ Ulcer

_____ Cholesterol   _____ Obesity   _____ Other: _____

_____ Diabetes

Figure 8.2   Client health history form.

Medications

Are you currently taking any medications? _____ Yes _____ No

If yes, please list the medication and for what condition.

Medication: _____ Condition: _____

Medication: _____ Condition: _____

Medication: _____ Condition: _____

Medication: _____ Condition: _____

Allergies

Do you have any allergies? _____ Yes _____ No

If yes, please list and indicate if medication is required.

Allergy: _____ Medication required: _____

Allergy: _____ Medication required: _____

Injuries

Do you have pain,
or have you injured
any of the following
areas?

_____ Neck   _____ Shoulder: R / L

_____ Upper back   _____ Elbow: R / L

_____ Lower back   _____ Wrist: R / L

_____ Hip: R / L

_____ Knee: R / L

_____ Ankle R / L

Please explain: _____

_____

_____

_____

Contact In Case of Emergency

Name: _____

Phone number: _____

Relation: _____

Family physician

Name: _____

City: _____

Phone number: _____

(continued)

Figure 8.2 *(continued)*

Lifestyle

	Always	Sometimes	Rarely
I get 7-8 hours of sleep per night	_____	_____	_____
I am physically active 3 times a week	_____	_____	_____
I have regular medical checkups	_____	_____	_____
I eat 3-5 servings of vegetables daily	_____	_____	_____
I eat 2-4 servings of fruit daily	_____	_____	_____
I eat 6-10 servings of grains and cereals daily	_____	_____	_____
I eat 2-3 servings of meats and nuts daily	_____	_____	_____
I make a conscious effort to eat healthy	_____	_____	_____
I follow a strict diet	_____	_____	_____
I have no stress in my life	_____	_____	_____
I am a very happy person	_____	_____	_____
I am highly motivated	_____	_____	_____

Comments: _____

_____

_____

Personal Trainer

By signing this form, I certify that I have asked for and understand the pertinent information required for me to make an informed decision.

Signature: _____ Date: _____

Client

By signing this form, I certify that I have fully disclosed all pertinent information in an honest and truthful manner.

Signature: _____ Date: _____

Figure 8.2 *(continued)*

want to use forms such as SMART goal-setting worksheets as useful tools in counseling a client and setting up an activity program.

Client Risk Stratification

From the combination of the answers on the PAR-Q and the health history questionnaire, you will have to determine the risk that clients will put themselves in when engaging in an exercise program and what appropriate precautions should be taken. This process involves risk stratification, or placing your client into one of three categories: apparently healthy, increased risk, or known disease—and basing your decisions on the risk profile as outlined in figure 8.3.

Apparently Healthy

An apparently healthy client is one who answered "no" to all questions on the PAR-Q, exhibits no signs or symptoms of disease, and has no more than one major cardiac risk factor. These people are able to start a moderate-intensity exercise program and undergo fitness testing without a referral from a medical practitioner. However, men over 45 years of age and women over 55 years of age in this category should undergo a medical exam as a precautionary measure before engaging in vigorous physical activity.

Increased Risk

Clients at increased risk will have two or more coronary risk factors but exhibit no signs (e.g., high

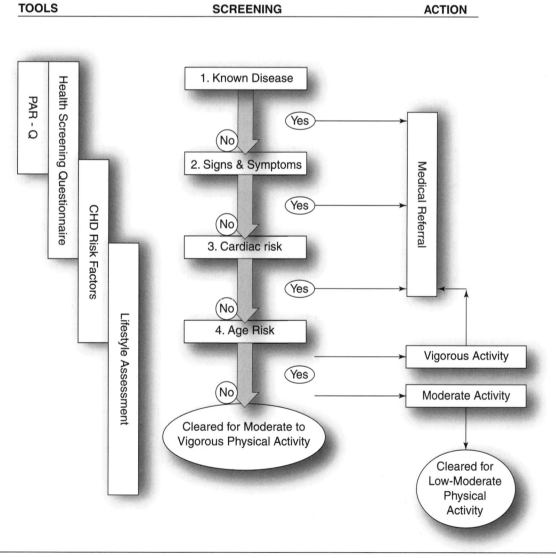

Figure 8.3 Preexercise screening guide.

Adapted, by permission, from T. Olds and K. Norton, 1999, *Pre-exercise Health Screening Guide* (Champaign, IL: Human Kinetics), p. 29.

BP) or symptoms (e.g., chest pain on exertion) of cardiorespiratory or metabolic disorders. These clients may start a progressive moderate-intensity physical activity program under close supervision (40%-55% HRR; 60%-70% HRmax). These clients should undergo clinically supervised maximal testing procedures before engaging in any vigorous physical activities.

Known Disease

Clients who have two or more coronary risk factors and exhibit positive signs (e.g., high BP) or symptoms (e.g., chest pain on exertion) or have known cardiac, pulmonary, or metabolic disorders should be referred to an appropriate health professional for testing and exercise guidance.

Referrals

After completing the health screening process, you will have a much better understanding of your client's current health status and medical condition. It is recommended that personal trainers not work with people who have serious medical conditions. Any clients who answer "yes" to a question on the PAR-Q or have two or more cardiovascular risk factors along with positive signs and symptoms should be directed to consult with their physician before engaging in a physical activity program. Any exercise guidance should only be done after a doctor provides clearance for **unrestricted physical activity** through the use of a form such as the PARmed-X (also available from CSEP at www.csep.ca/forms.asp). Clients who are not cleared for unrestricted physical activity should be referred to the appropriate health professional for exercise guidance.

Working with a client who is not cleared for unrestricted physical activity through either the screening process or medical referral leaves the personal trainer at risk of being liable in the case of personal injury or health problems associated with the client being active.

Summary of Important Points

1. Performing health screenings of clients is an essential component of the initial stages of the personal training process.

2. Each client should complete and sign a PAR-Q form annually.

3. The use of a second health screening form, such as a health history questionnaire, helps you collect additional information about a client's health history and current health status.

4. The information that clients share in health screening must be kept confidential.

Case Studies

Roger

Roger is a male over 45 years of age, has borderline hypertension, is overweight, and is previously sedentary. He has a high health risk for type 2 diabetes, hypertension, and coronary heart disease. Although he answered *no* to all of the questions on the PAR-Q, he has at least three cardiac risk factors and should obtain a doctor's referral and clearance before beginning his exercise program. Though not mandatory, Roger could benefit from completing a lifestyle questionnaire.

Molly

Molly is a young, previously active female who answered *no* to each question on the PAR-Q. She is overweight and at increased risk for type 2 diabetes, hypertension, and coronary heart disease, but does not appear to have any other health risks. Because of this, Molly is classified as apparently healthy. Molly is free to begin a moderate-intensity fitness program without any further screening. Filling out a health-screening form should be required, and a lifestyle questionnaire may help identify factors that should be addressed in order to help her obtain her goals.

Jennifer

Jennifer is a 40-year-old female with little health risk. She answered *no* to each question on the PAR-Q and is apparently healthy. She is able to begin a moderate-intensity activity program without any further screening, although filling out a health-screening form should be required, and a lifestyle questionnaire may help you make better suggestions for ways to increase her activity outside of the gym and help her obtain her goals.

CHAPTER 9

Fitness Assessment

Gregory S. Anderson, PhD
Brian Justin, MHK

CHAPTER OBJECTIVES

After completing this chapter, you will be able to

1. discuss the value and purpose of fitness assessments,

2. identify normal values for resting HR and resting blood pressure (BP),

3. explain how cardiovascular fitness is tested,

4. describe how to measure body composition using various methods,

5. discuss how muscular strength and endurance are evaluated, and

6. explain how to assess flexibility for most clients.

Many personal trainers use fitness assessments to complement their clients' fitness training. Performing a fitness assessment gives you a clear indication of clients' current health status and actual fitness level. This information is invaluable in fine-tuning exercise prescription. To follow best practices and allow for exercise prescription that has the greatest potential to improve clients' health and wellness, all personal trainers should start with baseline information derived from a quality fitness and lifestyle appraisal.

Fitness and lifestyle assessments can be useful for

- determining a client's current health status (using resting HR and BP);
- determining lifestyle factors that may be counterproductive to the client's fitness goals;
- identifying a client's actual fitness level for muscular strength, muscular endurance, cardiovascular endurance, body composition, and flexibility;
- determining the client's strengths and weaknesses for the purpose of goal setting and counseling;
- isolating significant injuries or risk factors that might affect the client's ability to exercise with a personal trainer;
- developing a unique, individualized, and accurate exercise prescription for each client that takes into consideration needs, desires, and lifestyle factors;
- establishing a baseline and setting a standard for the client to measure future progress; and
- motivating clients, thus increasing exercise adherence and compliance.

The question you must address is how much information you need in order to develop an accurate exercise program compared with your clients' desire to understand their current fitness level. For example, asking a very unfit client who is moderately overweight to perform difficult fitness tests may shake that client's self-esteem. On the other hand, a regular exerciser might desire a full battery of fitness assessments to evaluate personal progress and success. You must determine what the client's priorities are and then decide what fitness assessments are necessary and what tests are most

appropriate. Choosing tests wisely is of the utmost importance—a skilled personal trainer must know not only what tests are available, but also when each test may be most appropriate.

Before any exercise programming, it is important to evaluate the results of fitness assessments in order to determine appropriate exercise prescriptions for clients. It is important that you become skilled in taking both resting HR and BP, two basic screening tests for physical activity readiness.

Testing Procedures

Pretesting must always precede tests and measures. Before testing, clients should be told what to wear, when and where the test will take place, and to not exercise or drink caffeine or alcohol for 12 hours before the test. Once clients arrive, they should fill out a PAR-Q (see chapter 8), have the testing session explained to them, and then sign an informed consent document. Copies of the PAR-Q and informed consent should be kept on file.

Prescreening also includes some physical measures. Clients should have their resting BP and HR taken. To perform the active portions of the testing, a client's resting systolic BP must not exceed 140 mmHg and resting diastolic BP must not exceed 90 mmHg. Resting pulse must be less than 100 bpm. Because these are fundamental screening procedures, every trainer must be competent in taking their clients' resting HR and BP. Taking these two measurements gives a good indication of the client's current health status; thus, keeping track of these values at regular intervals is crucial.

Resting Heart Rate

Resting HR can be measured by placing the fingers on a pulse site (carotid artery or radial artery). To get the most accurate reading, you can instruct clients to measure resting HR for at least 30 seconds in the morning before getting out of bed. To determine bpm, multiply that value by 2. When taking HR measurements, it is important to count the first beat as zero. An HR monitor can also be used to measure both resting and exercise HRs.

As clients increase their cardiovascular fitness, their resting HR gradually decreases. Normal resting HR is approximately 70 bpm for men and 75 bpm for women. A resting HR of 100 bpm or higher is a warning sign to look more closely at the client's overall health and request a doctor's clearance before training the client. See appendix table C.1 for normative data on resting heart rate.

Resting Blood Pressure

Resting BP is measured using a stethoscope and a sphygmomanometer. Ask the client to sit comfortably with the left arm supported. Place the BP cuff on the client's upper left arm and pump to over 200 mmHg. Slowly release the pressure (2 mmHg per second) as you listen through the stethoscope (placed over the brachial artery). Listen for the first tapping sounds (following the same rate as heart beat); this is the *systolic pressure.* Systolic pressure is the amount of pressure on the walls of the arteries as the heart contracts, and it represents the work of the heart muscle. A normal resting systolic pressure is 120 mmHg.

Continue to let out the air from the sphygmomanometer. The tapping will get louder, then become muffled, and then disappear. When you can no longer hear the noise, this is the *diastolic pressure.* Diastolic pressure is the pressure on the walls of the arteries as the heart relaxes and fills again, and it indicates resistance to peripheral blood flow. A normal resting diastolic pressure is 80 mmHg.

Look for a normal resting BP of 120/80 mmHg. If the resting systolic BP is 140 mmHg or higher or the resting diastolic BP is 100 mmHg or higher, refer the client to a doctor for clearance to exercise. Resting systolic BPs of 85 mmHg or lower are also problematic, and these clients may be prone to dizziness and light-headedness, which must be taken into consideration when prescribing exercise.

Testing Order

Testing should occur in a logical, consistent order. Prescreening measures are always performed first, followed by the body composition analysis. After a light warm-up, cardiorespiratory fitness testing should precede muscular strength and endurance testing and flexibility measures. Always repeat the testing sequence in the same order for consistent results.

Evaluating Body Composition

Many clients come to a personal trainer because they want to lose body fat and change their body composition by gaining muscle. Shedding extra body fat is a common goal for clients and a constant challenge for personal trainers.

The purpose of assessing body composition is to divide the body into the primary tissue (muscle, fat, bone, and organ) and chemical (lipid and nonlipid) masses. However, when most of us think of assessing body composition, our thoughts turn immediately to body-fat content. Interest in body-fat content has grown over the past 50 years as it has become clear that obese people have a higher risk of heart disease, high cholesterol, high blood pressure and stroke, diabetes, several digestive and pulmonary disorders, degenerative joint diseases such as osteoarthritis, and even some cancers. However, although these relationships exist, recent research indicates that it is the distribution of adipose tissue (where fat is located on the body), and not the total amount of body fat, that determines the health risk of obesity. Fat carried internally in the trunk area carries the greatest risk, whereas peripheral fat under the skin carries a lower health risk. Hence, the lack of information on the distribution of adipose tissue in a measure such as percent body fat is a major limitation and links to health are not readily apparent. Percent body fat is an overrated measure and is often misunderstood by both trainers and clients. If performing assessments for health purposes, you must monitor where the fat is on the body, and thus percent body fat is of little use. The form in figure 9.1 can be useful for tracking a client's body composition.

Choice of Measures

Since the early 1940s, the field method of choice has been anthropometric measures of both skinfolds and girths. These tools help reduce the error of measurement, often fit the situation and client needs, and are useful in tracking changes in total amount and distribution of adipose tissue as well as changes in muscle mass. To track individual progress, plotting of basic anthropometric data is recommended. The median value of data taken in triplicate (the middle of three measures) reduces potential error in measurement. By comparing measures over time at regular intervals, you can then track values associated with reduced health risk and those associated with increased health risk, and you may offer the client a better platform from which changes can be explained.

Regardless of the measurement you use, you must understand that each assessment has room

Client Information

Name: _____   Date: _____

Appraiser: _____

Height (cm): _____   BMI (kg/m²): _____

Weight (kg): _____   Waist girth (cm): _____

Circle the appropriate risk based on BMI and waist girth.

CATEGORY	BMI (KG/M²)	Disease risk relative to normal weight and waist circumference	
		MEN ≤102 CM WOMEN ≤88 CM	MEN >102 CM WOMEN >88 CM
Underweight	≤18.5	—	—
Normal	18.5-24.9	—	—
Overweight	25.0-29.9	Increased	High
Obese I	30.0-34.9	High	Very high
Obese II	35.0-39.9	Very high	Very high
Extreme obesity	≥40.0	Extremely high	Extremely high

Bioelectrical Impedance Analysis

Fat-free mass (kg): _____   Fat mass (kg): _____

Goals

1. _____

_____

2. _____

_____

Figure 9.1   Body composition assessment form.

for error. In other words, they are only estimates of body composition. Use assessment results to track client progress as opposed to comparing one client with another. Ratios should be avoided in body composition assessment. Because predicting percent body fat through any method is imprecise and does not provide information concerning regional fat and fat distribution, it is not recommended. To date, the recommended practice is to take several girths and skinfolds and graph the data in order to track changes in body composition. These changes will allow one to monitor change relative to an anatomical location, and hence are more related to health risk and prevention.

Skinfolds and Girths

Skinfolds measure the thickness of a double fold of skin and underlying adipose tissue (fat). Using a skinfold caliper, the thickness is measured by lifting the skinfold between your thumb and forefinger along the length of a fat pad at predetermined locations. These locations have to be precise to be effective and require knowledge of anatomy and anatomical landmarks. Once raised, the skinfold caliper is applied at 90° to the skin over the skinfold, and the caliper is released so that is squeezes the skinfold gently. The measure is read from the skinfold caliper after 2 seconds.

Girths measure the total circumference of either a limb or the trunk at predetermined levels. Girths include skin, fat, muscle, and bone. They are very useful because if a skinfold measurement goes down but girth goes up, the muscle has grown in size; however, if the girth and skinfold measurements both increase, the girth has grown because of increased fat deposits.

A chart containing height, weight, girths, skinfold measurements, sum of skinfold measurements, sum of trunk skinfold measurements, and sum of peripheral skinfold measurements may be an appraiser's most valuable tool. From these data, you can identify distribution patterns of adipose tissue and track absolute change in skinfold thickness over time. This information can then be used to reflect health risks, such as that associated with a low sum of trunk skinfolds but high waist girth (i.e., more internal fat, which has a greater health risk). In this case, a reduced waist girth would be the most appropriate indicator of changes in health risk. However, in someone with a high waist girth and a high sum of trunk skinfolds, both a reduction in skinfold thickness and a corresponding reduction of the waist girth would be warranted.

Waist Girth Measurements

Waist girth is obtained to help identify fat distribution in the abdominal region which is associated with increased health risk. The waist girth is taken with the subject standing with even weight on each foot, with feet shoulder width apart. A flexible metal tape measure is placed so that it is level around the circumference of the waist at the level of greatest narrowing. Be sure to not indent the skin, but only have enough tension to hold the tape horizontal and in the proper location. If noticeable narrowing is not apparent, take waist girth at the midpoint between the lowest floating rib and the top of the hip bone (iliac crest), or in obese clients, 2 centimetres above the navel. See appendix table C.2 for normative data on waist girth.

Bioelectric Impedance Analysis

A popular method of measuring body composition is bioelectrical impedance analysis. In this method,

equipment sends a mild electrical current through the body from the wrist to the foot. The more lean tissue (muscle) the client has, the quicker the current travels because the water in the lean tissue provides little resistance; the fatter the client is, the slower the tissue conducts the current.

The benefits of bioelectric impedance analysis are that it is quick, easy, and noninvasive; no technician is required; the analyzers are relatively inexpensive; and the analyzers may provide a computer printout including fat-free mass, fat mass, the ratio of fat to total body mass (i.e., percentage body fat), and ideal weight. The drawbacks include the specificity of the equations (age, gender, obesity), the sensitivity of measured resistance to the placement of electrodes and hydration status of the client, and the variability among analyzers (even when made by the same company). Further, there is no indication of fat distribution using this method, and hence the health-related concerns related to increased or decreased body fat cannot be addressed.

When reporting data from bioelectric impedance analysis, report absolute weights of fat-free tissue (lean tissue) and fat mass. Changes in these values, and not the ratio of these values (i.e., percent body fat), should be encouraged based on clients' goals.

Predicting Health Risk

By using several measures that are related to fat distribution and the proportionality of the body (how heavy it is for its height), you can estimate the client's health risk. For example, a large waist girth indicates fat carried in the trunk, which carries a higher health risk than fat that is carried on the limbs. Hence, a waist girth of 1.0 metres or greater is considered a health risk for a female and a girth greater than 1.2 metres is considered a health risk for a male.

Using clients' height and weight, you can determine their body mass index (BMI), which indicates whether they are carrying an acceptable amount of weight for their height. BMI is calculated by dividing the weight in kilograms by the height squared in metres (BMI = kg/m^2). A BMI of less than 19 or greater than 25 puts clients at risk; a BMI greater than 30 often indicates obesity, although bodybuilders with a great deal of muscle will also fall above 30, so you must be careful in your interpretation. Using the sum of skinfold measurements will help you make this decision. A large sum of skinfold measurements, a large waist girth, and a BMI over 30 suggest that the client is overweight because of increased body fat and thus is at a health risk, so weight loss (reduction of fat mass) would be an important goal for health reasons.

To determine disease risk from centralized fat deposition, the National Institutes of Health (NIH) and the National Heart, Lung, and Blood Institute (NHLBI) endorsed a simple clinical guideline for the identification and evaluation of overweight and obesity in 1998. By using the classical BMI categories for overweight and obesity and super-imposing waist girth to determine the distribution of excess weight, they developed a prediction of health risk. Table 9.1 identifies those who are at increased health risk for diabetes, hypertension, and coronary heart disease.

Evaluating Cardiorespiratory Fitness

Cardiorespiratory fitness is defined as the efficiency of the cardiovascular, respiratory, and muscular systems at delivering and extracting oxygen for energy production and mechanical muscle work. There are a number of fitness assessments that measure cardiovascular fitness. The measurement of this fitness parameter is expressed as $\dot{V}O_2$max, also known as *maximal oxygen uptake* (see chapter 3).

The most accurate way to measure cardiorespiratory efficiency is through a direct measurement of oxygen uptake during a maximal graded exercise test. A more common approach in the fitness industry, however, is to estimate oxygen uptake, or $\dot{V}O_2$max. This can be done using a timed distance (e.g., 1.5-mile [2.5-kilometre] run or Rockport Fitness Walking Test), using distance per unit of time (e.g., 12-minute run), or evaluating the client's HRR to graded submaximal exercise. Many submaximal methods exist to evaluate cardiovascular fitness from an HRR, including the use of steps, a treadmill (walk or run), or a stationary bike or cycle ergometer. A graded exercise test (GXT) means that the intensity of the exercise is gradually increased (i.e., grade, resistance, speed).

In a submaximal GXT, the client performs the exercise at increasing intensities without exceeding 85% of the client's age-predicted HRmax (see chapter 3). The trainer evaluates how the client responds to the increasing difficulty by measuring the HR in bpm. At the conclusion of the test, the trainer evaluates how hard the client was able to exercise before reaching the 85% barrier. The harder the client can exercise, the higher the calculated $\dot{V}O_2$max and the fitter the client.

Rockport Walking Fitness Test

The Rockport Walking Institute has developed a walking test to assess cardiorespiratory fitness for men and women within the age range of 20 to 69 years. It is a safe test to administer and is useful for testing sedentary and older clients. To administer this test, instruct clients to walk 1 mile (4 laps around a standard 400-metre track on the most inside lane) as quickly as possible, then take their HR immediately at the end of the test along with the time in minutes it took them to do the walk. An HR monitor would be useful; however, if you are manually taking the HR, a 15-second pulse count using the radial pulse will do. Clients should warm up and actively stretch 5 to 10 minutes before the test, and they should wear good walking shoes and loose-fitting clothes.

TABLE 9.1 Criteria for Increased Health Risks

CATEGORY	BMI (KG/M²)	Disease risk relative to normal weight and waist circumference	
		MEN ≤102 CM WOMEN ≤88 CM	MEN >102 CM WOMEN >88 CM
Underweight	≤18.5	—	—
Normal	18.5-24.9	—	—
Overweight	25.0-29.9	Increased	High
Obese I	30.0-34.9	High	Very high
Obese II	35.0-39.9	Very high	Very high
Extreme obesity	≥40.0	Extremely high	Extremely high

Adapted, by permission, from J.C. Griffin, 2006, *Client-centered exercise prescription*, 2nd ed. (Champaign, IL: Human Kinetics), pp. 88-89.

To estimate $\dot{V}O_2$ max, you can use the following generalized equation:

$$\dot{V}O_2 \text{ max} = 132.853 - 0.0769(\text{BW}) - 0.3877(\text{age}) + 6.315(\text{gender}) - 3.2649(\text{time}) - 0.1565(\text{HR}).$$

BW = body weight in pounds; gender = 1 for males and 0 for females; time = minutes.

You can compare your results to those in table 9.2.

One important reason to have clients perform submaximal cardiovascular fitness tests is to educate them about the relationship between HR and to exercise intensity and to compare HR to RPE (see chapter 3). If you teach clients how exercise should feel at different intensities, they will have a better idea of how hard to exercise during cardiorespiratory training.

TABLE 9.2 Average Values for Maximal Oxygen Uptake

AGE	$\dot{V}O_2$MAX, MALES (ML $\cdot$ KG^{-1} $\cdot$ MIN^{-1})	$\dot{V}O_2$MAX, FEMALES (ML $\cdot$ KG^{-1} $\cdot$ MIN^{-1})
18-25	42-46	38-41
26-35	40-42	35-38
36-45	35-38	31-33
46-55	32-35	28-30
55-65	30-31	25-27

Adapted from the CPAFLA manual from CSEP.

Evaluating Muscular Strength and Endurance

Many personal trainers assess muscular strength and endurance to help them develop an effective and accurate resistance training program. It is very difficult to measure absolute strength because it is the maximum amount of force that can be exerted one time, or in the 1-repetition maximum (1RM). Tests for predicting muscular strength and endurance can be categorized into normative and nonnormative tests.

Normative Strength Tests

Tests with normative data have values that rate the level of performance (i.e., poor to excellent) of the item being tested. These values are based on specific age populations, and a large number of subjects have been examined in order to establish them, so it is easy to compare your clients' results with the rating to quantify their fitness level for the item you are testing. However, the exact protocol used to establish the norms must be used when testing clients.

Grip Strength

You can assess upper-body strength using a hand-grip dynamometer, where the client squeezes the handle with maximal effort using both the right and left hands. The results of this test show a good correlation with a client's actual upper-body strength because it requires grip strength to complete the lifts for the upper body and even in some lower-body exercises (e.g., deadlift). Following is the protocol for this test:

1. Have the subject grasp the dynamometer. Be sure it is adjusted so that the second joint of the fingers fit snugly under the handle. Lock the grip in place.

2. The dynamometer should be held in line with the forearm at the level of the thigh away from the body. The hand and dynamometer should not touch the body during the test.

3. Instruct the subject to forcefully squeeze the dynamometer while exhaling (to avoid buildup of intrathoracic pressure).

4. Alternate hands, performing two trials per hand.

5. Combine the maximum scores for each hand and record them. Compare with age-adjusted norms.

6. See appendix tables C.3-C.5 for normative data on grip strength.

10-Repetition Maximum Test

Instead of performing a 1RM test, which is a high-risk test, you can perform a 10RM test (resistance where no more than 10 repetitions can be performed) of a specific movement pattern. The 10 RM testing can be used with healthy adults who have lifting experience. Typically the bench press, leg press, squat, lat pull-down, and shoulder press are used, but you can use any resistance exercise that you want to test that your client is familiar with. To predict a 1RM from the 10RM, simply divide by .75. Following is the procedure for conducting a 10RM test:

1. Have the client warm up for 5 to 10 minutes to increase core temperature.

2. Instruct the client to perform 5 to 10 repetitions at 50% of perceived 10RM.

3. After a 1-minute rest and some light active stretching, the client performs 5 repetitions at 75% of perceived 10RM.

4. Increase the weight to the client's perceived 10RM.

You can also compare your clients' estimated 1RM to their body mass by simply dividing the 1RM load in pounds by their body weight in pounds. This will give you a ratio of strength to body mass that you can monitor and compare with future tests or normative data for applicable tests. Normative data for ratios of strength to body mass for the bench press and leg press are provided in Appendix C. Be sure to familiarize yourself with the exact protocols used during the development of the norms.

Nonnormative Strength Tests

Nonnormative tests do not possess any data for comparison and therefore there are no ratings. The data obtained is compared with a future performance to observe for improvements. You can set the protocol for your test as long as your procedures for future testing remain consistent.

Percent-Improvement Tests

Many of the muscular strength and endurance tests use traditional protocols that have little application to clients' daily movement and exercise patterns. Instead, you can use an approach to muscular strength and endurance testing made popular by exercise physiologist Douglas Brooks: the percent-improvement approach. The following procedure can be used with whatever exercise you decide to test:

1. Pick a movement pattern that you would like to test.

2. Find a resistance your client can perform for 10 repetitions (10RM) of that movement pattern as outlined in the 10RM test discussed previously.

3. Once the weight is found, record it on your data sheet.

4. Retest in 4 to 6 weeks to evaluate whether there has been any improvement by an increase in repetitions of that weight.

5. Calculate the percent improvement by dividing the difference between the previous and most recent tests by the initial test result and then multiplying the result by

100. For example, if your client improved by completing 15 repetitions, you would subtract 10 from 15, which equals 5. Then you would divide 5 by 10 (initial test result) to equal .5. Multiply .5 by 100 and you get a 50% improvement.

6. If you still want to track this movement pattern after the retest, complete another 10RM test to find the new strength level.

The drawback of this type of testing is that you do not have any normative data for comparison. The advantages of this type of testing are that you can create your own test parameters, test more specific movement patterns, and track changes in your clients' strength and endurance levels. If you want to test more on the endurance continuum, you can perform a 15RM test; if you want to test more on the strength continuum, you can complete a 6RM test. This type of testing puts the trainer in the driver's seat and allows you to test for meaningful data that you can use in your client's program.

Normative Muscular Endurance Tests

Clients can perform two tests for muscular endurance. One test measures endurance of the abdominal muscles by having the client perform a maximal number of curl-ups in 60 seconds. The more curl-ups clients perform, the better their muscular endurance. Keep in mind that you are primarily testing the muscle endurance of the rectus abdominis and external obliques in a trunk flexion pattern. This does not give the whole picture of abdominal endurance, which requires more specific and comprehensive testing beyond the scope of this manual. The other test is a push-up test, where the client performs as many push-ups as possible until muscular failure occurs. This test can be done with clients in a push-up position on their knees or toes, and it indicates muscle endurance in a pushing movement pattern. These tests are outlined next.

Push-Up Protocol

Standardization of the push-up hand placement and lever length allow you to compare results from one test to the next. Follow this standard protocol:

1. Instruct the client to perform a couple of push-ups to observe for proper execution.

2. Have the client lie on the stomach with hands pointing forward and positioned under the shoulders.

3. Have the client push up from the mat, fully straightening the elbows and using the toes as a pivot.

4. The upper body must be kept in a straight line and then returned to the start position with the chin touching the mat. The stomach and thighs should not touch the mat.

5. If the client cannot do a full push-up, the pivot should occur from the knees with the ankles plantar flexed and feet in contact with the mat.

6. The client performs as many repetitions as possible until technique breaks down over 2 consecutive repetitions or the client is seen to strain forcibly.

7. Compare results with the data provided in appendix table C.6.

Abdominal Curl-Up Protocol

Probably one of the most used tests of abdominal muscular endurance and part of a fitness test for the back, the abdominal curl-up test is difficult to set up and standardize at first. Practice setting up clients and watching for errors in repetitions so that you learn to standardize this measure.

1. Apply two pieces of masking tape on a mat 10 centimetres apart.

2. Have the client lie supine with the head lying on the mat and the knees bent to 90°.

3. The arms should be fully extended when the fingertips are at the zero mark. The client should keep the heels in contact with the mat throughout the test.

4. Set the metronome to 50 bpm.

5. Have the client curl up far enough that the fingertips touch the 10-centimetre mark while exhaling. During the curl-up, the palms and heels must remain in contact with the mat. On the return, the head and shoulder blades must touch the mat with the fingertips touching the zero mark.

6. The client performs as many curl-ups as possible to a maximum of 25 in the 1-minute time limit.

7. Terminate the test if the client experiences undue discomfort, is unable to maintain cadence, or is unable to maintain the proper curl-up technique over 2 consecutive repetitions.

8. Compare results with the data provided in appendix table C.7.

For nonnormative muscular endurance testing, you can use the percent-improvement approach outlined previously.

All of these assessments are easy to perform, and the results give you a good indication of the client's muscular strength and endurance. This helps you develop an appropriate starting place for resistance training and a method of comparison so you can see if your programs are increasing muscular strength and endurance in your clients.

Evaluating Flexibility

Assessing flexibility is useful because detecting muscle imbalances and joint instabilities helps you develop exercises that correct these weaknesses and reduce the risk of injury. This section outlines two general flexibility tests.

Sit-and-Reach Test

The sit-and-reach test is commonly used to measure forward trunk flexion. Sitting with legs extended and upper body upright, the client reaches toward the toes using a flexometer. The distance that the client can reach forward determines relative flexibility in the hamstrings and low back muscles. The results can indicate areas of inflexibility that might put the client at risk for low back pain. Following is the protocol for the sit-and-reach test:

1. The client warms up for 5 to 10 minutes and performs 2 modified hurdler's stretches for 20 seconds on each leg.

2. The client removes shoes and sits with the soles of the feet against a sit-and-reach box at the 26-centimetre mark. The inner edges of the soles are placed within 2 centimetres of the measuring scale.

3. The client should reach forward with both hands as far as possible, holding this position for approximately 2 seconds. Be sure that the hands are parallel and the client does not lead with one hand. The fingertips can overlap and should be in contact with the measuring device of the sit-and-reach box.

4. The score is the most distant point reached with the fingertips. The best of two trials is

recorded. To assist with the best attempt, the client should exhale and drop the head between the arms when reaching. Testers should ensure that the client's knees stay extended; however, do not press the knees down. Clients should not hold their breath at any time during the test.

5. Normative data is provided in appendix tables C.9-C.10.

If a flexometer is not available, a metre stick may be used. At this point, the normative data for the sit-and-reach test would no longer be valid but one could still get an accurate measurement of how a client was progressing from test to test.

Shoulder Flexibility Test

The shoulder joints are used in many different sport movements, work activities, and activities of daily living. The shoulder flexibility test measures internal and external rotation of the shoulders. Restricted rotation of the shoulder may lead to pain or injury. Following is the protocol for this test:

1. The client raises one arm, bends the elbow, and reaches down across the back as far as possible.

2. At the same time, the client extends the other arm down and then up behind the back, trying to cross the fingers over those of the other hand. Watch for clients trying to arch their back to improve their score; correct this and have them start the test again.

3. Measure the distance of finger overlap to the nearest half centimetre. If the fingers overlap, score a plus; if they fail to meet, score a minus.

4. Repeat with arms crossed in the opposite direction. Average the two scores and compare with those found in table 9.3.

TABLE 9.3   **Shoulder Flexibility Test Norms**

RATING	SCORE (CM, AVERAGE OF LEFT AND RIGHT SIDES)
Poor	<–2.5
Below average	–2.5 to –0.5
Average	–0.5 to 4.4
Above average	4.5 to 12.0
Excellent	≥12.0

Based on your comfort level with the various fitness assessment protocols that exist and the relevance to your client's needs, you must decide what fitness assessments to use on a regular basis. The test included in the Can-Fit-Pro battery of fitness assessments were chosen because of the relative ease to implement, the low cost to perform, the time needed for evaluation (see the Data Collection Form on p. 119).

Sources of Error in Fitness Testing

The validity and reliability of testing can be affected by client factors, the equipment, the personal trainer's skill, and the environment.

Client Factors

Before measuring your clients' muscular fitness, familiarize them with equipment and testing procedures. Some clients may have very little weightlifting experience and may need time to practice the lift. Have them try the lift while you give technique corrections. Additionally, motivate your clients during the test to encourage them to do their best by giving them positive feedback after each trial.

Equipment Used

The design of testing equipment may also affect your clients' test scores. Be sure equipment is calibrated and in proper working condition. Make certain that the equipment fits your clients' body dimensions.

Personal Trainer Skill

Observation skills, technique mastery, and familiarity with testing protocols will allow for accurate test administration and results. Be aware of the type of grip used and be sure to standardize starting and ending positions in accordance with a standardized or trainer-designed protocol.

Environmental Factors

Factors like room temperature, humidity, and people present may affect test scores. Ideally the room temperature should be 21 to 23 degrees Celsius to maximize client comfort. Aim for a clean facility with limited distractions (i.e., no overcrowding).

Name: _____   Date: _____

Location: _____   Appraiser: _____

Screening

Weight (kg): _____   Height (cm): _____

Resting systolic BP (mmHg): _____   Resting diastolic BP (mmHg): _____

Resting HR (bpm): _____

Cardiorespiratory Fitness

1,600 m walk time: _____   HR (bpm): _____

$\dot{V}O_2max = 132.853 - 0.1692(BW) - 0.3877(age) + 6.315(gender) - 3.2649(time) - 0.1565(HR)$

Note: BW = kg; Gender = 1 for male and 0 for female.

Strength and Endurance

Grip strength

Right   _____ kg   _____ kg   _____ kg
Left   _____ kg   _____ kg   _____ kg
Combined _____ kg   _____ kg   _____ kg

Percent improvement test

Exercise 1: _____   _____ pre   _____ post
Exercise 2: _____   _____ kg   _____ repetitions
Exercise 3: _____   _____ kg   _____ repetitions

Push up: _____ repetitions
Curl up: _____ repetitions

Flexibility

Sit-and-reach test

_____ cm   _____ cm   _____ cm   _____ cm   Best _____ cm

Shoulder flexibility

Right reaching down   _____ cm   _____ cm   _____ cm   Best _____ cm
Left reaching down   _____ cm   _____ cm   _____ cm   Best _____ cm

Figure 9.2 Data collection form.

Conclusion

You can decide with your clients whether to perform a full or partial fitness assessment. As a personal trainer, you can obtain useful information through fitness assessments. However, the clients must be interested in and motivated by the assessments and their results. If you and a client choose not to perform fitness assessments, you will not have detailed information to assist you in developing a program. As such, be especially conservative when developing initial workouts.

Summary of Important Points

1. The decision to perform a fitness assessment should be made by the client and the personal trainer.

2. All fitness assessments should be performed by a certified fitness assessor in order for the information to be valid, reliable, and reproducible.

3. A normal resting HR is 70 bpm for men and 75 bpm for women.

4. A normal resting BP is 120/80 mmHg.

5. Cardiorespiratory fitness can be measured by assessing HRR as the client performs an exercise that gradually gets more difficult (i.e., GXT).

6. Assessing body composition helps to identify if the client has a health risk due to excess body fat.

7. Using muscular endurance and strength testing, a personal trainer can develop an effective resistance training program.

8. An assessment of flexibility for all joints helps the trainer identify areas of weakness for each client.

PART III

Program Design

CHAPTER 10

Program Design Concepts

Rod Macdonald, BEd

CHAPTER OBJECTIVES

After completing this chapter, you will be able to

1. identify the *four elements* of good program design,

2. understand periodization and its application to program design,

3. understand the common principles of training, and

4. understand the five step process of program design and delivery.

Importance of Program Design

As a personal trainer, the programs you design for your clients are critical to their success. In every program, you will combine a diverse array of elements, resulting in the practical application of your combined theoretical knowledge, your experiences with other clients, and a little experimentation based on sound research and principles of training.

One measure of the success of your programs is if they deliver results. However, this success is dependant on numerous factors that occur before, during, and after you design the program. A personal trainer may spend hours creating a program tailored to the needs of a specific client. A well-designed program will not only help clients achieve their goals safely, it will also be a resource that the trainer can refer back to, assessing what exercises and approaches to training worked and are most likely to produce results for the same and subsequent clients.

Based on the information you have been introduced to in previous chapters, you can see how the concepts of cardiorespiratory, strength, and flexibility training, along with the information gathered through health and fitness screening, provide the information you need to create a sound program.

Four Elements of Good Program Design

Good personal training programs have four elements in common: They are safe, effective, efficient, and enjoyable. Creating a quality program is both an art and a science, and all four elements are required in equal parts before optimal results can be obtained. Like the legs of a table, if one element is missing or not strong enough, the client may become disillusioned or worse, injured, and the client–trainer relationship can collapse (see figure 10.1).

Safe: Although there is a measure of risk with any exercise, the program must not cause injury or exacerbate existing injuries.

Effective: The program must deliver the results it was intended to deliver; otherwise there will be a gap between the client's expectations and the end product.

Efficient: The program must respect the time commitment that the client has made.

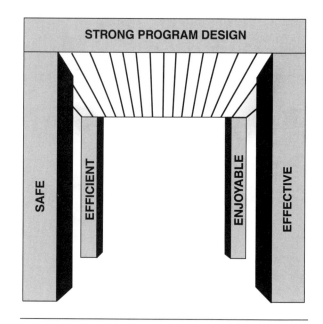

Figure 10.1   A strong program design should resemble a sturdy table.

Enjoyable: The program must have a measure of enjoyment (as defined by the client), leaving the client looking forward to repeating the program in future sessions.

Regardless of how much planning goes into any given program, there will inevitably be areas that need adjustment as the program is delivered for the first time, not to mention longer-term adjustments as the client progresses. To foresee the longer-term adjustments, you need to not only know what the client's long-term goals are but also have a plan for achieving them. The best way to create this type of plan is the scientific application of variation, also known as *periodization*.

Periodization

Periodization is the systematic organization of training periods (measured in time) to facilitate the most efficient path from goal setting to goal attainment. It allows the personal trainer to create a safe, easy-to-understand program that achieves short-term goals in the context of the client's longer-term goals. The ability to demonstrate to clients that you have a long-term plan for them will increase their confidence in you as well as ensure a long-lasting client–trainer relationship.

When clients stimulate their body through exercises, the body will undergo a reaction of some kind. If the stimulus is not sufficient, there will not be any noticeable change. If the stimulus is of the appropriate intensity and duration, the body will not only compensate, it will supercompensate (Bompa 1999), even from a single training session (see figure 10.2). Supercompensation is where the body not only returns to the previous level of performance (in a single bout of exercise the client will have a lower level of performance at the end of the session versus at the beginning), it actually increases in performance when given sufficient recovery.

In the case of multiple, successive training sessions, several scenarios may unfold. If the training stimulus is insufficient or there is too much recovery between training sessions, there may be little if any improvement (figure 10.3). If there is too much stimulus or not enough recovery between training sessions, the client is likely to see a decrease in performance (figure 10.4). If the stimulus is just right, the client will see successive improvements in performance (figure 10.5). Although the amount of improvement is not likely to be sustained over time, a well-designed program can optimize the improvements.

A real-life example of the *sum of training effect* is postal carriers. They are accustomed to walking hundreds of kilometres a week, sometimes up and down stairs and in challenging conditions. One might think postal carriers are extremely fit; however, because the stimulus never changes significantly, once their bodies become accustomed to their routes, their fitness quickly plateaus without further adaptation. However, an example of a decline in performance would occur if you were to take a deconditioned person along a postal

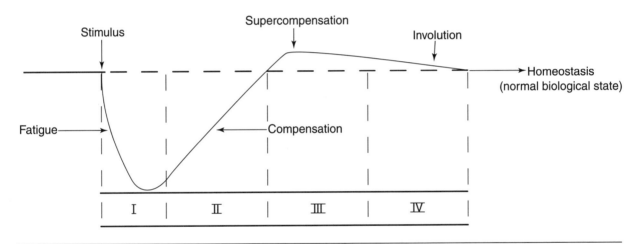

Figure 10.2   Supercompensation cycle of a training lesson.

Adapted, by permission, from N. Yakovlev, 1967, *Sports biochemistry* (Leipzig: Deutche Hochschule fur Korpekultur).

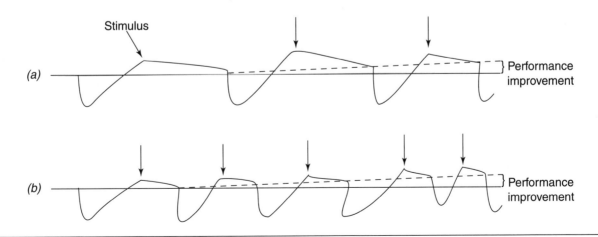

Figure 10.3   The sum of training effect.

Adapted, by permission, from D. Harre (ed.), 1992, *Trainingslehre*, (Berlin: Sportverlag).

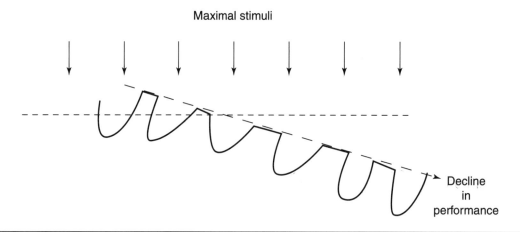

Maximal stimuli

Decline
in
performance

Figure 10.4   Decline in performance from prolonged maximal intensity stimuli.
Reprinted, by permission, from T.O. Bompa, 1994, *Periodization*, 4th ed. (Champaign, IL: Human Kinetics), p. 17.

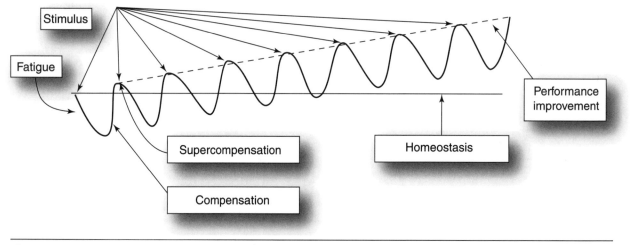

Stimulus

Fatigue

Performance
improvement

Supercompensation

Homeostasis

Compensation

Figure 10.5   Successive improvements in performance.

carrier's route You would find that within a few days the deconditioned person would be very tired, sore, and possibly injured because the stimulus was either too great or there was not enough rest between bouts of exercise.

Can-Fit-Pro Model of Periodization

Although there are multiple models of periodization, the Can-Fit-Pro model of periodization is adapted from the work of Tudor Bompa and streamlined to apply to fitness. Like most models of periodization, the Can-Fit-Pro model is built from the following components:

- **Macrocycle:** This is the largest component of the periodized program, usually consisting of several months to several years (e.g., an Olympic athlete's 4-year program).

- **Mesocycle:** This is the intermediate component of the periodized program, usually consisting of 1 to several months.

- **Microcycle:** This is the smallest component of the periodized program, usually consisting of 1 to several weeks. A microcycle would not usually be shorter than 1 to 2 weeks because it is difficult to measure progress in such a short period of time.

The purpose of using periodization versus a more instinctive or haphazard organization of training is that periodization both ensures more confidence in the expected outcome as well as provides a record to look back at after a certain amount of time and examine what worked and what did not. Periodization does not imply the creation of a rigid program that cannot be altered. On the contrary, a personal trainer using a periodized program is always able to substitute alternative exercises or methods of training based on the client's progress.

Differences Between Periodization Models

Traditional periodization is based on preparing for sport using multiple modes of training to improve technical skill, psychological stamina, and tactical training as well as fitness. Can-Fit-Pro's model of periodization focuses almost exclusively on fitness as developed through strength training, cardiorespiratory training, and flexibility training. Training for fitness is the domain of personal trainers, but the skills and abilities related to specific sports are best left to the qualified coaches of those sports. In other words, because the majority of personal training clients are either training for fitness or are using fitness to achieve other goals (e.g., weight management, health improvement), fitness is the focus of personal training periodization. Although the fitness gained through personal training would undoubtedly improve the client's athletic skills in a variety of sports, the sport itself is deemphasized and the technique of the fitness training is emphasized. Figure 10.6 demonstrates an overview of an annual periodized program showing both intensity and volume of training.

In figure 10.7, you can see a more detailed use of periodization, designed for a university rower. Because the athlete's competitions are mainly in the month of October, there is an increasing level of intensity as that time approaches. This does not

mean that the athlete only trains at this level of intensity, but rather that the overall focus of the training is primarily high intensity. As a result, the athlete will also perform an appropriate amount of low-intensity sessions as active recovery and as maintenance of the oxygen transport system. Each month has been broken into 2- to 3-week microcycles until September, when the next 8 to 10 weeks are broken into 1-week microcycles. This permits small adjustments to the program to accommodate adaptations required for competition.

Table 10.1 demonstrates how a client's program might be spread out over 12 months (macrocycle) with progressive increases of training (combined intensity and volume). Each 4-month period (mesocycles A, B, and C) represents periods where the client's program would focus on specific goals, building toward the larger goal. Each month (microcycles 1-12) allows for even more specific challenges fitting within the mesocycles. The 5th and 9th microcycles are slightly lower in training load to permit recovery from the previously higher levels.

Application of Periodization to Program Design

To apply periodization to program design, one must balance stress with recovery. This balance is based on the clients' fitness, nutrition, and commitment to recovery (e.g., going downhill skiing after a substantial leg workout is not a commitment to recovery). In addition, it is always best to err on the side of too much recovery rather than

TABLE 10.1   Sample Can-Fit-Pro Model of Periodization

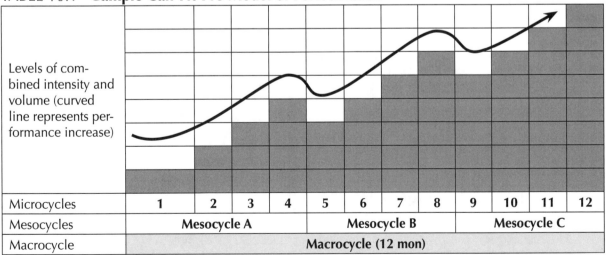

Levels of combined intensity and volume (curved line represents performance increase)												
Microcycles	1	2	3	4	5	6	7	8	9	10	11	12
Mesocycles	Mesocycle A				Mesocycle B				Mesocycle C			
Macrocycle	Macrocycle (12 mon)											

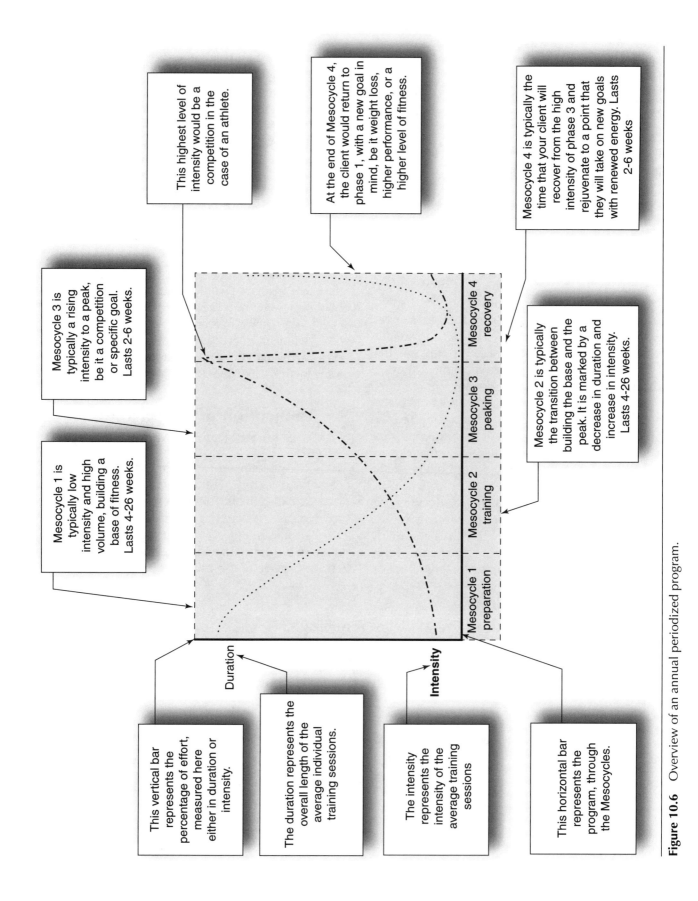

This highest level of intensity would be a competition in the case of an athlete.

At the end of Mesocycle 4, the client would return to phase 1, with a new goal in mind, be it weight loss, higher performance, or a higher level of fitness.

Mesocycle 4 is typically the time that your client will recover from the high intensity of phase 3 and rejuvenate to a point that they will take on new goals with renewed energy. Lasts 2-6 weeks

Mesocycle 3 is typically a rising intensity to a peak, be it a competition or specific goal. Lasts 2-6 weeks.

Mesocycle 1 is typically low intensity and high volume, building a base of fitness. Lasts 4-26 weeks

Mesocycle 2 is typically the transition between building the base and the peak. It is marked by a decrease in duration and increase in intensity. Lasts 4-26 weeks.

Duration

Intensity

Mesocycle 4 recovery

Mesocycle 3 peaking

Mesocycle 2 training

Mesocycle 1 preparation

This vertical bar represents the percentage of effort, measured here either in duration or intensity.

The duration represents the overall length of the average individual training sessions.

The intensity represents the intensity of the average training sessions

This horizontal bar represents the program, through the Mesocycles.

Figure 10.6 Overview of an annual periodized program.

Diagram of Periodization for a University Rower

Month	December	January	February	March	April	May	June	July	August	September	October	November
Competition												
Phase	Mesocycle A Preparation		Mesocycle B Training (transition from phase 1)			Mesocycle C Training (transition into peaking phase)				Mesocycle D Peaking		Mesocycle E Recovery
Emphasis	General Development		Specific Development		Transition	Technical/Specific Development			Transition	Competitive Development and Maintenance		Maintenance/ Recovery
Cardio System	Endurance		Endurance/ Power	Power			Power/ Endurance			Technical Endurance		Maintenance/ Recovery
Muscular System	General Strength		General Endurance			Specific Endurance				Maintenance		Maintenance/ Recovery
Flexibility	General Development					Specific Development				Maintenance		Maintenance/ Recovery
Technique			Simulation			General Development				Specific Development		Maintenance/ Recovery

Indicates competition

Graph of Intensity and Volume of Training by Month

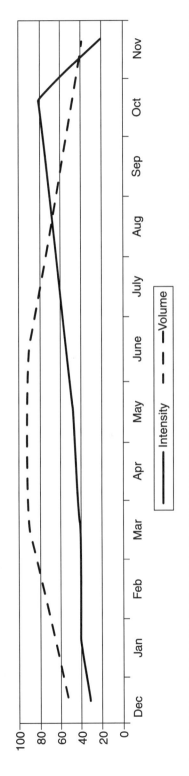

— Intensity   - - - Volume

Figure 10.7 Detailed use of periodization for a university-level rower.

too little. This becomes more challenging when the client is working out more than every other day. For example, if the client works with you on Monday, Wednesday, and Friday, but the client also runs on Tuesdays, Thursdays, Saturdays, and Sundays (which should have been revealed in the client's exercise history or in your ongoing communication), this could have dramatic implications for how you structure your program.

Though not an absolute necessity, clients should have at least 1 full day of either passive recovery (no exercise) or active recovery (walking or other low-impact, low-intensity exercise of short duration). In addition, clients should not be doing two hard workouts back to back, regardless of order. Ideally, they would perform a hard workout followed by an easy workout the next time.

Table 10.2 demonstrates how periodization of stresses can permit the combination of multiple modes of training with a lesser likelihood of injury. Without periodization, the combination of stresses might be too much and result in a chronic injury. Clearly, overall there must be a balance within the program, taking into account aspects of the client's training both within as well as outside the gym environment.

When designing the program, Can-Fit-Pro's principles of training should be considered as the foundational elements of periodization. Whether applied to strength, cardiorespiratory or flexibility training, these principles must be understood by both the personal trainer and their client (for complete descriptions of these principles refer to Chapter 1)

Can-Fit-Pro's Training Principles (revisited)

- **FITT:** This principle suggests that when designing a personal training program, the Frequency, Intensity, Time, and Type of exercise must be considered.

- **Individualization:** This principle suggests that programs and modifications to programs must be made to accommodate every person's individual needs.

- **Specificity:** This principle suggests that if clients want to improve an aspect of their performance, they have to train that aspect.

- **Progressive overload:** This principle suggests that to improve, clients must continually challenge their fitness.

- **Recovery:** This principle becomes increasingly important as the clients' workouts become more stressful. Recovery should not be seen as optional, but as a mandatory principle of training that must be considered for every program.

- **Structural tolerance:** This principle suggests that structural tolerance (the strengthening of tendons, ligaments, etc.) will result in the ability to sustain subsequently greater stresses in training, with a greater resistance to injury.

- **All-around development:** This principle suggests that people who are well developed through all components of fitness are less likely to sustain injury and more likely to perform better in sport and in life.

TABLE 10.2   Periodization of Stresses

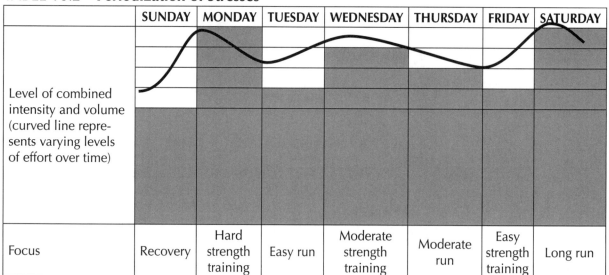

	SUNDAY	MONDAY	TUESDAY	WEDNESDAY	THURSDAY	FRIDAY	SATURDAY
Level of combined intensity and volume (curved line represents varying levels of effort over time)							
Focus	Recovery	Hard strength training	Easy run	Moderate strength training	Moderate run	Easy strength training	Long run

- **Reversibility:** This principle suggests that once training ceases, the body will gradually return to a pre-training state.

- **Maintenance:** This principle suggests that once a level of fitness has been achieved, it is possible to maintain it with less work than was needed to attain it.

How to Design a Program

Although there are a variety of ways to design a program, you will find that using a standardized process provides both a recipe to follow as well as opportunities along the way to ensure you are not missing any information that may be critical to the success of the program. Figure 10.8 is an overview of program design.

Step 1: Information Gathering

Before any program begins, the most important component is information gathering. These components are found in part II of this text and include the following:

- Health screening results
- Fitness assessment results

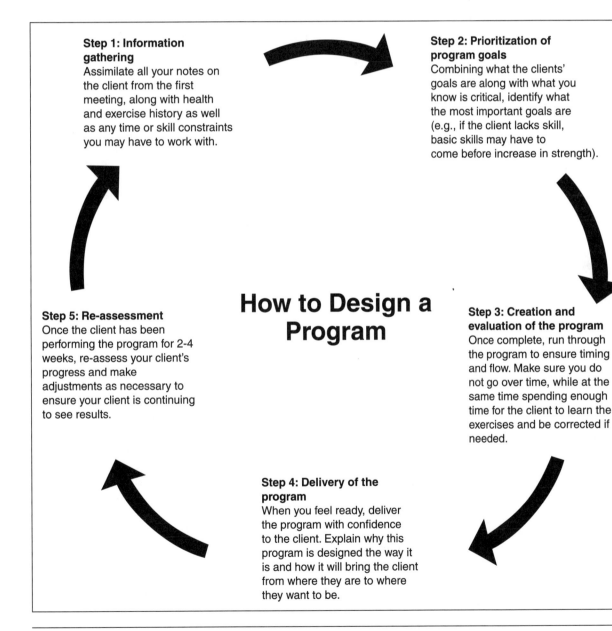

Figure 10.8   An overview of program design.

- Health history
- Exercise history
- Client preferences
- Client goals
- Predicted obstacles (time, client skill, and so on)
- Available equipment inventory
- Resources, if needed (exercise resources from books, articles, Web sites, and so on)

Without all of the information in this list, it is less likely that you will create as effective a program as possible. For example, if you are not aware of the client's preference to not use free weights and build a program solely using free weights, the client may feel intimidated and overwhelmed by the program. After acknowledging this preference, you might integrate one simple exercise using free weights until the client's confidence increases. Once you have gathered all of this information, you can integrate it into the program.

Step 2: Prioritization of Program Goals

Most clients will have multiple goals, and it is your responsibility to help prioritize them. By working with the clients, they will better understand the process, in addition to recognizing whatever obstacles may prevent them from achieving their goals. As well, many clients have a goal that is important to them but cannot be achieved without the establishment of certain skills and abilities. For example, if the client would like to lose 20 kilograms of adipose (fat) tissue but has never worked out before, strength training with cardiorespiratory training will have to be combined as a program focus. However, without a strong foundation of strength training skills, the client will not achieve the goal of weight loss as quickly as possible, so the program must first introduce strength training and bring the client's skills up to a level where the client can maximize the results.

Step 3: Creation and Evaluation of the Program

Because the content of the program depends on its duration, you must first start with the time constraints the client has given you. Based on these constraints, you need to factor in the basic components of a program, including the following:

- Warm-up
- Strength training

- Cardiorespiratory training
- Flexibility training and cool-down
- Breaks between exercises or modes of training
- Unforeseen interruptions (unavailable equipment, friends of the client wanting to chat, and so on)

Warm-Up

All programs must include a warm-up to make sure the body and mind are ready for the workout. Without a warm-up, clients may have a less effective or an injurious workout due to lack of diverted blood flow and lack of attention to the tasks at hand.

Strength Versus Cardiorespiratory Training After the Warm-Up

The choice to include cardiorespiratory versus strength training after the warm-up depends on a few things. From a time perspective, it is more efficient to continue the warm-up and move right into the cardiorespiratory training because the client is likely to already be on a piece of cardiorespiratory equipment. If you were to continue with strength training after the warm-up, the client would have to warm-up again before starting the cardiorespiratory training. However, if the client's goals include an emphasis on muscular development, the strength training should follow the warm-up so that the client has the most energy and enthusiasm for this component.

Optional Exercises

Although you will design a program for the total amount of time available, you can include optional exercises or ways to maximize time if the opportunity presents itself. For example, once clients are comfortable with a program, they could perform the warm-up and cool-down on their own. Going further, if you feel that the strength training component requires the most attention, you can have clients perform the cardiorespiratory training on their own (or vice versa) so you can increase the time spent on that training component.

Flexibility

Flexibility training is usually incorporated into the cool-down. The advantage to including the flexibility component directly after the cardiorespiratory component is that the client's muscles will be warmed up and more pliable; therefore the muscles will be more receptive to flexibility training compared with stretching when they are cold.

If flexibility follows strength training, the muscles will be pliable and receptive to flexibility training, but not to the same degree as after cardiorespiratory training.

Choosing Exercises

In choosing which exercises a client will perform, an infinite number of combinations are possible. For a new personal trainer this may seem daunting; however, there are a few simple steps you can take to find the exercises that are most appropriate for your client (see table 10.3). As you gain experience, exercise selection will become more instinctive and less process oriented.

Environmental Considerations

When designing the program, it is important to be mindful of the environment in which the program will be performed. These considerations should include physical obstacles or challenges that you may need to inform your client of (slippery floors, confined spaces, etc.) as well as climate-based challenges such as heat, humidity, or cold. For example, if the program will be performed in a very hot, humid environment, there may need to be more breaks, lower intensity, and encouragement to hydrate effectively. Conversely, if the program is to be performed in a colder environment, the warm-up may need to be extended and the workout may need fewer breaks to prevent the client from becoming chilled. If it is not readily apparent, ask the client where they will be working out so that you can make any necessary modifications to avoid putting your client at greater risk of injury or discomfort.

Terminology

When building a program, certain terminology is required for consistency, including the following.

- **Repetitions (reps):** A repetition is a single complete movement or exercise. For example, one rep of a dumbbell biceps curl consists of the concentric (muscle-shortening) motion and eccentric (muscle-lengthening) motion.

- **Sets:** A set is a combination of reps without rest. For example, a set of 12 reps of a dumbbell biceps curl is the full motion repeated 12 times.

- **Load:** This is the amount of resistance used for a given exercise. Keep in mind that the resistance provided by a dumbbell versus a machine versus tubing may vary significantly even if they are supposed to be the same. Always have the client attempt a new exercise with less load and then progress to the targeted load.

- **Tempo:** Tempo is the speed at which the exercise is performed. This usually consists of four numbers, counted in seconds, for each rep. For example, a 4:0:5:0 tempo for the biceps curl would mean a 4-second concentric movement followed by no pause before a 5-second eccentric movement followed by no pause before proceeding to the next rep. Pauses are sometimes used to hold a position to either eliminate momentum or increase voluntary contraction of the targeted muscle group.

- **Rest:** Rest is the time between sets or exercises. The amount of rest will dictate how much recovery

TABLE 10.3 Filtering Process for a New Personal Trainer (Chest Exercises)

FILTERING QUESTION	POTENTIAL CHALLENGE	POSSIBLE SOLUTION
What muscle group are you targeting?	There are thousands of chest exercises to choose from.	Select 5-10 exercises that you are confident teaching and that are effective.
What exercises can be performed where the client will be working out (equipment choice)?	If the client will be working out in a home gym, a program that includes a weight-stack chest press is not likely to be available.	Select 5-10 exercises, including both equipment-dependant and nonequipment-dependant exercises.
Is the level of risk acceptable for each exercise?	Some have higher risk (i.e., dumbbell chest press) and some have lower risk (i.e., machine chest press)	Rank the exercises by risk and required skill.
What potential challenges may I face in teaching this exercise?	The client may ask a question about the exercise or the client's reaction to it.	Prepare for potential questions as much as possible and only instruct exercises you can demonstrate with perfect technique.

the energy systems receive, potentially changing the focus of the exercises and ability to perform them with proper technique. For strength training, a beginner needs a minimum of 45 to 60 seconds between sets to continue; however 1 to 2 minutes are more likely to allow complete recovery for subsequent sets.

Open Versus Closed Kinetic Chain Exercises

When evaluating exercises, one continuing controversy is whether the focus of a strength training program should be on open kinetic chain exercises (OKCE) or closed kinetic chain exercises (CKCE). An OKCE is where the foot or hand is free to move in space, such as in performing a seated leg extension or a lat pull-down or kicking a ball. A CKCE is where the foot or hand is typically fixed and cannot move throughout the exercise, such as in performing a barbell squat or a chin-up or getting out of a chair. Research has shown that CKCEs produce less stress on the joints because they typically use more muscle and are therefore more stabilizing to the joints; however, real life is a combination of open and closed kinetic chain movements. Can-Fit-Pro's position is that a combination of OKCEs and CKCEs is the best approach for most programs.

Choosing Equipment

When deciding what type of equipment to use within a program, there are many factors to consider. These factors include where the exercises are to be performed (at home or in a gym), whether anyone else will be using the equipment (it might be unavailable at times), and above all how easy it is to perform the exercise correctly in the context of the client's skill and confidence.

Tables 10.4 through 10.6 demonstrate different types of equipment for strength, cardiorespiratory, and flexibility training and their advantages and disadvantages.

Set Performance

When creating the strength component of the program, you will have to decide how the client will perform the sets you have assigned. Most beginners will perform straight sets (where they complete the sets on an even tempo, one at a time), whereas more advanced clients will require more challenging ways to perform the sets. Table 10.7 lists a variety of approaches to set performance.

Step 4: Delivery of the Program

Once you have created the program, you must deliver it to the client. This aspect is what most people would consider to be a personal trainer's job; however, based on the preceding information you can see that much more goes into it. When you are ready to deliver the program, it is important to let the client know what to expect.

Establishing Expectations

Before the first training session with a new personal training client, you will presumably have had at least one conversation by phone, or preferably in person. This conversation may take place at the same time as a fitness assessment or even before that and will include information about the sessions, business policies, and other small talk.

Many clients will not know what to expect from these first communications, let alone from a health and fitness screening and subsequent training sessions. It is your responsibility to communicate clearly what they should expect of the process as well as what your expectations are of them and what expectations they should have of you. By setting the expectations ahead of time, you are creating an ideal setting for the first training session.

First Training Session

When you meet for the first training session, it is essential to be prepared. You should ensure that you have a few moments between clients to review the next client's file and history and know how you are going to take the client through the session, from first greeting them all the way to ending the session.

For example, if a client is lacking in self-confidence, you might tell him how pleased you are to see him and acknowledge that he should be proud of just being there. If, on the other hand, the client is always stressed and pressed for time, you can move more quickly into the session, and once you have started you can reduce her stress through slower movements and focused breathing.

The goal of the first session is to orient the client to the program and lay the foundation for future sessions by teaching correct technique and increasing the client's self-confidence. If you have designed a program that should take 50 to 60 minutes to complete, it will take you at least twice as long to properly go though the program the first time because you will have to demonstrate the exercises and make corrections throughout.

TABLE 10.4 **Strength Training Options**

STRENGTH TRAINING OPTIONS	ADVANTAGES	DISADVANTAGES	CLIENT SKILL LEVEL REQUIRED
Body weight	• No cost • Can be performed anywhere; very functional	• Can be difficult for deconditioned or overweight clients	Moderate to high
Free weights (dumbbells, barbells, kettlebells)	• Simulate real-world resistance • Relatively low cost • Versatile application	• Sometimes hard to control • Require specific training for correct technique	Moderate to high
Weight-stack or pulley machines	• Guides the client through a pattern of movement • Often includes photos or images to help the client remember technique • Deconditioned or weak clients do not have to change excessive weights; usually changes are made with a pin	• May not be made for shorter or taller clients • Can be complicated to use • Each machine usually is only practical for one or two exercises • Require more space	Low to moderate
Plate-loaded, leverage-based machines	• Less expensive than typical machines (uses manually loaded Olympic plates for resistance)	• Require more space than conventional machines due to swinging motion	Low to moderate
Pneumatic machines	• Pneumatic resistance allows the user to change the resistance with switches or foot pedals at any time • Permits explosive movement without momentum	• Do not accurately imitate real-world resistance • Very expensive • Require pneumatic compressor	Low to moderate
Elastic resistance	• Portable • Inexpensive • Can be used for virtually any exercise • Different tubing resistance permits a range of users	• Resistance increases through the ROM • Can encourage eccentric part of the movement to be too fast	Low to high
Water resistance	• Creates resistance in all directions • Resistance accommodates force applied	• Requires pool • Not appropriate for everyone • More time consuming	Low to high
Air resistance	• Resistance accommodates force applied	• Limited number of exercises currently available	Low to moderate

When you meet clients for the first session, greet them and start with small talk, such as about the weather, their kids, or simply how their day is going. To save time, have them start their warm-up if they have not already done so and go over what you are going to be doing throughout the session so they know what to expect. Ask them if anything has changed related to their health and remind them that they need to tell you if they have been injured outside of the training environment so you can make the necessary adjustments.

During the first session, you will have to orient clients to the program, showing them where the equipment can be found and how to adjust the equipment (seat height, how to remove and replace collars on a barbell, and so on). Your clients will likely be training without you from time to time, and they need to feel confident making all these adjustments by themselves. You should provide small illustrations or stick figures to help clients remember how to perform the exercise if the equipment does not have such illustrations (weight

TABLE 10.5 Cardiorespiratory Training Options

CARDIORESPIRATORY TRAINING OPTIONS	ADVANTAGES	DISADVANTAGES	CLIENT SKILL LEVEL REQUIRED
Stationary bicycle (upright)	• Usually easy to learn • Can be a less expensive option for home equipment • Low impact	• Many clients find it boring	Low
Stationary bicycle (recumbent)	• Usually easy to learn • Can be a less expensive option for home equipment • Recumbent bikes offer support to the lower back • Low impact	• Many clients find it boring	Low
Stair climber	• Low impact • Moderately expensive	• May not be appropriate for those with knee injuries	Low to moderate
Treadmill	• Usually easy to learn • Low to moderate impact	• Can be very expensive	Low to moderate
Rowing ergometer	• Provides nearly full-body workout • Less expensive than most cardiorespiratory equipment • Low impact	• Proper technique can be difficult to learn • Provides less feedback compared with other equipment • Not appropriate for those with shoulder injuries	Moderate to high
Elliptical machine	• Low impact • Easy to learn	• Stride length is normally fixed and may not be correct for some tall or short clients • Not all units have upper-body option	Low to moderate
Cross-country ski machine	• Provides almost full-body workout • Low impact	• Can be difficult to learn technique • Not appropriate for those with shoulder injuries	Moderate to high
Upper and lower climber	• Provides almost full-body workout • Low impact	• Many clients find it difficult and boring • Not appropriate for those with shoulder injuries	Moderate
Upper-body ergometer	• Works the often-underused upper body • Offers an alternative to those without the use of their legs • Low impact	• Most clients do not have the upper-body endurance to get a good workout • May be difficult to learn proper technique • Not appropriate for those with shoulder injuries	Moderate
Tread climber	• Interesting new option • Low impact	• Can be disconcerting at first • Not a good option for frail clients with less coordination	Moderate

TABLE 10.6 **Flexibility Training Options**

FLEXIBILITY TRAINING OPTIONS	EXAMPLE	ADVANTAGES	DISADVANTAGES	CLIENT SKILL LEVEL REQUIRED
Use of minimal equipment	Mat or floor exercises	• Portable • Inexpensive • Can be used for virtually any position	• Requires clients to get on the ground • Possible sanitation concerns	Low to high
Equipment based (machines designed for stretching)	Precor stretch trainer	• Does not necessitate getting on the ground • Gives diagrams for stretches to be performed	• Expensive • Does not work for all muscle groups	Moderate to high

machines typically do, whereas free weights do not). There should also be space on the program card where adjustments can be noted in a logical way.

With the first and subsequent exercises, once clients understand the equipment, you will have to demonstrate correct technique using cues that they will easily remember and then allow the clients to perform the exercise on their own. It is critical that they be able to perform the exercise correctly without added challenge (i.e., increased resistance or intensity) before applying any additional challenges. Before proceeding to the next exercise, summarize the exercise and reinforce the effort the client has put forth.

After going through the entire program, ask clients if they have any questions and finish the session on a positive note like, "Great work! You really understand the need for good technique, especially on the squat. Do you have any questions before we wrap up?"

Table 10.9 provides a sample exercise demonstration.

Subsequent Training Sessions

In subsequent training sessions, it is important to continue to correct exercises and reinforce proper technique. Continually challenge clients by introducing new exercises or variations of existing exercises every few sessions. Always make sure the client is ready for the challenge, and if the change is significant, have the client try the exercise with little or no resistance first and then add resistance slowly.

TABLE 10.7   Approaches to Set Performance

TYPE OF SET PERFORMANCE	DEFINITION	RATIONALE	EXAMPLE
Supersets	Two or more sets are combined with little or no rest for the same or different muscle groups.	Supersets maximize efficiency and increase intensity.	Same muscle group: cable chest crossovers immediately followed by barbell bench press Opposing muscle groups: leg extensions followed immediately by leg curls
Drop sets (also known as running the rack or strip sets)	The weight used for a given exercise is reduced when exhaustion is reached to permit continued exercise.	By reducing the weight, stress of muscle fibres can continue beyond the point that was possible at the starting weight.	Biceps curls with 10 kg dumbbells dropping to 8 kg, 6 kg, and 4 kg
Pyramid sets	Multiple sets are combined in an ascending or descending (or both) fashion.	By modifying the weight and reps completed, one may be able to stimulate both slow- and fast-twitch muscle fibres more completely.	Combination of sets of the following reps: 15, 10, 8, 6, 4, 6, 8, 10, 15
21s	Superset whereby you stimulate the upper half of the movement, the lower half of the movement, and the full movement.	By splitting the movement, it is believed that you can reduce weak spots in the strength curve.	Biceps curls using the lower half of the movement for 7 reps, the upper half of the movement for 7 reps and the whole movement for 7 reps, for 21 reps total
Staggered sets	A set or exercise is performed between sets for a particular muscle group.	By using this downtime, you can maximize efficiency and accomplish more during the session.	Performing a set of abdominal crunches between 3 sets of shoulder presses; stretching a tight area of the body between every set of the program
Circuit training	Sets of strength, cardiorespiratory, and flexibility training are combined in a circuit with little or no time between sets.	Maximizing use of time allows for more volume of training.	Completing 1 set each and repeating full circuit three times: Chest press, seated row, 2 min jump rope, biceps curl, triceps extension, crunches, 2 min jump rope, leg extension, leg curl, and 2 min jump rope
Slow	Increasing time under tension, slow training dramatically increases either the concentric or eccentric (or both) parts of the rep.	Increased time under tension has been shown to be safe (momentum may be almost zero) and effective.	Tempo of 5:0:15:0 or other combination whereby momentum is reduced
Split training	Muscle groups are split up based on the goals of the client, number of days they can work out, and personal preference.	Allows for more total volume or intensity in a single session and an increased focus on specific muscle groups.	See examples in table 10.8

TABLE 10.8 **Common Split Training Combinations**

SPLIT	SUNDAY	MONDAY	TUESDAY	WEDNESDAY	THURSDAY	FRIDAY	SATURDAY
3 days	—	Whole body	—	Whole body	—	Whole body	—
4 days	—	Chest Shoulders Triceps Core	Legs Back Biceps	—	Chest Shoulders Triceps Core	Legs Back Biceps	—
5 days	—	Chest Shoulders Triceps Core	Legs Back Biceps	—	Chest Back Core	Shoulders Triceps	Legs Biceps Core
6 days	—	Chest Triceps Core	Legs Shoulders	Back Biceps Core	Chest Triceps	Legs Shoulders Core	Back Biceps

TABLE 10.9 **Sample Exercise Demonstration**

WHAT TO DO	WHAT TO SAY	EXAMPLE
Bring the client to the location of the exercise.	Introduce the exercise verbally, mentioning the name, the muscle groups worked, and the purpose as it is relevant for the client.	"This is the leg press. It mainly works the thighs and is great for improving jumping, picking up heavy objects, and overall fitness (relate the exercise to whatever is most relevant to the client)."
Demonstrate the adjustments of the exercise.	Show the client where the adjustments are made and why.	"The adjustment on the leg press allows for a person of almost any height to use it. It is located here, and to adjust it, just pull on this lever and move up or down until your thighs are parallel to the platform."
Demonstrate the exercise.	Explain how to perform the exercise, including cues and things to avoid.	"Make sure your back is stable and your eyes are facing forward. Start by pressing through the heels, making sure your knees track over your toes. As you press, exhale throughout the movement and pause slightly at the end of the movement without locking your knees. Return to the start position by slowly lowering yourself and inhaling throughout the movement. Continue without pause until you cannot maintain technique or are otherwise uncomfortable, bring the weight to the platform, and get off the equipment."
Allow the client to try the exercise.	Talk the client through the movement, asking how and where the client feels the exercise.	"Where do you feel the most work being done? Are you pressing through the heel? That looks great. Continue breathing and I'll let you know when to stop."

CHAPTER 11

Typical Personal Training Programs

Rod Macdonald, BEd

CHAPTER OBJECTIVES

After completing this chapter, you will be able to

1. be comfortable with a typical personal training program,

2. know when to change the program, and

3. understand the difference between changing the exercise or the performance of the exercise.

Thousands of different programs could be created for any client with a specific goal. Table 11.1 includes just a few of the programs possible for achieving a variety of common goals. These are not the only way to create a program of this sort; rather, they provide a reference point as to what a safe and effective program might look like.

Balancing the Program

When designing a program, there is often a focus on balance of exercises. Balancing of components is critical, but only within the context of the individual client. When clients come to you, they are bringing with them a variety of needs and goals that are often out of balance. This usually requires you to have the creativity to design a program that is actually unbalanced in order to help balance the needs and goals of the client.

For example, if a client comes in with slightly forward leaning posture not related to an injury or skeletal deformity and he can return to a neutral posture if he tries, as a trainer you will be able to help him. What will be required, however, is the deemphasis of chest and anterior shoulder exercises and an emphasis on rhomboid, posterior deltoid,

and trapezius exercises until the client returns to neutral posture. This unbalanced approach would be used to help restore balance.

This type of unbalanced approach is also applicable to flexibility, such as where a client is more flexible in the upper versus lower body, and to cardiorespiratory training, such as deemphasizing cardiorespiratory exercise if the client continues to be a lifelong runner.

What Should I Do When . . . ?

When delivering a program, there are inevitably times when something occurs that you are not expecting. As the saying goes, expect the unexpected, and even if you do not know exactly how to deal with the situation, you will be prepared to react in a calm and professional manner.

In general, when something unexpected comes up, remain calm, assess the situation, and without reacting too quickly, respond with the most appropriate action. It can sometimes be helpful if you imagine what the most experienced and professional personal trainer would do in the same situation.

The following are some common scenarios.

What Should I Do When . . .

My Client Is Having Chest Pain During the Program?

If your client is having chest pain during the program or other symptoms of a heart attack, follow the emergency procedures established at your facility and call 9-1-1 immediately. The client may act embarrassed and ask you not to, but it is better to err on the side of caution when dealing with this type of situation.

My Client Is Complaining of Her Toes Falling Asleep or Going Numb on the Treadmill?

This sometimes occurs when clients lean too far forward, their shoes are too small or tied too tightly, or in the case of the treadmill, when they are not landing in a heel-to-toe fashion. As the tread of the treadmill rolls backward, it encounters the foot moving in the opposite direction. When in contact with the treadmill, the shoe typically stops moving or begins moving backward while the toes momentarily continue to move forward, sometimes jamming

in the toe box of the shoe. Ask the client to try to keep up with the movement of the treadmill and roll from the heels to the toes.

My Client Is Always Getting Into Conversations With Friends, Compromising the Workout?

Take 5 minutes after the session to express your concern about the effectiveness of the sessions. Explain that you want the client to see the results you can deliver, but the constant interruptions may prevent this. If the client persists in chatting during sessions, you can either accept it or change the sessions so the client is so busy that she has less opportunity to be interrupted (e.g., use a water bottle instead of going to the water fountain; use staggered sets or circuit training).

The Equipment I Want to Use Is Always Busy?

If you design your client's program to include popular equipment, you may find yourselves constantly running into a delay. Depending on how long the equipment is occupied, you may need alternative exercises. For example, you might ask your client to complete a stretch for a particularly tight muscle group between exercises or when delayed. For every exercise you include, you should have either documented options or alternatives in mind that you can use.

My Client Doesn't Want to Try New Exercises?

Clients who are resistant to change make it challenging to achieve success. One tip is to compromise—ask that they try an exercise for 1 or 2 weeks and if they still do not like it, you can go back to the original exercise. If you've made a good choice, the client will likely see the benefit of the exercise and want to keep it in the program.

My Client Complains of Back Pain During Certain Exercises?

If your client experiences back pain or any other abnormal (unexpected) discomfort during exercise, discontinue the exercise immediately.

Double-check the technique, reduce the load, and have the client try again. If the pain persists, choose an alternative exercise that does not produce the pain and have the client seek a diagnosis from a sports medicine physician.

My Client Refuses to Complete the Parts of the Program He's Supposed to Do on His Own?

If your client will not consistently complete the homework you assign, such as cardiorespiratory training and stretching, change the program so everything is included in the sessions. That way, if the client does any more work outside the sessions, it is extra, but at least you know he is completing everything when he's with you.

My Client Can't Stay Focused Enough to Use Any Stability Training Equipment?

Whether for stability training or any exercise, if the client cannot focus enough to maintain good technique, choose an easier exercise. Technique is the most important aspect of training and must be upheld at all times.

Modifying Programs

To ensure optimal success, great personal trainers not only plan variety within their programs, they also anticipate when and where their clients will need variation. This section will provide a toolbox of methods by which you can modify any exercise to make it more interesting and more challenging or alternatively easier and less challenging on those days when clients may be feeling a little less enthusiastic.

When to Change the Program

There is no strict rule as to when to change your clients' programs, but the rule of thumb is approximately every 2 weeks, depending on how often the clients are exercising and what their skill level is. Keep in mind that you need not change everything in the program, but you should change some aspects on a regular basis. For example, if your client is finding the squat challenging but the chest press easy, you might leave the squat as is and modify the chest press to make it more challenging.

Table 11.2 shows the different variables and

examples of how they can be incorporated into a program, along with examples and cautionary notes. To make changes, follow these steps:

1. Tell clients when you first begin to train them that you will be making changes on a regular basis as necessary to ensure their progress toward their goals.

2. When clients are ready, inform them that you will be making a change to the program.

3. Based on their current level of ability and fitness, make changes slowly and incrementally (always underestimate rather than overestimate).

4. Anticipate areas of difficulty or risk given the changes and plan for them.

5. Assess results from the implemented changes.

6. Be flexible and make adjustments as necessary, possibly returning to the previous level of challenge until clients are more prepared.

7. Ask clients for feedback and make any necessary adjustments.

TABLE 11.1 Sample Program Designs*

PROGRAM COMPONENT	BEGINNER	OLDER ADULT	TIME CONSTRAINED/ INTERMEDIATE
Frequency	1-3 days/week	2-3 days/week	1 day/week
Total volume	Low-moderate	Low	Low
Intensity	Low-moderate	Low-moderate	Moderate
Sessions/day	1	1	1
Strength training			
Sets	1-3	1-2	1
Reps	8-12	12-15	10
Recovery	60 s	60-120 s	30 s
Set performance	Straight	Straight	Straight
Speed of motion	Slow-super slow	Slow-super slow	Moderate
ROM	Full	Full	Full
Stability	Full	Full	Full
Sensory perception	Full	Full	Full
Types of exercise	Mostly machines	Mostly machines	Machines
Number of exercises	5-10	5-10	5
Sample exercises	Chest press Seated row Lateral raise Leg press Leg curl Abdominal curl Back extension	Chest press Seated row Leg press Abdominal curl Back extension	Chest press Seated row Leg press Abdominal curl Back extension
Cardiorespiratory exercise			
Duration	15-30 min	20-45 min	20-45 min
Intensity	40%-60% HRM	40%-60% HRM	60%-80% HRM
Type	Stationary bicycle Walking Swimming Aqua fitness Basic group fitness	Stationary bicycle Walking Swimming Aqua fitness Basic group fitness	All previous types, plus the following: Stair climber Intermediate group fitness classes Cycling classes Elliptical machines

* = Each program would require individualized modifications as the client progresses and would include a thor-

NOT TIME CONSTRAINED/ INTERMEDIATE	HYPERTROPHY/ ADVANCED	ATHLETE/ADVANCED
5-6 days/week	5-6 days/week	5-6 days/week
Moderate	High	Moderate-high
Moderate	Moderate-high	High
2	2	2
Strength training		
3-5	5-15	4-5
Varied	8-12	Varied
30-60 s	60-120 s	Varied
Varied	Varied	Varied
Varied	Moderate	Varied
Varied	Varied	Varied
Varied	Full	Varied
Varied	Full	Varied
Machines and free weights	Mostly free weights	Mostly free weights
~15	20-30	10-15
Chest press	Flat bench press	Choice of exercises would
Chest fly	Incline bench press	be sport specific, adapted
Seated row	Decline bench press	to increase functional trans-
Lat pull-down	Shrugs	fer or to reduce imbalances
Lateral raise	Bent row	(i.e., dumbbell chest press on
Posterior raise	Back extension	stability ball versus machine
Biceps curl	Shoulder press	chest press)
Triceps press	Front raise	
Leg press	Lateral raise	
Leg curl	Posterior raise	
Leg extension	Biceps curl	
Abdominal curl	Preacher curl	
Reverse abdominal curl	Wrist curl	
Back extension	Reverse wrist curl	
	Triceps press	
	Overhead extension	
	Lying extension	
	Squat	
	Leg curl	
	Leg extension	
	Hip extension	
	Calf raise	
	Seated calf raise	
Cardiorespiratory exercise		
30-60 min	45-60 min	60+ min
60%-80% HRM	65%-75% HRM	70%-90% HRM
All previous types	Most exercise for this group is maintained at low-moderate intensity to prevent hypotrophic adaptations	All previous types, plus advanced classes

ough warm-up and cool-down.

TABLE 11.2 Program Modifications for Beginner to Advanced Clients

COMPONENT	HOW TO MAKE THE COMPONENT MORE CHALLENGING	EXAMPLE
Making a strength training workout more challenging		
Speed of motion	Go faster or slower.	Use a 14 s count instead of 6 or 7.
ROM	Use partial ROM or full ROM.	Focus on sticking point ROM.
Set performance	Use supersets, drop sets, giant sets, and so on.	Combine biceps curl and triceps extension.
Stability	Gradually remove stability.	Perform seated biceps curl on ball rather than bench.
Sensory perception	Gradually remove sensory feedback.	Close eyes during set.
Recovery	Reduce recovery time.	Take 30-45 s rest instead of 60.
Reps	Increase or decrease reps.	Drop reps to 5 (and increase weight) from 15 reps.
Sets	Increase sets.	Increase sets from 1 to 2.
Base of support	Narrow or widen the base of support	Wider hands with push-ups or sider stance for squats
Lever length	Lengthen or shorten the lever used in the exercise	DB side raises with arms extended vs. bent or push-ups from the toes vs. knees
Making a cardiorespiratory workout more challenging		
Speed	Go faster or slower.	Increase rpms, rate, or speed.
ROM (rower, VersaClimber, treadmill)	Focus on different aspects of the ROM.	Take partial strokes on the rower in different phases of the stroke.
Resistance (incline on treadmill, level on bike and cross-trainer, wind damper on rower)	Increase resistance.	Increase incline on the treadmill instead of speed.
Direction of movement (treadmill, cross-trainer)	Change direction.	Walk sideways on the treadmill or move backward on the cross-trainer.
Work–rest ratio (if using intervals)	Increase work time or decrease recovery time.	Instead of working for 1 min and taking 1 min rest, try 2:1 or 1:.5.
Making a flexibility workout more challenging		
Speed	Go faster or slower.	Move into a position dynamically.
Stability	Reduce stability.	Do stretches on one foot.
Transition	Move from one stretch to the next.	Move from a posterior deltoid to a triceps.
Duration	Hold the stretch longer.	Try 45 s instead of 15.
Breathing	Focus on breathing.	Inhale and exhale according to length of stretch.

Making a strength training workout more challenging

WHAT THIS DOES	THINGS TO AVOID
Increases or decreases the effect of gravity or momentum, thereby increasing or decreasing work that the muscle completes.	Don't go too fast or too slow (dangerous versus boring).
Creates angle-specific adaptation.	Don't neglect other ROMs.
Modifies intensity, variety, and time.	Don't undermine technique on either exercise.
Involves additional synergistic muscle groups.	Don't remove too much stability too soon.
Increases the challenge by decreasing sensory feedback.	Don't let clients injure themselves.
Increases intensity by allowing less repletion of ATP stores.	Don't exhaust the client.
Modifies results from endurance to strength.	Don't sacrifice technique for fewer or more reps.
Increases volume and therefore total amount of work.	Don't lose track of time (doubling work).
Increase or decrease need for balance	. . . make it so challenging the client's risk is unacceptably high.
By altering the lever length you can change the effective resistance without changing the actual resistance	. . . sacrifice technique just to use a longer lever (for example, swayed back during full push-ups)

Making a cardiorespiratory workout more challenging

Can modify energy system used.	Don't go too fast or too slow (incorrect technique).
Allows you to focus on one aspect of the movement.	Don't spend too much time on a small part of the movement.
Requires additional work and therefore additional calories.	Don't make radical changes, potentially overloading the client.
Uses undertrained muscles and motor pathways, increasing caloric output.	Don't use too high a speed or awkward movement.
Can modify energy system used.	Don't prevent adequate recovery or overstress the client with too long of a work interval.

Making a flexibility workout more challenging

Creates dynamic flexibility.	Don't let clients move too quickly or bounce.
Improves awareness of balance while using flexibility.	Don't lose the effect of the stretch.
Creates a more fluid movement.	Don't focus too much on transition and not enough on the stretch.
Allows muscle to relax more.	Don't lose point of tension.
Integrates mind and body more completely.	Don't let clients hold their breath or lose focus on the muscle.

The Program Card

If your clients are going to be working out on their own, it is important for you to provide them with a comprehensive program card to follow in your absence. A good program cards need not be complicated, but it does need to give the client enough information to complete the program with minimal questions. Some program cards simply outline the exercises to be performed, whereas others may provide space to record progress, while others may include illustrations to remind the client of the exercise. While you can create a program card to suit your needs, the most important elements are the following:

- The client is somehow identified on the card (if multiple cards are used in one facility)
- The exercises
- The sets and set performance
- The reps and tempo of the reps
- The rest between sets
- Any cues or comments to remind the client on how to perform the exercise

The weight is not as important as the reps (the reps will dictate the weight) to avoid ego getting involved, but can be added to the comments section for beginners as a reminder.

We have included a completed sample program card (figure 11.1) as well as a blank program card (figure 11.2) if you wish to use it. Keep in mind that there are many different versions of program cards available, and if you work in an established facility, they may have a card they prefer you to use. If you work independently, you may wish to customize or create your own program card.

Changing the Exercise Versus Changing the Performance

You don't have to necessarily change the exercise that the client is performing; you may be able to simply change how it is performed. For example, new clients who are performing a machine chest press may not need to progress to a barbell bench press if they are feeling intimidated by free weights. Instead they could perform the same machine exercise but increase the challenge by modifying the sets, reps, or tempo of the exercise or even how the body

is positioned during performance (e.g., lift the feet off the ground to engage more core stabilizers).

To ensure that your clients' training sessions will be safe, effective, efficient, and enjoyable, the programs you build must be dynamic. By applying a periodized approach to program design based on constant modifications for variety and injury prevention, your clients will achieve their goals and you will have a long-lasting and successful relationship with them.

Case Studies

The previous chapters have addressed many of the specific programming options for Roger, Molly, and Jennifer. As such, the following are overall recommendations to consider when designing their programs. They follow the four elements of program design: safe, effective, efficient, and enjoyable.

Roger

When designing Roger's program, remember that he is a business administrator nearing retirement, so he will likely respond best to a program that is a no-nonsense approach to exercise, giving him what he needs without any wasted time. This approach will give him fewer excuses to skip a workout, thereby increasing the likelihood that he will adopt fitness as a lifestyle.

Roger's program must focus on weight loss for two reasons—being overweight is a contributor to his health risk, and losing weight is one of his goals. By reducing his weight as quickly and safely as possible, Roger will be more likely to justify the additional effort it takes to integrate exercise into his life.

Since Roger is only willing to commit to 45 to 60 minutes, at least initially, efficiency comes second to safety in his program. Although his initial workouts may be shorter, you will need to increase both the intensity and duration of his cardiorespiratory workouts as quickly as possible, though not at the same time. Due to his time constraints and your need to monitor Roger, his time commitment might look like this:

- Warm-up—5 minutes
- Cardio—25 minutes
- Strength—15 minutes
- Flexibility—5 minutes

Client name: _____ Date: _____ Update: _____

YOUR LOGO

555-123-4567
www.yourcompany.com
info@your company.com

Training Guidelines

Always warm up (~10 minutes full-body cardio).

Always stretch after working out.

Program Breakdown

Two days/week: Complete exercises 1-12, alternating between day 1 and day 2.

Four days/week: Complete exercises 1-6 on days 1 and 3 and exercises 7-12 on days 2 and 4.

SUNDAY	MONDAY	TUESDAY	WEDNESDAY	THURSDAY	FRIDAY	SATURDAY
Off	Off	Day 1	Off	Day 2	Off	Off
Off	Day 1	Day 2	Off	Day 3	Day 4	Off

EXERCISE	GROUP	SETS	SET PERFORMANCE	REPS (DAYS 1 AND 3)	REPS (DAYS 2 AND 4)	TEMPO	REST(S)	COMMENTS
1. Push-ups off stability ball	Chest, shoulders, triceps	2	Straight	Max	Max	4-0-4-0	45-60	Toes on ball, one foot at a time
2. Wide-grip lat pull-down to front	Lats, rear deltoids, biceps	2	Straight	12-15	8-10	4-0-4-0	45-60	Focus on scapular retraction
3. Full cable row with scapular retraction	Rhomboids, trapezius, rear deltoids	2	Straight	12-15	15	4-0-4-0	45-60	Keep arms straight and squeeze shoulder blades together
4. Squatting dumbbell shoulder press	Legs, anterior deltoids, triceps	2	Straight	12-15	8-10	3-0-3-0	45-60	Combine deep squat with standing shoulder press (two-part movement)
5. Seated lateral raise on ball	Medial deltoids	2	Straight	12-15	8-10	3-0-3-0	45-60	Bring legs closer together to progress
6. Seated dumbbell biceps curl on ball	Biceps	2	Straight	12-15	8-10	3-0-3-0	45-60	Superset with triceps
7. Lying dumbbell triceps press on ball	Triceps	2	Straight	12-15	8-10	3-0-3-0	45-60	Keep arm at 45° to floor
8. Stationary lunge with ball	Quads, glutes	2	Straight	12-15	8-10	4-0-4-0	45-60	Keep rear foot on ball to lunge; use support if necessary
9. Supine leg curl on ball	Hamstrings, glutes	2	Straight	Max	Max	4-0-4-0	45-60	Start with one leg and finish with both

(continued)

Figure 11.1 Sample client program form.

149

EXERCISE	GROUP	SETS	SET PERFORMANCE	REPS (DAYS 1 AND 3)	REPS (DAYS 2 AND 4)	TEMPO	REST(S)	COMMENTS
10. Kneeling prone forward ball roll	Core	2	Straight	Max	Max	4-0-4-0	45-60	
11. Single-leg back extension	Erector spinae, glutes, hamstrings	2	Straight	12-15	8-10	4-0-4-0	45-60	
12. Twisting hanging leg raise	Abdominals	2	Straight	Max	Max	3-0-3-0	45-60	
13. 45° dumbbell twist on ball	Core	2	Straight	Max	Max	4-0-4-0	45-60	Start with 3 lb (1 kg) dumbbell; bring legs closer together to progress

Cardiorespiratory Training Guidelines

Choose from among the following programs, performing at least two per week, never repeating the same program two sessions in a row.

Workout 1

Intervals: 15-20 min at 1:1 ratio (1 min high intensity followed by 1 min recovery or low intensity on any equipment)

Workout 2

Fartlek training: 20-30 min at varying intensity every 2 min (change variable every 2 min, maintaining 75%-85% HRmax on any equipment.)

Treadmill example:

2 min at 0% incline at 6 mi/h (9.5 km/h)   2 min at 5% incline at 5 mi/h (8 km/h)

2 min at 10% incline at 3.5 mi/h (5.5 km/h)   2 min at 15% incline at 3 mi/h (5 km/h)

Workout 3

Steady state: 30-45 min at 75%-85% HRmax (continuous training on any equipment)

Flexibility

____ Standing pectoral stretch ____ Cobra stretch ____ Modified hurdler's stretch

____ Overhead triceps stretch ____ Cat stretch ____ Calf stretch

____ Cross-body posterior deltoid stretch ____ Lying quad stretch ____ Soleus stretch

Figure 11.1 *(continued)*

Client name: _____ Date: _____ Update: _____

Training Guidelines

_____

_____

_____

_____

Program Breakdown

_____

_____

SUNDAY	MONDAY	TUESDAY	WEDNESDAY	THURSDAY	FRIDAY	SATURDAY

EXERCISE	GROUP	SETS	SET PERFORMANCE	REPS (DAYS 1 AND 3)	REPS (DAYS 2 AND 4)	TEMPO	REST(S)	COMMENTS

Your logo here

(continued)

Figure 11.2 Blank client program form.

EXERCISE	GROUP	SETS	SET PERFORMANCE	REPS (DAYS 1 AND 3)	REPS (DAYS 2 AND 4)	TEMPO	REST(S)	COMMENTS

Cardiorespiratory Training Guidelines

Workout 1

Workout 2

Workout 3

Flexibility

Figure 11.2 *(continued)*

This program time flow will deliver the workout in 50 minutes, including breaks and transitions, and result in measurable outcomes.

Molly

In contrast to Roger, Molly is not going to be a hard sell and in fact needs to restrict her enthusiasm to ensure she does not burn out or negatively affect her studies. Molly will probably respond well to being pushed (assuming her departure from team sports was not a negative one). You will likely be able to challenge her physically and mentally, but make sure you reward her with praise and positive reinforcement.

If Molly commits to attending 2 group fitness classes per week in addition to volleyball 1 to 2 times per week, you can focus on lower duration, higher intensity cardio training and strength training to increase lean muscle tissue slightly during her session with you and the additional 2 workouts on her own. She would not start at this level, but rather add one element per week. After about 4 to 5 weeks, her workout would flow accordingly:

- Warm-up—5 minutes
- Cardio—25 minutes (high intensity, such as intervals)
- Strength—40 minutes (circuit training or combinations of sets)
- Flexibility—10 minutes

Jennifer

In further contrast to Roger and Molly, Jennifer has already been working out, so she will not require the same induction into a program that the others might. Jennifer's major challenges will probably be time, focus, and energy due to her substantial work and family responsibilities.

Because she is looking for an easy workout, it would be best to stay away from interval training or high-intensity strength training. Jennifer's schedule might look like this:

- Warm-up—5 minutes
- Cardio—15 minutes (high-intensity)
- Strength—15 minutes (circuit training or combinations of sets)
- Flexibility—5 minutes

Roger's Exercise Schedule

	SUN	MON	TUE	WED	THURS	FRI	SAT
Personal training sessions or workouts on his own		X		X		X	X

Note: Choice of days based on the assumption that Roger has communicated these as the best days to exercise. Saturday's workout could be a low- to moderate-intensity cardio workout with a longer flexibility component (no strength training).

Molly's Exercise Schedule

	SUN	MON	TUE	WED	THURS	FRI	SAT
Personal training sessions or workouts on her own		X		X (on own)		X (on own)	
Volleyball			X		X		
Group fitness classes				X			X

Note: Choice of days based on the assumption that Molly has communicated these as the best days to exercise.

Jennifer's Exercise Schedule

	SUN	MON	TUE	WED	THURS	FRI	SAT
Personal training sessions or workouts on her own			X			X (on own)	

Note: Choice of days based on the assumption that Jennifer has communicated these as the best days to exercise.

Client name: __Roger__ Date: __May 7, 2007__ Update: __May 21, 2007__

Strength Training Guidelines

Always warm up (~10 min full-body cardio).

Always use a neutral spine and never lock the joints.

Always stretch after working out.

Program Breakdown

2-3 days/week: Perform all exercises on 2 nonconsecutive days of the week, adding another day if time permits.

SUNDAY	MONDAY	TUESDAY	WEDNESDAY	THURSDAY	FRIDAY	SATURDAY
		X		X		X

ABC FITNESS

555-123-4567
www.abcfitness.com
info@abcfitness.com

EXERCISE	GROUP	SETS	SET PERFORMANCE	REPS	REPS	TEMPO	REST	COMMENTS
1. Machine chest press	Chest, front of shoulders, back of arms	1-2	Straight	12-15	N/A	0:3:0:4	90 s	Keep shoulders low and use steady range of motion. Don't lock out the elbows.
2. Seated cable row	Upper and mid-back, back of shoulders, front of arms	1-2	Straight	12-15	N/A	0:3:0:4	90 s	Let weight pull shoulder blades forward at start and begin movement with retraction of shoulder blades. Finish with elbows pulled back as far as possible.
3. Machine leg press	Thighs, glutes	1-2	Straight	12-15	N/A	0:3:0:4	90 s	Keep glutes in contact with seat and press through heels.
4. Leg curl	Back of thighs	1-2	Straight	12-15	N/A	0:3:0:4	90 s	Keep body in full contact with bench. Complete flexion of knee.

#	Exercise	Muscle group	Sets		Reps		Tempo	Rest	Notes
5.	Back extension	Lower back	1-2	Straight	12-15	N/A	0:3:0:4	90 s	Keep slight bend in knees. Feel extension through the entire spine from base to head.
6.	Twisting crunch	Abdominals	1-2	Straight	12-15	N/A	0:3:0:4	90 s	Knees bent, curl from the neck, gradually flexing the spine and decreasing the distance from ribs to hips. Do not strain neck.
7.									
8.									
9.									
10.									

Cardiorespiratory Training Guidelines

Pick one workout for each workout day, but never repeat the same workout twice in a row.

Workout 1

Steady state: After warm-up, 15 min at 65%-75% HRmax (continuous training on any equipment). Add 1 min every workout up to a total of 30 min. Follow with 5-10 min cool-down.

Workout 2

Light interval training: After warm-up, alternate between 1 min at 75% HRmax and 2 min at 60% HRmax. Repeat 4-5 times, adding 1 interval per week up to 10 intervals. Follow with 5-10 min cool-down.

Flexibility

Perform each stretch for a minimum of 45 s, preferably repeating 2-3 times.

___ Standing chest stretch

___ Overhead triceps stretch

___ Cross-body posterior deltoid stretch

___ Cobra stretch

___ Cat stretch

___ Lying quads stretch

___ Modified hurdler's stretch

___ Calf stretch

Client name: _Molly_   Date: _June 11, 2007_   Update: _June 25, 2007_

ABC FITNESS

555-123-4567
www.abcfitness.com
info@abcfitness.com

Strength Training Guidelines

Always warm up (~10 min full-body cardio).
Always use a neutral spine and never lock the joints.
Always stretch after working out.

Program Breakdown

4 days/week: Perform exercises 1–5 on Mondays and Thursdays and 6–10 on Tuesdays and Fridays.

SUNDAY	MONDAY	TUESDAY	WEDNESDAY	THURSDAY	FRIDAY	SATURDAY
	X	X		X	X	

EXERCISE	GROUP	SETS	SET PERFORMANCE	REPS	REPS	TEMPO	REST	COMMENTS
				THURSDAY	FRIDAY			
1. Barbell bench press	Chest, front of shoulders, back of arms	2	Straight	12–15	N/A	0:1:0:4	30–60 s	Keep spine neutral, pressing the bar to arm's length without locking out. Lower the bar until arms are at a 90° angle.
2. Dumbbell pullover	Chest, lats	2	Straight	15–20	N/A	0:1:0:4	30–60 s	Go through full range of motion until arms are perpendicular to the floor.
3. Barbell bent-over row	Upper and mid-back, back of shoulders, front of arms	3	Straight	12–15	N/A	0:1:0:4	30–60 s	Keep spine neutral and pull the barbell up to the navel.
4. Upright row	Shoulders, upper back	1	Straight	12–15	N/A	0:1:0:4	30–60 s	Keep knees soft and lead with elbows. Go no higher than shoulder height.

#	Exercise	Target	Sets	Set type	Reps		Tempo	Rest	Notes
5.	Dumbbell lateral raise	Side of shoulders	1	Drop set	12-15 × 3 drops	N/A	0:1:0:4	30-60 s	Raise dumbbells to shoulder height.
6.	Barbell back squat	Thighs, glutes	1	Straight	6-8	N/A	0:1:0:4	30-60 s	Keeping spine neutral, lower weight until legs are parallel to floor. Keep heels down.
7.	Dumbbell walking lunge	Thighs	3	Straight	15-20	N/A	0:1:0:4	30-60 s	Keep knees and hips at 90° angles, head up, and shoulders back.
8.	Standing calf raise	Lower legs	3	Straight	20-30	N/A	0:1:0:4	30-60 s	Rise evenly across all toes for full range of motion.
9.	Back extension on ball	Lower back	3	Straight	20-30	N/A	0:1:0:4	30-60 s	Use wall to brace and extend spine gradually.
10.	Twisting crunch on ball	Abdominals	3	Straight	20-30	N/A	0:1:0:4	30-60 s	Spread feet for base and brace against wall. Curl up gradually without straining neck.

Cardiorespiratory Training Guidelines

Use workout 1 on Mondays and Thursdays and workout 2 on Tuesdays and Fridays.

Workout 1

Steady state: After warm-up, 45 min at 75% HRmax (continuous training on any equipment). Follow with 5-10 min cool-down.

Workout 2

Interval training: After warm-up, alternate between 30 s at 90% of HRmax and 3 min at 70% HRmax. Repeat 8-10 times. Follow with 5-10 min cool-down.

Flexibility

Perform each stretch for a minimum of 45 s, preferably repeating 2-3 times.

— Standing chest stretch

— Overhead triceps stretch

— Cross-body posterior deltoid stretch

— Cobra stretch

— Cat stretch

— Lying quads stretch

— Modified hurdler's stretch

— Calf stretch

— Soleus stretch

Client name: _Jennifer_   Date: _January 22, 2007_   Update: _February 5, 2007_

ABC FITNESS

555-123-4567
www.abcfitness.com
info@abcfitness.com

Strength Training Guidelines

Always warm up (~10 min full-body cardio).

Always use a neutral spine and never lock the joints.

Always stretch after working out.

Program Breakdown

2–3 days/week: Perform all exercises on 2 nonconsecutive days of the week, adding another day if time permits.

SUNDAY	MONDAY	TUESDAY	WEDNESDAY	THURSDAY	FRIDAY	SATURDAY
		X		X		Optional

EXERCISE	GROUP	SETS	SET PERFORMANCE	REPS	REPS	TEMPO	REST	COMMENTS
1. Machine chest press	Chest, front of shoulders, back of arms	1	Straight	8–10	N/A	0:2:0:3	60 s	Keep shoulders low. Use steady range of motion. Don't lock out the elbows.
2. Seated cable row	Upper and mid-back, back of shoulders, front of arms	1	Straight	8–10	N/A	0:2:0:3	60 s	Let weight pull shoulder blades forward at start and begin movement with retraction of shoulder blades. Finish off with elbows pulled back as far as possible.
3. Machine leg press	Thighs, glutes	1	Straight	8–10	N/A	0:2:0:3	60 s	Keep glutes in contact with seat and press through heels.
4. Back extension	Lower back	1	Straight	15–20	N/A	0:2:0:3	60 s	Keep slight bend in knees and feel extension through the entire spine from base to head.

5. Back extension	Lower back	1	Straight	15-20	N/A	0:2:0:3	60 s	Keep slight bend in knees. Feel extension through the entire spine from base to head.
6.								
7.								
8.								
9.								
10.								

Cardiorespiratory Training Guidelines

Pick one workout for each workout day, but never repeat the same workout twice in a row.

Workout 1

Steady state: After warm-up, 20 min at 70%–80% HRmax (continuous training on any equipment). Follow with 5-10 min cool-down.

Workout 2

Interval training: After warm-up, alternate between 2 min at 80% HRmax and 2 min at 65% HRmax. Repeat 5 times. Follow with 5-10 min cool-down.

Flexibility

Perform each stretch for a minimum of 45 s, preferably repeating 2-3 times.

___ Standing chest stretch

___ Overhead triceps stretch

___ Cross-body posterior deltoid stretch

___ Cobra stretch

___ Cat stretch

___ Lying quads stretch

___ Modified hurdler's stretch

___ Calf stretch

PART IV

The Professional Personal Trainer

CHAPTER 12

Psychology of Personal Training

Mike Bates, MBA

CHAPTER OBJECTIVES

After completing this chapter, you will be able to

1. understand the personal trainer's role as it relates to client psychology,

2. understand the stages of change and how to work with clients based on the stage they are in,

3. identify the major variables that determine exercise adherence,

4. explain how to set effective goals,

5. understand how to deal with different personalities,

6. list some of the negative perceptions or challenges that new exercisers have toward exercising, and

7. explain the concept of lifestyle coaching.

In order for personal trainers to be truly effective, they need to have a keen understanding of the clients they are working with. This means they need to go beyond the physical components of the exercise program and understand what motivates the clients, what scares them, what frustrates them, and what gets them excited, and they need to know what types of questions to ask in order to get this information. This chapter will review critical psychological concepts as they relate to personal trainers working with their clients. This chapter will also show you that working with a client involves much more than simply designing an exercise program. If the program is going to be effective in the long run, you must take into account the psychology of personal training.

Personal trainers need to have a wide array of skills in order to be effective. They must not only have the subject knowledge, but they must also be comfortable delivering it effectively. Knowledge without comfort in explaining it to someone else should be a signal to trainers that they need to practice more or refer the client to someone else who has the comfort and expertise.

Working With Clients

Personal trainers are asked to provide feedback and advice throughout the client–trainer relationship. This occurs during assessments, exercise prescription, and ongoing monitoring of the client. Communication skills are at the heart of an effective client–trainer relationship. The trainer must be able to listen effectively and respond empathetically. If these skills are lacking, it will be very difficult for trainers to build the kind of relationships they need with their clients.

Some qualities of effective personal trainers are as follows (adapted from Howley and Franks 2003, p. 360):

- **Knowledgeable**—Trainers should know about the subject matter they are discussing and will be discussing with their clients. This also means they should be knowledgeable enough to know when they are giving advice that is outside of their scope of practice.

- **Supportive**—Trainers should support clients and their goals.

- **Model of healthy behaviour**—If trainers do not practice what they preach, it will be very difficult to convince their clients that the program is worth the sacrifice.

- **Trustworthy**—Clients should feel comfortable sharing information related to their health and well-being so that the trainer can make the most informed decision about that client's program.

- **Enthusiastic**—The trainer should be motivating and show a keen and genuine interest in clients and what they are doing inside and outside of the fitness centre.

- **Innovative**—The trainer should be constantly looking for ways to add variety and improve their clients' programs and ultimate results.

- **Patient**—Trainers will work with many different types of clients; some will be similar to them and some will be very different. Regardless of the personalities and level of motivation, it is critical that the trainer exhibit a high degree of patience with all clients as they progress toward their goals. Some will move quickly and others will move slowly; they both need the trainer's patience to be successful.

- **Sensitive**—As a trainer, you will need to be sensitive to clients' needs and characteristics. Whether you can relate to them or not, it is critical that you show compassion and understanding.

- **Flexible**—Each client is unique and will require you to be flexible in your approach. One style will definitely not fit all of your clients.

- **Self-aware**—As a trainer, you need to be aware of your own strengths and weaknesses and how others perceive you. It will be impossible for you to grow personally and professionally without a strong sense of who you are and how others view you.

- **Able to access material resources and services**—It is unlikely that you will have all of the answers to all of your clients' questions and concerns, so you must be able to refer your clients to other professionals or other resources.

- **Able to generate expectations of success**—You will need to convince your clients that they are capable of many things that they initially believe they are unable to do. All of the skills mentioned in this list will help in this area.

- **Committed to providing timely, specific feedback**—Clients need to know how they are doing as they progress toward their goals. Immediate feedback is essential to keeping your clients focused and motivated. The more specific the feedback is, the more valuable it will be to the client.

- **Capable of providing clear, reasonable instructions and plans**—As a trainer, you have a vast knowledge base, most of which your client does not need to hear about in detail. Your job is to communicate your message in a way that clients will understand, retain, and find motivating.

As you can see, there are many skills that personal trainers need to bring to the table in order to work effectively with their clients. These skills will develop over time and are constantly being upgraded as the trainer gains experience. The best trainers are able to adapt their skill set to the client they are working with. We will talk more about how trainers need to adapt their style later in this chapter.

Appropriate Behaviours for Personal Trainers

As a certified personal trainer, it is your responsibility to act in a professional manner and in a way that reflects positively upon the profession. The following are a few behaviours to be aware of:

- Maintain a strictly professional relationship with all clients.
- Only give exercise-related advice to clients in areas in which you have received formal training.
- Only design programs for clients who are relatively healthy and free of any special conditions or diseases unless you have been trained to work with this type of client.

It is important to draw a clear line between what you are trained to do and what you are not. The Can-Fit-Pro scope of practice (see chapter 7) elaborates on this, but there are also situations where you will need to use your professional judgment as to how you should proceed.

Behaviour Change

The most popular way to look at behaviour change is the transtheoretical model, also known as the stages of change model. This model describes behaviour change as a constantly changing process that follows specific steps. The model tells us that the approach should be different based on what stage the person is in. For example, your approach would be very different with someone who has been exercising regularly for the past 6 months compared with someone who has not been exercising regularly and has failed at many previous attempts. This model provides specific strategies for each stage.

The traditional stages of change applied to an exercise setting would look like this:

1. **Precontemplation**—The person is not seriously thinking about changing or starting an exercise program.
2. **Contemplation**—The person has started to think about exercising or changing behaviour and has most likely identified a course of action.
3. **Preparation**—In this stage, the person has actually begun to plan for the change and may have made some minor changes in behaviour.
4. **Action**—At this stage, the person has taken action and has begun to make the necessary changes, but it has been less than 6 months since the person started making these changes.
5. **Maintenance**—This stage begins 6 months after the person has successfully adhered to an exercise program.

Regardless of which stage your client is in, the potential for relapse always exists. You need to recognize that relapses will occur and have a strategy for dealing with them. Each client has a different exercise history and needs to be treated individually. Only after you have assessed which stage your client is at can you determine which intervention strategies to use. The following are intervention strategies that can be used at each stage.

1. Precontemplation
   - Increase awareness of the importance of exercise and stress the benefits.
   - Make a list of pros related to exercising regularly.
   - Provide general education one on one or through print or electronic publications.
   - Discuss health risks.
   - Discuss myths and fears related to exercise.

2. Contemplation
- Continue with education and discussion of benefits.
- Provide clear and specific recommendations for the exercise program.
- Identify social support system (family, friends, coworkers, or other exercisers).
- Increase self-confidence.

3. Preparation
- Evaluate support system and barriers.
- Provide personalized exercise prescription.
- Work on goal setting and action plan.

4. Action
- Talk to client about self-monitoring.
- Talk to client about self-reinforcement.
- Enhance self-efficacy.
- Try to prevent relapses.
- Deal with relapses.
- Provide encouragement.

5. Maintenance
- Review and revise goals and exercise program.
- Try to prevent relapses.
- Provide social support.

The majority of the clients that personal trainers work with will be in the preparation, action, or maintenance stage, so this is where the majority of your focus will be. It will be difficult for you to identify people who have not yet begun to take any sort of action (precontemplation or contemplation)

To determine the stage your client is at, you can use the questionnaire in figure 12.1.

For each of the following questions, please circle Yes or No. Please be sure to read the questions carefully.

Physical activity or exercise includes activities such as walking briskly, jogging, bicycling, swimming, or any other activity in which the exertion is at least as intense as these activities.

	NO	YES
1. I am currently physically active.	0	1
2. I intend to become more physically active in the next 6 months.	0	1

For activity to be regular, it must add up to a *total* of 30 minutes or more per day and be done at least 5 days per week. For example, you could take one 30-minute walk or take three 10-minute walks for a daily total of 30 minutes.

	NO	YES
3. I currently engage in *regular* physical activity.	0	1
4. I have been *regularly* physically active for the past 6 months.	0	1

Note: You may want to cover the following scoring algorithm before reproducing this questionnaire for a client.

Scoring Algorithm

If (question 1 = 0 and question 2 = 0), then you are at stage 1.

If (question 1 = 0 and question 2 = 1), then you are at stage 2.

If (question 1 = 1 and question 3 = 0), then you are at stage 3.

If (question 1 = 1, question 3 = 1, and question 4 = 0), then you are at stage 4.

If (question 1 = 1, question 3 = 1, and question 4 = 1), then you are at stage 5.

Figure 12.1   Physical activity stages of change questionnaire.

Reprinted, by permission, from B.H. Marcus, J.S. Rossi, V.C. Selby, R.S. Niaura, and D.B. Abrams, 1992, "The stages and processes of exercise adoption and maintenance in a worksite sample," *Health Psychology* 11: 386-395.

Following are some general motivational strategies (taken from Howley and Franks 2003, p. 354).

- Provide positive behavioural feedback.
- Encourage group participation and group support to offer the opportunity for social reinforcement, camaraderie, and commitment.
- Recruit spouse and peers to support the behavioural change.
- Provide a flexible routine to decrease boredom and increase enjoyment.
- Provide periodic exercise testing to give information about progress toward goals and the opportunity for positive reinforcement.
- Use behavioural change strategies, such as personal goal setting, contracting, and self-management, to foster personal control and perceived competency.
- Chart progress on record cards or graphs. Note and record progress daily to give immediate, positive feedback.
- Recognize goal achievement in newsletters and bulletin boards.
- Make fitness and exercise fun.

Determinants of Exercise Adherence

Many factors affect whether or not someone will stick to their exercise program. We'll examine each of the major factors in table 12.1.

TABLE 12.1   Factors Associated With Participation in Supervised Exercise Programs

DETERMINANT	POSITIVE	NEGATIVE	NEUTRAL
Personal factors			
Demographics			
Age		✓	
Blue collar occupation		✓	
Education	✓		
Gender (male)	✓		
High risk for heart disease		✓	
Income/socioeconomic status	✓		
Overweight/obesity			✓
Cognitive/personality variables			
Attitudes			✓
Barriers to exercise		✓	
Enjoyment of exercise	✓		
Expect health and other benefits	✓		
Intention to exercise	✓		
Knowledge of health and exercise			✓
Lack of time		✓	
Mood disturbance		✓	
Perceived health or fitness	✓		
Self-efficacy for exercise	✓		
Self-motivation	✓		

(continued)

Table 12.1   *(continued)*

DETERMINANT	POSITIVE	NEGATIVE	NEUTRAL
Personal factors			
Behaviors			
Diet			✓
Past unstructured physical activity during childhood			✓
Past unstructured physical activity during adulthood	✓		
Past program participation	✓		
School sports			✓
Smoking		✓	
Type A behavior pattern		✓	
Environmental factors			
Social environment			
Class size			✓
Group cohesion	✓		
Physician influence			✓
Past family influences	✓		
Social support friends/peers	✓		
Social support spouse/family	✓		
Social support staff/instructor	✓		
Physical environment			
Climate/season		✓	
Cost			✓
Disruptions in routine		✓	
Access to facilities: actual	✓		
Access to facilities: perceived	✓		
Home equipment			✓
Physical activity characteristics			
Intensity		✓	
Perceived effort		✓	
Group program	✓		
Leader qualities	✓		

Adapted, by permission, from R. Weinberg and D. Gould, 2003, *Foundations of Sport & Exercise Psychology*, 3rd ed. (Champaign, IL: Human Kinetics), pp. 409-410.

Demographic Variables

Demographics have traditionally had a strong relationship with exercise. In particular, education, male gender, and higher income or socioeconomic status have all been positively related to physical activity.

Cognitive and Personality Variables

When we look at all of the cognitive variables that have been tested over the years, the ones that have been the best predictors of physical activity are self-efficacy and self-motivation. By self-efficacy, we mean people's belief that they are capable of doing a particular exercise program. A person's level of motivation toward exercise is also a major determining factor of success in an exercise program. The more confident and motivated clients are, the more likely they are to be successful in the exercise program. You can facilitate this process by giving them feedback on how they are doing, setting realistic goals, and reassuring them that they can do it.

Behaviours

With respect to behaviour, the best predictor of someone's likelihood to participate in an exercise program is previous experience in an exercise program. There is little evidence to support that participation in sport in and of itself will predict future physical activity patterns, and there is also little evidence to support that physical activity patterns in childhood or early adulthood are indicators of future activity patterns. The key factor to look at is the recent history of physical activity. However, note that when children have a solid social support system that encourages physical activity and have role models to look up to, they are much more likely to be physically active when they are older. This emphasizes the importance of parental involvement in a child's future patterns of physical activity.

Environmental Factors

Environmental factors play a major role in predicting the likelihood of success. These factors include the social environment (e.g., family and peers), physical environment (e.g., weather, time, and distance from facility), and characteristics of the physical activity (e.g., intensity and duration).

Social Environment

Social support is a critical aspect of the social environment and plays an important role in the likelihood of someone sticking to an exercise program. A spouse in particular has a great influence, and in some cases the spouse's influence can be even stronger than the actual exerciser. As a personal trainer, you should identify your client's social support system to determine if it is going to help or hinder the exercise routine. If this social support system is not adequate, consider ways to help the client. One simple approach would be to make sure the client is introduced to others within the club. Although these introductions will not replace the client's long-established social network, it is a step in the right direction.

Physical Environment

The location of the fitness facility is another important factor when looking at the exercise program of a client. The closer the clients' home or workplace is to the exercise setting, the more likely they are to stick to that program.

Studies have shown (King et al. 2000) that women prefer to exercise on their own and in their own neighbourhoods. This is not to say that women will not exercise in your fitness facility, but it is something to keep in mind when you are designing a program. You might want to consider adding a couple of workouts outside the facility if this kind of exercise is something clients enjoy and it keeps them motivated. You should not be worried that they will leave you as a client. Your first concern should be what is best for them. If you are doing that, then everything else will fall into place.

The most popular reason people give for not exercising is lack of time, and this is unlikely to change in the foreseeable future. Lack of time is normally related to how people prioritize what they need to get done, and exercise is not normally as high on the list as it should be. If you can convince people that the benefits are worth the time sacrifice, you are much more likely to be successful. Additionally, you should be designing programs knowing that most people are time starved. If clients are regularly spending more than an hour at a time in your facility, you should take a serious look at their program and how long they are going to be able to maintain their commitment. You need to look at scheduling appointments that are convenient for the client, and you may need to consider shortening some sessions from 1 hour to 30 minutes.

Physical Activity Characteristics

The success of an exercise program depends on several structural factors. We will focus on the most important ones, which are exercise intensity, whether the exercise is done in a group or alone, and personal qualities of the trainer.

Exercise Intensity and Duration

The higher the intensity of the exercise, the greater the potential discomfort for the exerciser. This is especially true for those clients who are starting an exercise program from a relatively sedentary lifestyle. Research has shown that dropout rates are greater for people in high-intensity exercise (running) compared with low-intensity exercise (walking). The challenge is to find a moderate intensity with the appropriate duration so that the pain is minimized and the results are maximized for the client. If trainers follow the intensity and duration guidelines in this manual, their clients are much more likely to be successful. Higher intensity exercise also increases the chance for injury, which is another reason to prescribe moderate-intensity exercise programs for the majority of clients.

Group Versus Individual Exercise Programs

Group exercise programs have consistently shown better retention rates when compared with people exercising on their own. Reasons for this include social support, overall enjoyment, increased sense of personal commitment to continue, and opportunity to compare progress and fitness levels with others. Group exercising is not for everyone, but you should consider it for anyone you are working with.

Leader Qualities

A strong leader with likeable and knowledgeable qualities can often make up for many of the deficiencies in a program, like lack of equipment or space.

Setting SMART Goals

A key part of successful trainers' tool kit is their ability to set SMART goals. This approach to goal setting should be used whenever you are helping clients set short- and long-term goals.

SMART Goals

S—specific

M—measurable

A—action oriented

R—realistic

T—timed

Specific

Goals should be as specific as possible so that people can picture exactly where they need to be going. Questioning skills are essential to setting specific goals. When a client comes to you and says she wants to get in shape and feel better, what exactly does she mean by this? She could mean she wants to run a marathon, play with her kids, walk up stairs without getting out of breath, or lose weight—the possibilities are endless. The only way to really find out what she wants is to ask more questions, such as the following:

- What exactly do you mean by "get in shape" and "feel better"?
- How do you want to feel?
- What do you want to change?

Once you have asked these questions, you should have a better idea of what this person wants to do.

Measurable

Using measurable goals is a great way to give people feedback on their progress. Let's say your client wants to lose some weight and have more energy. Once you know how much weight he needs to lose, you can set a specific goal. Setting a goal for energy is a little different. When you are confronted with a goal that is difficult to measure, it is a good idea to use a rating scale. For example, ask the person where he is at on a scale of 1 to 10, where 10 is the point at which they have all the energy they desire. If this person says he is at a 5, you could tell him that by his next assessment he will increase his energy level to a 7 or an 8. If you can't set a specific numeric goal, then you will need to get your client to describe how he will feel when he has achieved his goal. For example, if someone wants to get in shape, she might say she will have achieved this goal if she can play with her kids for more than 10 minutes and walk up the two flights of stairs at work without getting out of breath. If you are not able to set a measurable goal, the goal is probably not worth setting.

Action Oriented

When you are setting a goal for your clients, you should associate a specific action with it. For example, if your client's goal is to lose 9 kilograms, an action associated with this might be to meet with you three times a week and get in one session on their own, with each session lasting at least 30 minutes.

Realistic

In order for a goal to be motivating, it must be believable to the client. If clients do not think they will be able to reach the goal you have set for them, the goal is not going to be very motivating for them. Alternatively, if you have set a goal that clients are motivated to achieve but the goal is too aggressive, they will eventually lose motivation because the goal is not realistic for them. You may need to educate your clients on what is actually realistic for them. If a client has a goal to lose 14 kilograms and get her weight down to 55 kilograms in 6 weeks, you are going to need to educate her on safe and effective ways to lose weight as well as the problems with quick-fix programs.

Timed

The last component to setting an effective goal is the time frame. Any goal you set should have a date associated with it. The time frame can be long term, short term, or a combination of each. For example if a person wants to lose 18 kilograms, you might tell him that he will be able to do this in 10 months, but you should also tell him that he will be able to lose 2 to 3 kilograms in 6 to 8 weeks. It is critical to break down long-term goals into short-term goals. Short-term goals are a great way to keep clients motivated and allow you to give them feedback as they progress toward their long-term goal. A long-term goal by itself may seem too far away, and it may not be as motivating since clients know that it will take so long to get feedback.

Working With Different Personalities

You will need to adjust your approach depending on the type of client you are working with; the same approach will definitely not work with all clients. That is not to say that the core competencies of being a good trainer change, however. All trainers need to be empathetic, have good listening and coaching skills, and be professional at all times. The degree to which you focus on each of these areas will change from client to client, and you will likely need to bring in some new skills depending on who you are training that day. For example, you may have one client who needs a lot of follow-up, so you must constantly keep in touch with him to keep him motivated and on track with his goals, whereas another client may simply want a lot of variety in her program and enjoy reading articles you bring in for her. One client may need you to be very motivating when you come in, whereas a different client may prefer that you not be quite as enthusiastic because the client himself is much more subdued.

Table 12.2 provides some additional examples of different personalities and how you might adjust your approach.

A great way to assess clients' personal preferences and thus their personality is to use a form like figure 12.2.

TABLE 12.2 Personality Styles and Treatment Strategies

PERSONALITY STYLE	CLIENT CHARACTERISTICS	TREATMENT STRATEGY
Technical	Systematic Analytic Questioning Organized Reflective Theoretical	Explain pros and cons of choices Be accurate Allow time—moderate pace Provide tangible evidence (educate) Follow up
Sociable	Friendly Attentive Supportive Amiable Relationship-oriented Demonstrative	Address the whole person Maintain relaxed and moderate pace Be a partner in the change Be a good listener Make eye contact Invite feedback
Assertive	Leader Controlling Pragmatic May be competitive May be energetic Opinionated	Be stimulating Increase pace, once successful Be businesslike May need to limit options but incorporate input Find the client's dreams or hidden agenda

Reprinted, by permission, from J.C. Griffin, 2006, *Client-centered exercise prescription*, 2nd ed. (Champaign, IL: Human Kinetics), 20.

Activity Preferences

What type of training activity (e.g., jog, cycle, hike, ski) do you prefer? _____

_____

What method of training (e.g., interval or continuous) do you prefer? _____

_____

Do you prefer group or personal training? _____

_____

Do you enjoy competitive or noncompetitive activities? _____

_____

What type of location do you prefer? _____

_____

What is your favorite type of equipment? _____

_____

What aspects of a past prescription did you enjoy? _____

_____

Is there anything in your type or level of current activity that you want to maintain? _____

_____

Special Interests

Do you have any current or past skills that you want to pursue? _____

_____

Do you want more information or resources on particular activities, health, or lifestyle topics? _____

_____

Do you definitely want to avoid anything? _____

_____

Are you interested in accomplishing something specific or being challenged? _____

_____

Are you looking for something new or some variety in your prescription? _____

_____

Expectations

Do you have any objectives that are particularly important? _____

_____

(continued)

Figure 12.2 What do you want?

Reprinted, by permission, from J.C. Griffin, 2006, *Client-Centered Exercise Prescription*, 2nd ed. (Champaign, IL: Human Kinetics), 21.

How will we know when you have reached your objective (be specific about measurable areas of improvement)? _____

_____

Are there any major behaviors that you wish to change (e.g., eating habits)? _____

_____

Do you have expectations for changes in a medical condition? _____

_____

Do you have any performance or sport-specific expectations? _____

_____

Do you want to know your status or improvement with respect to population standards or in comparison with your own previous efforts? _____

_____

Can you set priorities for your expectations? _____

_____

Figure 12.2   *(continued)*

Dealing With Clients' Fears and Perceptions

It is critical that you understand your clients' perceptions and fears before starting the exercise program. This is sometimes difficult for a trainer because the trainer's background and experiences are likely different than the clients'. In most instances, the trainer has a wide variety of experiences with exercise and is very confident in an exercise setting. This is probably in direct contrast to the client, who has either not had a lot of experience or has had experiences that have not been positive. These situations may have caused the client to be fearful of many things related to exercise, including fitness facilities, the people who work and workout in them, and even the exercise program itself. If you expect everyone to view exercise the same way as you, you will be in for a major shock. It is important that you understand and address your clients' previous experiences and current perceptions toward exercise. Only after this has been done can you get down to the business of designing an appropriate program for the client.

Some other common beliefs or perceptions that your clients might have are as follows:

- Unrealistic expectations for themselves
- Fear of failure
- Fear of not knowing what to do
- Perception that everyone will be looking at them
- Belief that they are the only ones who feel the way they do

Lifestyle Fitness Coaching

Lifestyle fitness coaching takes into account the fact that today's personal trainers need to take a holistic look at their clients. This process is defined as the following:

An ongoing and guided process of dialogue between a client and a health fitness professional that is

- *informed by comprehensive fitness-related data about clients needs, interests, and personal orientations, and*
- *directed toward broad-based goals of personal and health gains that are attained through sustained involvement in physical activities, which are adjusted periodically according to the clients' evolving life agendas (Gavin, 2005, p. IX).*

Lifestyle fitness coaches understand that there is more to the program than simply the exercises. As discussed previously in this chapter, if trainers want their clients to be successful in the long term, they need to take into account many factors. Lifestyle coaching is one approach to this, but it is a discipline unto itself that requires further study, certification, and practical experience.

In general, it is best to deal with the types of situations described below ahead of time so that clients know what their boundaries are before starting a program with you. When situations occur afterward (which they inevitably will), they should be dealt with immediately. Any lack of feedback can be construed as saying the actions are acceptable, which only makes them more difficult to deal with later on. These problems should always be dealt with in a one-on-one meeting so that clients are not made to feel more uncomfortable than they probably already do.

Summary of Key Points

1. Many of the qualities of an effective personal trainer are intangible things like trustworthiness, patience and self awareness.

2. The stages of change model is a great way for personal trainers to assess their clients and then prescribe exercise based on the individual's positioning within the various stages.

3. There are many variables that will determine the level of adherence to a client's

What Should I Do When . . . ?

My Client Exhibits Unprofessional Behaviour?

In this situation, it is best to address the behaviour right away in a one-on-one setting. Explain to the client why the behaviour was not appropriate and the impact it has on you and others. If the behaviour persists, you may need to ask the client to leave the fitness centre.

My Client Exhibits Negative Behaviours or Attitudes?

In this situation, the trainer will need to educate the client on the importance of having a positive attitude and how the negative attitude can affect the client's workouts and others around them. This client will also need encouragement and support from the trainer since this is not likely something that will change right away.

My Client Doesn't Adhere to the Program Outside of Personal Training Sessions?

A one-on-one conversation will need to occur where the trainer explains to the client how these activities are negatively affecting the workout and the client's ultimate goals. If the client does not change these behaviours, results are less likely to occur. If the trainer cannot get the client to the goal because of these behaviours, the trainer will need to consider terminating the relationship. If the client and the trainer can both deal with the negative activities outside of the session, then the decision to continue might be appropriate as long as the client understands the impact they will have on the results of the training program.

My Client Comes to a Session Under the Influence of Alcohol or Drugs?

In a one-on-one meeting, the trainer needs to tell the client that this behaviour is inappropriate and unsafe. The trainer should not continue with the workout if the client is under the influence. This should be taken very seriously and if it continues, the client should be told that you will have to end the relationship.

My Client Talks Too Much About Personal Matters?

Trainers need to use their judgment as to when the client is going too far in this area. They will need to communicate that they are uncomfortable with where the conversations are going and that the conversations are taking away from the workouts. It should be clearly communicated that the trainer cares about the client and wants to hear how the client's day has gone and if anything is affecting the workouts, but if that discussion goes beyond a brief conversation, it is not something that the trainer is professionally comfortable with.

My Client Tells Inappropriate Jokes?

The trainer needs to clearly communicate to the client why this is inappropriate and the impact that it can potentially have on others, including the trainer. This should be done in private in a one-on-one setting.

exercise program. The variables can be broken down into demographic, cognitive, environmental and the characteristics of the actual activity.

4. Successful personal trainers need to understand how to adapt their own style to the individual characteristics of their clients personality.

5. As a personal trainer it is important for you to understand the common beliefs and perceptions that a client comes to you with.

6. Lifestyle coaching is a holistic way for trainers to work with their clients and their individual psychosocial needs.

Case Studies

Roger

Upon completion of a lifestyle questionnaire, you find that Roger is in the preparation phase of the stages of change model. You might decide that your major focus with Roger will be to evaluate his support system since it is clear from the questionnaire that he does not have many people around him who are regular exercisers. In this case it would be a priority to introduce Roger to other people who have a similar exercise background. This will not only help him build a support system, it will also show him that he is not unique with respect to his age and fitness level. Since Roger works long hours, you might get his permission to occasionally contact him at work to see how he is feeling and to gauge his progress toward his goals.

Molly

Despite the fact that Molly has been active in the past, she is currently at the preparation phase of the stages of change because she has not been active for a couple of years. You determine that her major barrier will be the unrealistic expectations she has put on herself. Her initial feedback stated that she would work out with you or on her own 4 to 5 days per week and play volleyball a couple times per week. It is clear to you that she will not be able to maintain this based on her busy school schedule and the fact that she has not exercised much since starting university. You should thus discuss this challenge with her and convince her that a more realistic goal is to work out with you once per week and follow the program you have designed for her 1 to 2 times per week on her own. You can give her the option of missing one of these workouts if she plays volleyball twice that week. Also point out that although volleyball has many benefits, the recreational league she will be joining may not play a major role in helping her achieve her weight-loss goals due to the low level of intensity she will be playing at.

Jennifer

After completing the lifestyle questionnaire, you find that Jennifer is at the action phase. She has been working out regularly for the past month but has not been doing it long enough to make it a habit. Your major focus with Jennifer is to make sure she is aware that she can get a great workout in 30 to 45 minutes. The information she has been reading has convinced her that she needs to work out longer than this. Your entire focus with her is about making the workouts quick and convenient, so you should design her home workouts to meet these needs as well. Her home workouts should be designed to involve her kids while she is exercising. This allows her to spend time with them and also allows the whole family to get exercise together. From a lifestyle perspective, the more activity she can get with her family, the easier it will be for her to stick to her program.

CHAPTER 13

Business of Personal Training

Mike Bates, MBA

CHAPTER OBJECTIVES

After completing this chapter, you will be able to

1. identify and explain the 4 Ps of marketing,

2. identify various pricing structures,

3. explain the pros and cons of various types of promotional efforts,

4. explain the benefits of referrals and identify the various types of referrals,

5. explain the steps you can take when selling your services,

6. identify the key aspects of your professional image,

7. explain the best way to terminate a relationship,

8. identify the key aspects of risk management,

9. understand when you need to have insurance, and

10. explain policies and procedures.

As a personal trainer, you are running your own business. Whether you are working inside or outside of a fitness club, it is ultimately your responsibility to market your services, make your sales pitch, keep your records and paperwork in order, develop and enforce policies and procedures, manage risk, and present yourself in a professional manner. It is true that some clubs will assist you in many of these areas, but your success will eventually come down to your ability to master them yourself. This chapter will provide an overview of what you need to know in order to be successful in the business side of personal training.

Career Opportunities

Personal trainers work in many different capacities and are compensated in many different ways. Each path has its pros and cons.

One of the most popular ways to get started in the fitness industry is to work as a personal trainer within a fitness centre. In this role, trainers are either paid by the hour or split their revenue with the club (i.e., club takes 50% and trainer takes 50% on any money collected from the trainer's clients). This is an ideal starting point for most entry-level trainers for the following reasons:

- It provides access to the established clientele of the club.
- Working at an hourly rate can often allow you to get paid before you have your own clientele.
- It provides access to a large amount and variety of equipment.
- There is minimal financial risk for you.
- The club will assist in marketing and selling your personal training services.
- Administrative support (e.g., scheduling, bookkeeping) is normally offered by the club.
- Insurance should be provided if the club is paying you.

Some of the disadvantages of working for a fitness club include the following:

- Revenue is normally split with the club.
- You may have others duties at the club.
- Hours may not be as flexible as you would like.

- You are accountable to your coordinator.
- You are competing with other trainers for business.

A second potential job position would have you working within a personal training studio. In this situation the only people who use the studio are those who are paying a personal trainer. These locations are normally smaller than the average fitness club and only cater to people who are interested in personal training. Some of the advantages of this type of situation are as follows:

- The company helps you attract clients.
- The studio already has the equipment you will need.
- Insurance is provided if the studio is paying you.
- Training might be offered by the company.

Some of the disadvantages of working in a personal training studio are as follows:

- You have to split your profits with the company.
- Equipment is limited due to space limitations.
- Someone else is boss.
- Hours may not be as flexible.

A third option for personal trainers is to work as a contract or freelance trainer. In these situations, you are running your own business. This might be in a private studio of your own, in clients' homes, or in a fitness club that you pay rent to in order to use its facility. Some of the advantages of this approach include the following:

- You are self-employed.
- You can set your own hours.
- You don't have to share your revenue.
- You are in control and can decide how you want to run your business.

Some of the disadvantages include the following:

- You must pay startup and ongoing expenses.
- You need to find your own clients and do your own marketing.
- You have to assume some financial risk.

- You need to have some business skills or pay someone who has them.
- You need to purchase insurance.

As you can see, there are many options when it comes to working in the fitness industry as a personal trainer. You need to decide what is best for you and your particular situation. If you are unsure where to start, you can always ask people who are working in the field for their thoughts.

Marketing Your Services

When you get started in the fitness industry, clients will not be walking up to you offering to pay you for your services. In order to gain clients, you will need to market your services so that potential clients are aware of you and what you can offer them. The traditional way to look at marketing is to break the process into four areas—product, price, promotions, and place. Also known as the *4 Ps of marketing*, these areas will form the core of your marketing plan. The marketing plan is the comprehensive action plan that will generate clients for your business. In this chapter we will take a closer look at the 4 Ps of marketing and how you can apply them to your personal training business.

Product

For our purposes, the product is actually you and your services. Based on the work of Mullin, Hardy, and Sutton (1999), we will look at three factors to consider when looking at your product: differentiation, development, and positioning.

Differentiation refers to your ability to separate yourself from other personal trainers and make yourself unique. Examples of this would be a trainer who has some special educational experiences (e.g., university degree or specialized training), a unique workout, a focused client base (e.g., seniors, people looking to lose weight, people with no time), or special personal characteristics (e.g., being a great motivator). The more you can differentiate yourself, the more likely you are to be remembered. The concept of differentiation is a key starting point for all personal trainers as they consider what it will take for them to be successful.

In terms of **development,** it is critical that you are constantly looking for ways to offer new programming ideas or information that will keep clients motivated and working toward their goals. There

are lots of ways to come up with new ideas. Here are just a few:

- Attend conferences and workshops.
- Ask your clients what they are looking for.
- Join industry associations to keep up on trends and to network.
- Look at other industries to see what is working for them and then determine if you can use similar ideas in your business.

The fitness industry is constantly changing, and we are continually finding new and better ways for people to work out. Generating new ideas for you and your clients is critical to your long-term success in the industry. Most successful trainers would agree that the one of the keys to their success is their ability to continually reeducate themselves and then incorporate this new information into how they work with their clients.

Positioning is the perception that people have about you and your business. What image do you want to set and what message do you want to communicate? It is crucial to make sure that you are consistent in your approach to positioning. People need to know what to expect and are looking for consistency. If one day you are conducting an advanced sport conditioning program with an athlete and the next day you are working with seniors on a functional exercise program, you may be sending an inconsistent message to potential clients. This is not to say that personal trainers can't work with a wide variety of people; however, if your goal is to attract the average sedentary adult and your marketing pieces all include finely chiseled bodies, you may not be sending the right message.

The point is that you need to keep in mind how you want people to perceive you. Each of these factors will leave an image in a potential customer's mind. It is critical that you spend time thinking about the image you want people to have of you. Every aspect of marketing that follows is done with this image in mind.

Price

There are many ways to price your services. Pricing for personal training will vary based on many different factors, including geographic location, your experience and education, and the number of other personal trainers available. Generally speaking, you will be able to charge more for personal training in certain areas based on the cost of living and the economy in those areas. Trainers with more experience and education are also able to charge more for their services; the only stipulation is that you need to show people what they will get with this added experience and education. Don't expect to be able to charge a premium price without putting some thought into what your clients will be getting for the added education and experience.

The last factor to consider when setting a pricing structure for your services is the amount of competition you have, or the number of options potential clients have for personal training services. As with any other service or product, the fewer options customers have, the more they will have to pay. This is an example of demand outpacing supply. If there are more clients demanding personal training than there are personal trainers, the few trainers that are available will be able to charge a premium for their services. If you are competing against other trainers, you will need to take into consideration their rates and their services. As competition increases, clients will be able to consider all of the personal trainers available. A highly competitive market for personal training will normally force trainers to charge similar prices since clients often shop around for the best value. In these situations it is critical that you are able to sell yourself and differentiate yourself from other trainers.

Most personal trainers will sell their services as either individual sessions or in packages of 10 or 20 sessions or sometimes more. Most of the time clients receive a discount based on the number of sessions that they purchase. A potential pricing structure is listed next.

1 session	$50
10 sessions	$450 ($45 per session)
20 sessions	$800 ($40 per session)

Traditional sessions are 45 to 55 minutes in duration, but many trainers also offer 30-minute sessions that appeal to time-strapped clients. Since these sessions are less expensive, they may also help you address clients' concerns about the costs of higher priced sessions. If the previous pricing structure were used, a 30-minute session could be priced in the following way:

1 session	$35
10 sessions	$300 ($30 per session)
20 sessions	$500 ($25 per session)

In theory, trainers should be able to make more money if they have clients training in 30-minute intervals because they are able to train more people and generate more income per hour.

Although these have traditionally been the most common ways to price sessions, they are not the only pricing structures. Group training is another approach to personal training that has increased in popularity in recent years. These types of sessions are normally conducted in small groups (2-4) but can be organized however the trainer wants. In small-group sessions there is normally a lower price per person, but overall the trainer will be generating more money than in a single-person session. Group training works best when

- clients know each other,
- clients have come together or have organized themselves, and
- clients all have similar fitness goals.

One way to price group sessions would be the following:

| 2 people (20 sessions at 45-55 minutes per session) | Each person pays $300 ($30 per session) for a total of $600. |
| 4 people (20 sessions at 45-55 minutes per session) | Each person pays $250 ($50 per session) for a total of $1,000. |

Pricing by the session is the most common way to sell personal training, but again, it is not the only way. One challenge with this approach is that you constantly need to sell clients new packages as they use up their purchased number of sessions. Additionally, in these situations people are able to use the sessions as they see fit. If they want to take a couple of days off or a couple of months off in the summer, they can do so, leaving trainers with a gap in their schedule and in their expected income.

There are personal training studios that have had success pricing their sessions by the month. In these situations, clients agree to a set amount each month and also commit to a specific number of sessions in a week. If clients miss a session, they have no way to get their money back. On the positive side, clients may be more committed to their programs knowing that they can't use the sessions at a later date. Clubs may also offer a greater discount to clients who agree to longer contracts with monthly payments. There are many ways to set up monthly payment plans; the one described here is just an example.

As you can see, there are many ways to structure the price of your sessions. In the end it will come down to you and your club deciding what is best based on your situation and the marketplace you are in.

Promotions

You can promote your business in many ways. The most popular ways for personal trainers to promote themselves include the following:

- Direct mail
- Print or space ads
- Electronic media
- General networking
- Guerilla marketing
- Media outreach
- Referrals

When determining which methods are the most appropriate for you, always consider who your target market is. Potential target markets for personal trainers include seniors, athletes, people who have exercised in the past, current exercisers, businesspeople, people who belong to certain organizations, people who subscribe to certain publications, and any other group you can identify. Understanding how your target audience feels about exercise is important as you consider your marketing message. For example, if you work at a downtown fitness club with a large business crowd, your message to this audience will be very different compared with the message that would be targeted to a residential area with a higher proportion of seniors and families.

Regardless of the method you choose, keep in mind that people may need to see your message numerous times before they will actually remember it and take action. If you are not able to send out numerous messages to your market, then you will need to make sure you have a unique message that will get people to take action right away. For example, you might give a special offer to the first 20 people who call you or give a special discount to anyone who mentions they saw your ad.

Your potential clients are bombarded with marketing messages from thousands of companies each day. What is going to make you stand out? What is going to cause your audience to take action by calling you or coming in to see you? These are the questions you need to ask before deciding which type of marketing you will choose.

Direct Mail

Direct mail is a form of marketing that is sent directly to potential clients. In general, the more focused or specifically targeted the direct mail is, the better. In this text, we will consider direct mail to be anything sent via regular mail, and the actual flyer, letter, or document you design will be referred to as a *marketing piece*. This type of marketing is very effective because you are able to focus on specific characteristics. An example of a targeted piece of direct mail would be one that is sent to all the area codes within an 8- to 12-minute drive of your location. If you look at a map of your area and determine how far you can get in all directions in 8 to 12 minutes, you have just found what is referred to as your *isochrone*. Your isochrone is where you will get the majority of your clients. Experts agree that prospects will not normally drive more than 8 to 12 minutes to join a fitness club. Specifically, your primary market is normally within 8 minutes and your secondary market is within a 12-minute drive. Keep in mind that isochrones are based on travel time. If you are in a downtown area where people are going to walk, then it is an 8- to 12-minute walk.

The isochrone allows you to send marketing pieces to the clients who are most likely to join your club. Experienced personal trainers might argue that they have clients who travel much farther than this. The reality is that the relationship a trainer has with clients is a unique one. Once you are established, you might find that people do come from much farther, but the isochrone is still the best place to start your marketing efforts.

Other potential targets of direct mail include the following:

- People at a certain income level
- People who belong to a particular group (e.g., downtown business association or employees of a hospital)
- People who attended a particular event (health and wellness show at a local convention centre)
- Past members of a fitness club
- Teachers, lawyers, and so on

The key to direct mail is to get the right offer to the right person. You will need to carefully consider the characteristics of your potential clients as you decide on the most appropriate offer for them.

Advantages

- You can target your message as much or as little as you want.

- You decide how many people you want to send your marketing piece to.

- Marketing pieces can be sent in many different ways, from an insert with newspapers to a separate piece mailed through the postal service.

Disadvantages

- Postage and mailing costs can be high if you want to send mail to a large number of people. The more people you send mail to, the higher the cost.

- If you are not comfortable designing your marketing piece, you will need to get help from someone who is.

- If the piece is included as an insert with other material, it may not get enough attention because it is competing against other marketing pieces.

Print Ads

Print or space ads are a form of advertising normally found in newspapers, magazines, and newsletters. With this form of advertising, you have a dedicated space that is normally priced based on size. The bigger the ad, the more expensive it will be. In addition, colour ads are also more expensive than black-and-white ads. Discounts are normally given to those who commit to advertising over a period of time; that is, it's cheaper per ad if you commit to six ads as opposed to just one ad. When advertising in larger newspapers becomes cost prohibitive, you may want to consider smaller magazines and neighbourhood newspapers. These smaller publications might not get your message to as many people, but they might actually be more beneficial. Smaller publications are normally more focused in their content or geographic area, so depending on your goals, they might be more appropriate for you.

Advantages

- Space ads reach a larger number of people at a lower price than direct mail. The larger the audience, the more cost-effective space ads become.

- May establish a certain level of credibility for your business if you advertise in publications that are well respected.

- May be very targeted if you choose a subject-specific magazine (e.g., fitness and health).

Disadvantages

- Costs can be significant for larger publications.

- Marketing research tells us that people need to see an ad numerous times before they will actually respond to it.

- Ads may get lost when someone is looking at a page with many different things on it.

- You need to have a message that is going to attract people's attention right away; otherwise, they will simply turn the page.

Electronic Media

In this text, the term *electronic media* refers to anything that uses technology. We do not have enough space in this section to cover all of the potential ways to use technology to market your services, so we will focus on the most popular methods.

E-mail is a great way to market your services if you are able to obtain reliable e-mail lists of potential customers. In this way, e-mail is similar to direct mail since you are choosing who you want to send your message to and then catering that message specifically to them. The major difference between direct mail and e-mail is that e-mail is normally much quicker as well as much more cost effective since you are not paying for postage. On the other hand, e-mail has its limitations since potential prospects and customers likely have software programs known as *spam filters* that limit incoming e-mail from unknown sources. Some very good e-mail marketing companies and software programs are available that can be used at a reasonable price for those who are not technologically savvy. E-mail and traditional direct mail both have the same challenge of overcoming a barrage of competing messages in their given medium.

Developing your own Web site is also a great way to use technology in your business. Many great programs are available for those who are not comfortable designing their own Web pages. Web sites are a great way to provide an unlimited amount of information. Most of the formats we have talked about thus far have space limitations, but space is not an obstacle when it comes to the Internet. We are not saying that you should have so much information on your Web site that people feel overwhelmed, but you do have many more options with respect to the amount and type of information you can include.

Web sites are a great way to post updated information about your business. Many people use their Web sites as an educational tool to keep their clients motivated and informed. Your options are unlimited when it comes to developing your own site. In the beginning, it is best to keep the site relatively simple. This will allow you to see what your clients are interested in and how they will use the site. One challenge with Web sites is making sure the information is up to date and accurate. This is your responsibility. If you want people to use your site for specific reasons, then you will need to make sure those areas are constantly kept up to date. For example, if you are trying to educate people on good eating habits by posting articles every 2 weeks, then you will need to make sure you do this. You clients will quickly move away from your site if certain areas are not updated as you intended. As with e-mail, many companies and software programs are available that can help you with Web site design and ongoing maintenance.

Advantages

- Cost effective.
- Allows for quick delivery.
- Responses are easy to track.

Disadvantages

- Spam filters may prevent your message from ever being read.
- Approximately 20% of e-mail users change their address each year.
- Design elements are limited due to spam filters.

General Networking

Making yourself known within your community is another important element of promoting your business. Personal trainers should not feel nervous about letting friends and acquaintances know what they do for a living. This is a great (and free!) way to promote yourself. Close friends and acquaintances are a part of what is known as your *circle of influence,* the group of people that you have some sort of contact with or influence over. This influence may be very minor in most

situations, but these are still people that you know and will most likely want to help you if they can. In these situations it is critical that you have business cards. It is a good rule of thumb to always carry a supply of business cards because you never know when you might be able to get a new customer or simply get the word out about what you are doing.

A common technique to help identify everyone in your circle of influence is to list all friends, family, people you do business with, and so on. Figure 13.1 is a form you can use to help identify those people you are closest with.

This list is simply a starting point for you to think about all the people you come into contact with. The majority of these people will be more than happy to tell others about what you are doing. If you don't come into personal contact with all of these people regularly, it would be a good idea to send out a letter letting them know what you are now doing.

Although the focus of this section has been on people you come into contact with regularly, do not hesitate to mention your services to anyone you meet, if the time and place are appropriate. You are working in a field that everyone needs to be able to access. Many potential clients are nervous because they have no idea where to start and they have negative images of exercise and fitness clubs in their minds. If you can make them feel comfortable, you will both have the opportunity to be successful—you because you are getting a new client and them because of the results they will see.

Advantages

- Costs are minimal.
- People in your circle of influence will normally pass the word on to their own circle of influence.
- People are normally more comfortable purchasing from someone they trust, so this obstacle should already be taken care of if you are working within your own group of contacts.

Disadvantages

- Your circle of influence may not be receptive to your business.
- Some people may feel you are crossing the line in your relationship with them by trying to sell them something.

Your circle of influence

Fill in the names of each person listed below.

Mother: _____

Father: _____

Brothers: _____

Sisters: _____

Aunts: _____

Uncles: _____

Cousins: _____

Friends: _____

Friends of family members: _____

Neighbours: _____

Current and former coworkers: _____

Physician: _____

Chiropractor: _____

Massage therapist: _____

Dentist: _____

Real estate agent: _____

Lawyer: _____

Insurance agent: _____

Accountant or tax planner: _____

Financial adviser: _____

Bank manager or person you deal with: _____

Current and former coaches: _____

Current and former classmates: _____

Current and former teachers: _____

Postal carrier: _____

Dry cleaner: _____

Church members: _____

Personnel at restaurants: _____

Members of other groups you belong to: _____

Personnel in businesses you regularly patronize: _____

Other: _____

_____

Figure 13.1 This form will help you identify the people in your circle of influence.

Guerilla Marketing

Guerilla marketing is a type of nontraditional marketing that normally you do not have to pay for. The possibilities are only limited by your imagination and the message you want to send to prospective clients. Here are a few examples of what we are talking about.

Guest Passes

Guest passes are a great way to get people to come into your establishment for the first time. They are normally given free of charge and allow the person to work out with you for free. It is generally suggested that you include a reasonable expiration date on these passes to create a sense of urgency in the potential clients' mind; otherwise, the pass is likely to be put aside and forgotten. Take care in the types of guest passes you use for general marketing and the type of passes you give out to actual clients. If too many of the same guest passes are given out, they will eventually lose their value because people will feel they are getting something that anyone can get. One way to overcome this problem is to give one type of pass to prospects and save some special passes for friends of current clients. You should place a higher value on guest passes given to your current clients, partly as a thank-you to them but also because your clients will probably bring a potential client who is more likely to pay for your services after using the guest pass since your current client has most likely spoken highly of you.

Information Tear-Off Sheets

These are simple information sheets with phone numbers that can be torn off at the bottom. The sheets will promote your business in some way and encourage people to call you if they want more information. They can be posted in all kinds of locations, like grocery stores, schools, or any other place that has a community events board. Owners may have restrictions on what they want posted, so it is always a good idea to check with them before posting anything.

Joint Marketing

Finding other businesses that can help to promote your business is a great way to attract new clients. Some examples of complementary businesses might be nutrition stores, weight loss clinics, massage therapists, and chiropractors. Other businesses might include grocery stores or other retail outlets.

They promote your business (by giving out flyers, posting signage, giving out free passes, and so on), and you in turn promote their business to your clients in some way. In the beginning when you do not have any clients, you may choose to give people some free personal training sessions in exchange for helping you. It's a good idea to implement some type of reward system for the businesses you are working with. For example, whenever someone comes to you based on seeing your information in another business, you could give that business owner a free personal training session. What you give them is not really that important, and you may choose not to give them something every time. The idea is that you are thanking them for helping you so that they are encouraged to keep promoting your business.

These are just a few examples of what you can do outside traditional forms of marketing avenues. Some forms of guerilla marketing may leave potential customers with a negative image of you and your business, so you will need to carefully consider this possibility when deciding what approach to take. In addition, some forms of guerilla marketing may border on being ethically questionable. Do not be so focused on attracting new clients that you turn people off your business altogether because of your marketing approach.

Lead Boxes

Lead boxes are often used in joint marketing initiatives and are a great way to get a high volume of prospects. They are normally placed on countertops at other businesses. Prospects fill out a ballot for a chance to win something, such as 10 free training sessions. Everyone who fills out a ballot is offered something, such as 10% off or one free training session. The more closely the business is aligned with yours, the better. For example, a weight loss clinic might give you better prospects than a dry cleaner. Either way, you will get a lot of ballots that are difficult to read or that have been filled out by people who are not interested in your service. Be prepared to make lots of phone calls and know that you will need to make many calls to get a few people who are interested in your services.

Advantages

- Low cost.
- Large number of potential clients available.
- Unlimited number of potential marketing ideas available.

Disadvantages

- Potential clients may perceive some approaches negatively (for example, leaving guest passes in phone booths or on windshields).
- Most options will require constant follow-up to ensure your partner business is keeping up with their end of the agreement.

Media Outreach

Similar to guerilla marketing, media outreach is normally done for free or at a low cost. The key to successful media outreach is getting your name in the media or in front of a large audience. This can be done in many ways, but here are a few:

- Send out a press release to all media in the area about a particular event.
- Establish yourself as an expert by writing in local publications, speaking on the radio, or getting interviewed on TV.
- Hold open houses and invite the media and influential people from the area.
- Work with well-known people who are in the local news regularly. You might consider giving some of these people free sessions and promoting your program to the media.
- Testimonials from clients are a great way to generate publicity when done correctly.

Advantages

- Should normally come with little cost.
- Potential to reach a large audience.
- Information about your business may be presented by a respected person in the media.

Disadvantages

- May be difficult to establish yourself with local media.
- If events are not planned properly, negative publicity may result.
- May not see immediate results if publicity is not on a large scale.

Referrals

The key to long-term success in the fitness industry is the ability to generate referrals from your clients. If you are able to take care of your clients and help them reach their goals, they will help you build your business. The most successful trainers do not actively seek new clients; instead, they have a waiting list of clients who are interested in being trained by them. This waiting list was not created by some great marketing piece that was sent out or that someone saw in a newspaper. It occurred because the trainer's clients were happy with the service. In general, referral sources can be organized into internal (current clients, past clients, other members) and external (friends, family, other health professionals, coaches) sources.

It is true that clients often will send you referrals without you even asking for their assistance, but more times than not you will need to ask your clients for some help in this area. The easiest way to do this is through guest passes (see page 185). Anytime is a great time to ask a client for a referral, but the best times are when clients first start and when they are happy with the results they have been getting, normally after 6 to 8 weeks. If you want to be proactive, you can even ask people to leave the names and phone numbers of their friends so you can call them to personally invite them. You may not be comfortable with this at first, but when presented properly it can be very effective. The purpose of asking for this information is that it allows you to follow up with people. When you simply give guest passes to clients, they may get forgotten or lost.

Here are some things to keep in mind when asking for referrals outside your fitness centre or client base.

- Think of everyone as a potential client, but respect people's time and space.
- Build partnerships whenever you can. People will be more likely to refer others to you if they are getting something in return, such as a free session or a program designed for them.
- Use the marketing techniques mentioned previously in this chapter to come up with creative ways to work with people.

Whenever you are asking for referrals, keep the following in mind:

- No one wants to be sold, so look at this as an opportunity to share some information or educate the person on what you are doing.

- Focus on the person's goals and then tailor your conversation around them.
- Let the person know that it would be helping you.

There are lots of creative ways to get referrals from your clients. As long as you ask in a professional manner and in a way that respects your clients, you are going to be successful.

Advantages

- Low cost.
- Buying decision is made easier for potential clients because of the referral.

Disadvantages

- You may need to get out of your comfort zone if this is not something you are comfortable doing.

Tracking Your Promotional Efforts

All good marketers track the results of their promotional efforts. How else will you know if the time and money you have invested have been well spent? When people call you or come in to see you, you should always ask how they heard about your business.

Each month you should have a running total of where your new clients are coming from. If all of your clients are coming from referrals and the yellow pages, is it really necessary to spend a lot of money on direct mail or newspaper ads? If you have been working as a trainer for more than a year and you are not getting at least 75% of your new clients from referrals, you are not doing what you should be in this area of marketing.

Place

The fitness industry is not unlike many other retail industries in that the location of your business will play a major role in your initial success or failure. You already know that people will not normally drive more than 10 to 15 minutes to join a fitness club. Other factors to keep in mind when choosing a location include traffic flow, parking, signage, perception of the neighbourhood, and future potential for expansion. Whether you are looking at opening your own personal training studio or working within a fitness club, your choice of location is an important one.

Successful trainers would agree that once you have a dedicated client base, your location is not as important. If your clients have been with you for a long time, they are going to be willing to drive a little farther to stay with you. This might sound contradictory to the earlier statement about people not being willing to drive more than 10 to 15 minutes. This is true of new clients, but if you have a loyal group of clients, the regular rules do not always apply when it comes to location. However, this is not to say that people will be willing to drive an extra hour to an area of the city with no parking and a high crime rate.

Selling Your Services

When most new personal trainers hear that they have to sell their services, the initial reaction is normally a negative one, and images of pushy, insincere salespeople come to mind. The good news is that if you are going to be successful as a personal trainer, the high-pressure sales approach is not something you need to worry about. This approach might work in the short term, but it will eventually turn people off and hurt your business.

Marketing will bring people to you, but you need to be comfortable selling your services if you want to make a living in this industry. The key to being comfortable with sales is getting people to trust you. If you know and believe in your product and can show prospective clients how it will benefit them, then you have the potential to be good at sales. Luckily, exercise is something that everyone needs, so you do not have to worry about trying to sell people something that they will not benefit from.

The following are some great ways to approach people about personal training:

- If you are approaching someone you do not know, it is always a good idea to introduce yourself and tell the person that you are a personal trainer.
- Next, ask about the person's reasons and goals for working out.
- With this information, you should then be able to determine whether this is someone who might be interested in personal training.
- Once you have a sense of whether the person might be interested, ask if you can

tell the person about what you do and how you might be able to help out. Be careful not to assume that people are not interested in your services. We are not suggesting that you be pushy, but you should be optimistic about the prospects of this person becoming a potential client.

- Once you have opened the discussion and you are confident that the person is interested in what you have to say, you can move to the next step, selling your personal training services.

Here is an example of the steps you can follow when selling your services:

1. Focus on the prospective clients and what they want.
2. Show them how you can help them achieve their goals.
3. Develop an action plan that outlines what you will do and the results they will see.
4. Ask for feedback on the plan.
5. Present your prices.
6. Overcome any objections.
7. Follow up.

Focus on Potential Clients and What They Want

Your first priority should be the prospective clients and what they want to achieve. You need to find out as much as you can about them before trying to sell them anything. This not only includes their specific fitness goals but also their perceptions, fears, and expectations. Throughout this information-gathering stage, you should focus on building trust and getting the client to feel comfortable with you and the surroundings. Remember, people are much more likely to buy from someone they like or trust. Once you have collected all of this information and gotten to know the person, you are ready to talk about your services.

Show How You Can Help Them Achieve Goals

The key to this step is differentiating between features and benefits. Features are characteristics that are specific to you, your services, or your facility, such as a 20-minute workout, five treadmills, quali-

fied staff, and so on. These characteristics are the same regardless of the potential client. Benefits are those characteristics that are specific to the person. A benefit of a 20-minute workout for busy people is that they will be able to fit in their workout. A benefit of qualified staff is that clients do not have to worry about starting a program that will hurt them or that will not work. Benefits should be specific to the information you gathered in step 1. People will buy from you because of the benefits they perceive they will get. If you build trust with people and show them how they will benefit by working with you, you are well on your way to gaining new clients.

Develop an Action Plan

Once you have communicated the benefits of your program to prospective clients, you will need to tell them exactly what you will do and the results they can expect. When developing this action plan, it is best to use SMART goals. Remember from chapter 12 that SMART stands for the following:

S—specific

M—measurable

A—action oriented

R—realistic

T—timed

Use this acronym when setting goals for prospective clients. It is always best to break long-term goals into smaller short-term goals. For example, if your client wants to lose weight, you could set the following goal: Lose 3 to 4 kilograms of body fat in 6 weeks by exercising 4 times a week with a personal trainer. For someone who wants to lose 10 kilograms, this would be a realistic and attainable short-term goal. As another example, here's a goal for a person whose energy level is presently at a 5 on a scale of 1 to 10 and who wants to have more energy: Get to an energy level of 8 in 6 weeks by exercising for at least 30 minutes 4 times a week.

Ask for Feedback

Once you have described the action plan, ask if the client has any questions about it. Several techniques can be used at this point. Many experts will tell you that you should never ask a question that you don't know how the client will answer. Some experts suggest only asking questions where "yes" is the answer, such as "Wouldn't you feel great if you lost those 4 kilograms in 6 weeks?" It is up to you to use whatever techniques you are comfortable with. You want to make sure you have answered any major concerns or questions before moving on to the next step.

Present Your Prices

Once you have answered all of the questions related to the action plan and your program, it is time to present your prices. It is important that you do not review your prices before this step because people will not have any idea what they are getting for the price. People are much more likely to buy from you if they trust you and understand the benefits of what you can offer them. If you give your prices right away, you have not addressed the most important parts of the sale process. When presenting your prices, many techniques are available. Following are just a few.

Alternate Close Method

In this situation, you present two options and then ask which is best for the person. The idea is that you are letting potential clients choose the package, but you are also not allowing them to easily say no. By asking which is best for the client, you are taking "no" out of the possible answers.

Assumptive Close Method

In this technique, you are assuming the person will purchase from you. Examples of questions you could ask after presenting your prices would be, "When can we get you started?", or, "How would you like to pay?" Both of these questions assume the person is going to buy from you.

Suggestive Close Method

In this method, you are suggesting what the person should purchase. The logic is that you are the expert and you should know what is best for the client since you are the one with the knowledge and experience.

Trial Close Method

This method is normally used before the actual sales presentation and before asking for the sale. The idea behind this method is that you are asking people what they think of things throughout the process. This allows you to gauge whether or not the person is likely to purchase from you. Following are some examples of trial closes:

- Could you see yourself working out in this fitness club?
- Could you fit in a 30-minute workout three times a week?
- Is your wife (or husband) in favour of you purchasing personal training sessions?

If the person answers "no" to any of these questions, you want to be able to address these obstacles before the presenting the prices.

Asking for the sale is difficult for many people. These are popular techniques that can make the process a little smoother for many new personal trainers; however, there are many other methods that can work for you. As long as you are giving your prices in a confident but sincere manner that is consistent with how you have been communicating with the person, the prospective client is going to be receptive.

Overcome Objections

Once you have presented your prices, many people will not respond favourably at first. Some of the most common objections are as follows:

- I want to think about.
- It's too much money.
- I need to talk it over with someone.

As a personal trainer getting started in the business, you need to accept that objections are going to happen. If you view objections as someone simply needing more information, then you will be comfortable dealing with them. Some experts suggest that potential clients may give up to five objections before they make a purchase from you. If you are not comfortable dealing with objections, you will be missing out on potential clients. There are many ways to deal with objections, but we will consider a very simple method to start with.

The majority of objections can be dealt with ahead of time through the use of proper trial closes. Asking people how long they have been thinking about working out and whether or not they are ready to get started is a great way to deal with the "I want to think about it" objection. Asking people if their spouse or significant other is in favour of them doing this is another good way to address a potential objection ahead of time.

Assuming you have covered these questions before giving prices, the first thing to do when you hear an objection is clarify it. You can do this by asking *why* or *what* types of questions. An objection normally comes from people who aren't ready to buy because they do not have all the information they need to be confident in their decision. If someone says, "I want to think about it," one potential response is, "What is it you want to think about?" This clarification will normally get the person to tell you something else, such as "I'm not sure I can afford it" or "I'm not sure I can make the time." The idea is not to be pushy but to find out exactly what it is you have not answered or what you need to focus on. Whether or not the person buys from you is not the major concern. The point is that you want to make sure you have answered all of the person's questions and concerns and discussed all of the possibilities you have to offer. For example, if potential clients say that they can't afford your services and you don't tell them about a payment plan you offer that allows them to pay over the next 3 months, you may have lost clients simply because you didn't understand what their objection really was. It wasn't that they couldn't afford your training, it was that they couldn't afford to pay for it all at once.

How you deal with objections is up to you. The approaches you use need to be ones that you are comfortable with. The techniques given previously are just a few examples of how you can close the sale.

Follow Up

Whether someone purchases from you or not, it is important to follow up with that person. There are many different ways this can be done, such as the following:

- Call to thank new clients for trusting you with their business.
- Call them to see if they have any questions and to find out what needs to happen to get them back in.
- Call them to see how they are feeling after their first workout.

Your Professional Image

One sure way to fail in the industry is to look and act the way many people perceive personal trainers—that is, muscle bound, unprofessional, not normal, intimidating, and unrelatable to the average person. This is still the perception that many potential clients have of the industry. It is your job to change this perception, which you can do by following these guidelines:

- Dress appropriately—This means tuck your shirt in, wear shirts with collars and sleeves (short or long), iron your clothes, don't wear a hat, limit the amount of jewelry you wear, don't wear your regular workout clothes, and don't wear clothes that are too big or small. In general, look professional, not like someone who works out in a gym.
- Establish proper grooming—This means shave, have well-kept hair, and avoid body odour.

When you are training a client, that person should be your entire focus. You should not be having conversations with other people around you, and you should not answer phone calls. All of your energy should be focused on your client. This means giving feedback and encouragement on how the person is doing and physically getting close to help with certain exercises.

Client–Trainer Relationship

Your relationship with your clients is another key to long-term success in the personal training field. As discussed, referrals can have a major impact on your business.

One of the keys to a good client–trainer relationship is that both parties know what to expect from each other. A great way to formalize these expectations is in an agreement. This document outlines the important business components of the trainer–client relationship. Common topics in this agreement include the following:

- **Term of the agreement**—Establishes how long the agreement is for or what is included.
- **Fees and payment structure**—What methods of payment will you accept and over what amount of time will clients be able to pay you? It is up to you whether you want people to pay in full or in installments.
- **Cancellation policy**—It is strongly recommended that you include and enforce this policy. If you do not follow through on it, your clients will assume it is acceptable to cancel appointments without appropriate notice.

- **Late policy**—Similar to the cancellation policy, this is an area that needs to be enforced before it becomes a common occurrence.
- **Refund policy**—Many trainers will provide a money-back guarantee for the unused portion of their sessions.
- **Informed consent**—This common stipulation ensures the client understands the risk of exercising.

Figure 13.2 is a sample personal training agreement.

Client–trainer agreements can be formatted in many different ways. The example in figure 13.2 covers the key elements, but you may need to modify it to suit your needs. The formal part of the client–trainer relationship is only one of the many areas that need to be considered. Some other areas that you need to pay attention to are as follows:

- **Professional image**—If you want to be treated and paid like a professional, you need to look and talk like a professional. Many people who purchase personal training sessions are professionals who are accustomed to being around certain types of people. If you want to attract this crowd, you need to keep these expectations in mind. Your professional image does not only apply to professional clientele. Anyone who is paying you for your services deserves the same level of service and attention to detail.
- **Integrity**—Do what you say you are going to do and keep your promises. The formal agreement will spell out many areas, but there are still many things not mentioned in it. For example, if you tell clients you are going to bring in an article on cutting calories, do it. If you tell clients you are going to follow up with them if they miss a session, do it. And, if you tell clients you are going to help them get healthier in all aspects of their life, do it! At the time it may seem like a minor event if you forget to do something, but the reality is that your clients will notice and will eventually lose faith in your ability to do the things you have promised.
- **Motivation and attitude**—Your clients are paying for you. They can most likely go anywhere to get a program. If you are not in a peak state each time you are with clients, then they are not getting what they paid for. If you are easily put off by people or certain types of situations and you can't overcome this when you are with clients, then

personal training is not for you. When you are with your clients, you need to be 100% present. This means all of your energy needs to be focused on them. Anything else that is going on in your life or at work needs to be put on hold.

- **Personality types**—Most of us are comfortable around people who are like us. In our personal lives, we will normally choose our friends this way. Unfortunately, you will not always be able to choose your clients as a personal trainer, so you must be able to adjust your personality style to that of your clients. The same approach will not work for every client. You will need to be flexible in your approach, but there may also be times when you choose not to take on new clients based on their personality because you will have to act in a way that you are not comfortable with. Regardless of the situation, it will normally be up to you to decide whether the client is compatible with your style.
- **General communication**—Clients need to feel comfortable with you so that they are willing to share any thoughts or concerns that are going to affect their session and their overall results. Listening is a key skill that all personal trainers need to master. This means listening without the intent of responding, trying to understand what people are saying and why they feel a certain way. When you do this, you not only listen to what they are saying, you also watch body language and potentially find out even more information. There are times when clients simply need someone to talk to. They may not need or want you to give them a solution. With experience you will become a good judge as to when you should respond and when you should simply be a sounding board.

The bottom line is that it is always less expensive to keep an existing client than it is to find a new one. You do not need to spend any money or time marketing to current clients and you don't need to spend a lot of time trying to convince them that you are the right trainer for them. They are already your clients; you simply have to take care of them and give them what they want.

If you place as much focus on the relationship as you do on the actual program, you will develop loyal clients who will bring all of the future clientele you will ever need. This will not happen immediately since building any relationship takes time, but if you take the time to focus on all of the people you are training and taking care of them and their needs, you will reap the benefits.

Personal Training Agreement

This agreement is made this date _____, by and between _____
_____ (hereinafter "the Trainer") and _____ (hereinafter "the Client"), an individual residing at _____.

Whereas _____ has a great deal of knowledge and expertise in the area of physical fitness and personal training, and whereas the Client wishes to benefit from _____
_____ services, advice, and programs during the term of this agreement. _____ is willing to offer such services upon the terms and conditions set forth in this agreement. The parties listed hereto agree to the following.

Term

The Client hereby hires and retains the Trainer for a period of _____ beginning _____
and ending_____. The Client shall be entitled to _____ sessions with the Trainer to be attended within such time period. (_____Initials)

Fees

For all services to be rendered by the Trainer under this agreement, the Trainer shall be paid at a rate of $_____
____ per session. The fees for all above sessions shall be paid in full upon execution of this agreement. The Client may elect to pay such fees on a monthly basis where all payments will be made by the _____ of each month with the charge for late payments being $_____. (_____Initials)

Cancellations

Cancellations must be made at least 24 hours in advance of scheduled sessions. Sessions cancelled less than 24 hours in advance will be charged in full to the Client. (_____Initials)

Late Arrivals

Sessions shall be _____ minutes in length and shall start at the scheduled time. Sessions will not be extended due to the tardiness of the Client or due to interruptions made by the Client. Any Client who has not arrived within 15 minutes after the scheduled time shall be deemed cancelled and will be charged for that session. (_____Initials)

Refunds

In the event that a medical problem or prolonged circumstances prevent completion of the contracted sessions within the time period set forth in this agreement, the Client may take an extended period of time, not to exceed 1 year, to complete said sessions. There shall be no cash refunds. (_____Initials)

Consent

I, the Client, have been informed, understand, and am aware that strength, flexibility, and aerobic exercise, including the use of equipment, are potentially hazardous activities. I also have been informed, understand, and am aware that fitness activities involve a risk of injury and that I am voluntarily participating in these activities and using equipment with full knowledge, understanding, and appreciations of the dangers involved. (_____Initials)

This agreement may not be changed except by written amendment duly executed by all parties.

Executed this _____ day of _____, 20____.

Signed,

Trainer: _____   _____   _____
                  Print name   Signature   Date

Client: _____   _____   _____
                  Print name   Signature   Date

Figure 13.2 Using a personal training agreement will keep your clients informed of their responsibilities.

Terminating the Relationship

Unfortunately, some client–trainer relationships need to come to an end before reaching all of the client's goals. There are many reasons for this, but a major one is some sort of incompatibility between the two people. As we stated earlier, it is critical that the trainer seriously assess potential clients' personality and whether they are the right fit for one another. Even when this is done, however, things can still go wrong.

When it comes time to end the relationship, great care should be taken in ensuring that the client is treated with respect and with a genuine interest in what is best for both of you. It might be a good idea to suggest another trainer, assuming you know of another trainer who would be suited for the client. It is also important to explain the reasons for the termination. If the person wants to see results and you are not the best trainer to help with this, then it is in both of your best interests to get this out in the open. If the client is the one terminating the relationship, then it is important for you to find out exactly why so that you can incorporate this feedback with future clients. Whether you agree with the reasons or not, you should act professionally and thank the person for working with you. In either of these scenarios, the personal trainer and client must reach a mutual agreement on a refund for any prepaid sessions that have not been delivered.

Risk Management

As a personal trainer, your clients place a great deal of trust in you. It is your professional responsibility to be aware of the risks your client and yourself are exposed to. In order to protect your clients and yourself, adhere to the following guidelines:

• Always act within the Can-Fit-Pro scope of practice for personal trainers, which is found on page 86 in this book. The Can-Fit-Pro PTS certification has given you the ability to work with your client in certain ways, as outlined in this manual. Anytime you start to move outside of these abilities, you are getting outside of your scope of practice as a Can-Fit-Pro PTS, and you could be held liable if a problem occurs unless you have received further education or certifications.

• *Negligence* is the failure to act as another reasonable, prudent professional would have acted in a similar situation. As a PTS, it is your responsibility to act in a reasonable and prudent manner.

• Ensure that all of your clients have filled out a comprehensive health history (PAR-Q) questionnaire (see chapter 8).

• Ensure that all clients have signed a waiver. This waiver is very limited in terms of its actual protection of the personal trainer, but it is still a good idea to use it.

• Ensure that you have followed up with your clients on any areas within the health history that are of concern and make sure that clients get written authorization from a physician when you are not able to assess the severity of an injury or condition.

• Ensure that your clients are always safe and working within their own capabilities and that you are prescribing an exercise program that is specific to their unique background and goals.

• After the initial assessment and program design, it is your responsibility to continually reassess your clients to make sure that they are able to make changes to their program and to ensure that they can handle increased intensities or new exercises.

• Ensure that your cardiopulmonary resuscitation (CPR) certification is always up to date.

• If you are not an employee of a company, you are required to have your own liability insurance. Please read the following section to get further information on insurance needs.

Insurance

Personal trainers often work as employees within the confines of a health club where coverage should already be provided by the insurance policy of the club. If trainers are doing any training outside the club or on their own time, they are not covered by the club, so they will need to purchase their own insurance. What determines whether personal trainers are employees of a club or are working on their own is who collects the money. Normally, if a personal trainer is being paid directly by the club for providing services, they are covered under the policy of the club as an employee or subcontractor. If this is your situation, check with the club owner to make sure that you are covered. If, on the other hand, you are being paid directly by the client, you are working as an independent contractor and the club insurance does not cover your personal training, even if you use the club facilities to do the workouts.

Litigious Situations

Following are some situations that could lead to litigation:

- Working outside of your scope of practice
- Prescribing exercise for clients who have an injury or a condition that you are not trained to work with
- Designing meal plans, analyzing nutritional plans, or giving specific nutritional counseling
- Exposing clients to unsafe or overly risky exercises based on their level of experience and capabilities
- Making false claims that cannot be supported by research

Policies and Procedures

The purpose of developing policies and procedures for your business is to identify potential problem areas ahead of time so that everyone is aware of what will be done in specific situations. The following is a list of policies that Can-Fit-Pro recommends all trainers follow:

- Establish a fixed pricing policy and don't sway from this unless it is absolutely critical.
- If clients cancel their appointment with you with less than 24 hours notice, they should be charged for that session.
- All clients should be offered a money-back guarantee if they are not happy with the results or level of service they are getting. This guarantee would only apply to the unused remaining sessions.

Case Studies

Roger

If you would like to increase your client base with people who are similar to Roger, here are some things to keep in mind:

- You will need to take a professional approach to these clients since they are most likely

accustomed to this kind of approach in their everyday business activities.

- Ensure that you have your personal trainer's agreement in good order and that you are well organized.
- Let potential clients know about your credentials and what makes you different from other trainers.
- You will need to make yourself available before or after work or potentially at lunch. These clients will not likely want to come back later at night once they have gone home.
- Since time is a major concern, you will need to be efficient with your time and consider offering 30-minute workouts.
- When selling your services, make sure you are confident in what you will be presenting and have lots of information ready if they ask for it.

Molly

If you would like to attract more clients like Molly, here are some strategies:

- These clients most likely want to see lots of variety in their programs and are not afraid of challenges.
- Make sure you set realistic goals and action plans. This is important for everyone, but Molly came to you with some especially aggressive goals.
- Consider adding sport conditioning drills to your routines, which may be exciting to this younger audience.
- Keep these clients focused on their goals and why they are coming to you, especially when you know they are struggling with the program outside of the gym.

Jennifer

If you would like to attract more career-oriented women who juggle a busy family life, here is what you are going to need to do:

- Recognize that they have a busy schedule and congratulate them on their commitment to exercise.
- Market a working mom's program that might get together a group of people with similar interests.

- Consider small group training so that Jennifer can benefit from the social support of others.

- Many of the same approaches that were used with Roger could also work with Jennifer since they are both working professionals.

Exercises

Mike Bates, MBA

UPPER BODY

CHEST

BARBELL CHEST PRESS

Movement—Horizontal adduction and elbow extension
Primary muscles worked—Pectoralis major, anterior deltoid, triceps group

How to perform

Starting position

- Hold the bar with a common grip, so that elbow is at approximately 90 degrees and upper arm is parallel to the ground
- While lying supine eyes should be roughly in line with barbell
- Ensure 5 points of contact (left and right foot, lower back, upper back and back of head) while keeping natural arch in back
- Retract the scapulae and hold throughout movement

Concentric phase

- Lift bar straight up
- Bend elbows and lower bar so that upper arm is approximately parallel to the ground

Eccentric phase

- Push the arms back to start position, straightening arms but not locking them out and without rotating the shoulders

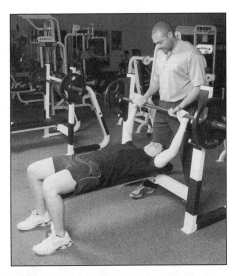

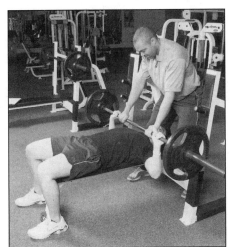

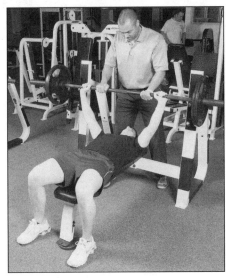

How to spot

- Trainer should be positioned at the head of the lifter so that they can assist with the lift off and monitor movement throughout the lift. Spotter should have hands close to bar at all times
- Ensure 5 points of contact at all times and look for changes in alignment of spine, arms and head

Variations

- Machine chest press (seated)

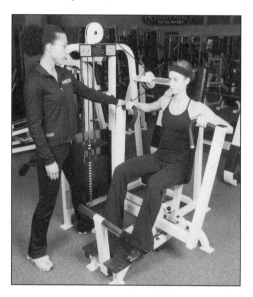 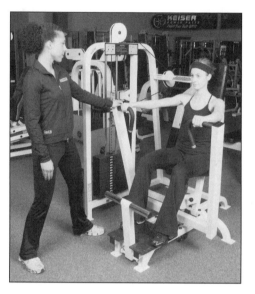

- Incline barbell chest press (wide grip)
- Decline dumbbell chest press

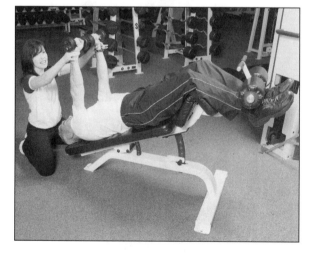 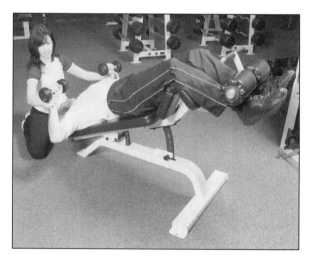

DUMBBELL CHEST FLY

Movement—Horizontal adduction
Primary muscles worked—Pectoralis major and anterior deltoid

How to perform

Starting position

- Retract the scapulae
- Hold dumbbells with a pronated grip
- Align the arms straight up from the shoulders
- Arms should be slightly bent at the elbows, with wrists in a stable position

Concentric phase

- Lower the arms down to about parallel to the floor, keeping them slightly bent throughout the entire movement
- Pull the arms up and together while contracting the chest

Eccentric phase

- Bring the arms back to the original starting position without extending the arms or rotating the shoulders

How to spot

- At head of bench in a kneeling lunge position. Spotting should be at the elbows. If the lifter becomes unstable the spotter may need to move the hands up to the wrist or as close to the weight as possible without obstructing the movement
- Monitor 5 points of contact and proper alignment

Variations

- Machine chest fly

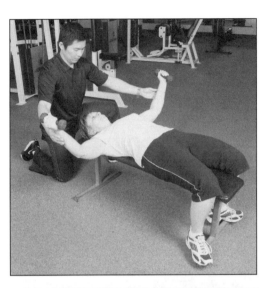

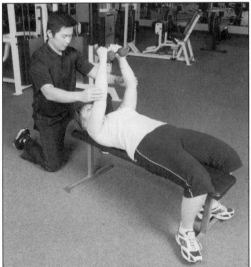

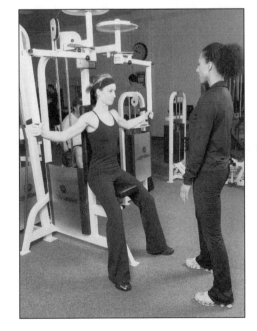

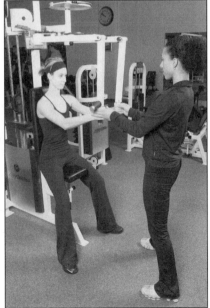

- Decline dumbbell chest fly

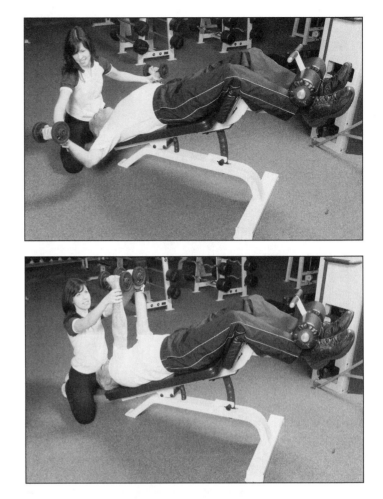

- Incline cable crossover

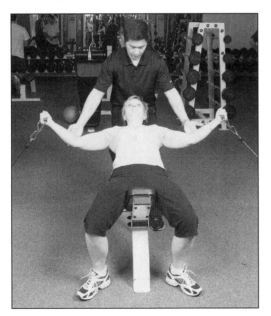
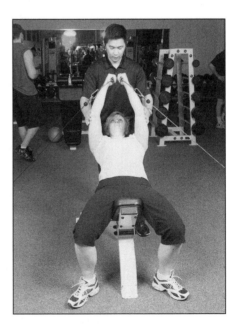

PUSH-UP (HANDS AND TOES)

Movement—Horizontal adduction, elbow extension, spine extension
Primary muscles worked—Pectoralis major, anterior deltoid, latissimus dorsi, triceps group, hip flexors, and core/trunk stabilizers

How to perform

Starting position

- In a supine position, with torso and legs off the floor, the exercisers hands should be wider than shoulder width and feet should be about hip width

Concentric phase

- Push up with your hands while maintaining good posture throughout.
- Push up until elbows are fully extended

Eccentric phase

- Lower back to original position, nose should be slightly above the floor while maintaining proper alignment

How to spot

- Trainer is in a kneeling lunge position next to the exerciser watching for proper alignment

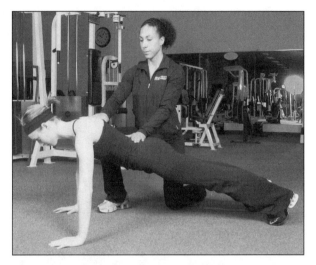

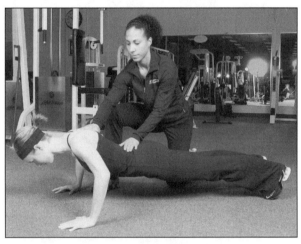

Variations

- Push-up (narrow hands, on knees)

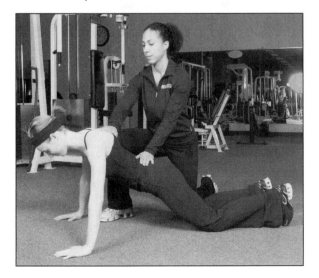

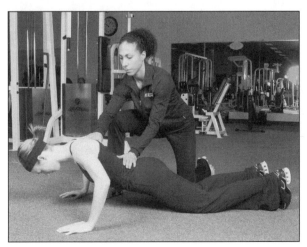

- Push-up (wide hands, feet elevated)

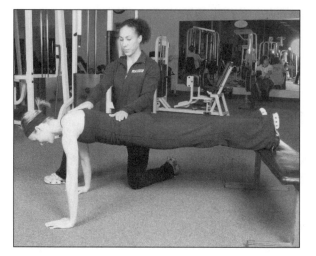
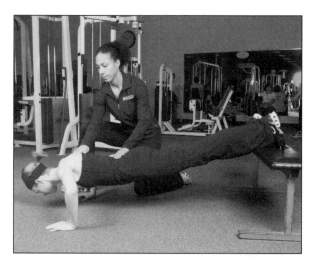

- Push-up (standing, against wall)

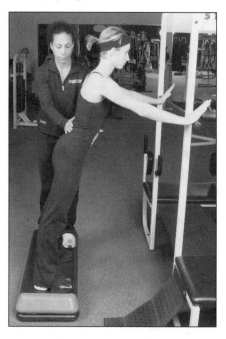
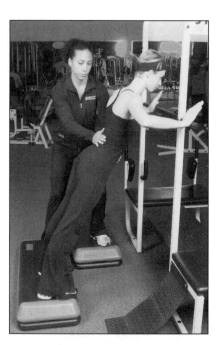

BACK

CABLE LAT PULLDOWN (WIDE GRIP)

Movement—Combination of shoulder adduction and horizontal shoulder abduction, scapular retraction and downward rotation, elbow flexion

Primary muscles worked—Latissimus dorsi, teres major, posterior deltoid, rhomboids, mid- and lower trapezius, levator scapulae, biceps group

How to perform

Starting position

- Wide, pronated grip, so that when the upper arms are parallel to the ground they form an approximately 90 degree angle
- Knees should be secure under pad and there should be a slight lean back (15-45 degrees)

Concentric phase

- Pull the bar toward chest until arms are about parallel to the ground
- Pull the scapulae down and together, creating a natural arch in the lower back
- Keep the scapulae depressed and retracted

Eccentric phase

- Let the arms back up slowly to the original starting position while keeping tension on the lats
- There should be no change in the angle at the hips once original degree of lean is established

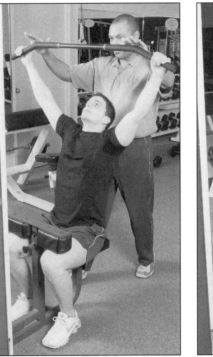
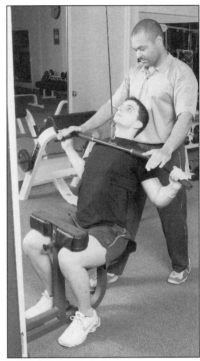

How to spot

- Spotter should be behind lifter with both hands on the bar
- Pulling the bar behind the head can be stressful on the shoulder joint and is not advised

Variations

- Cable lat pulldown (narrow supinated grip)

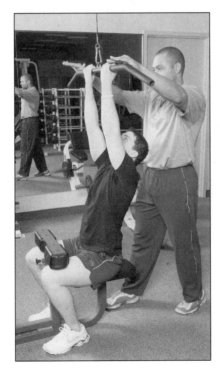
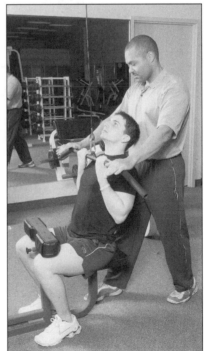

- Cable lat pulldown (medium grip)

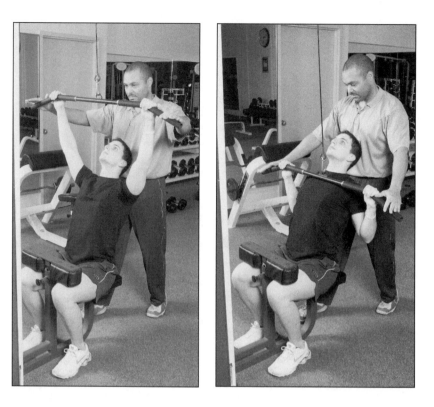

- Double cable lat pulldown

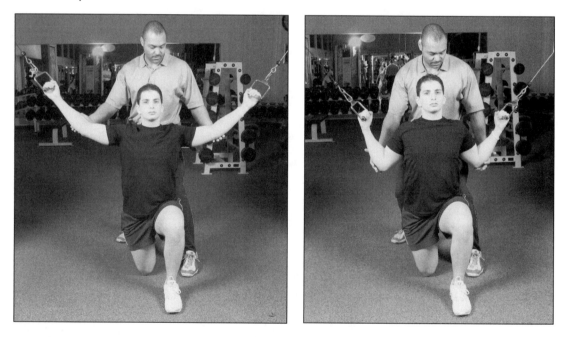

CABLE LAT ROW (SEATED WITH V-BAR)

Movement—Scapular retraction, shoulder extension, elbow flexion
Primary muscles worked—Rhomboids, mid-trapezius, latissimus dorsi, teres major, posterior deltoid, biceps group

How to perform

Starting position

- Plant feet firmly against machine with knees slightly bent
- Lean back slightly and keep natural arch in lower back
- While holding handles, keep wrists in a neutral position and elbows slightly bent

Concentric phase

- Keeping the arms slightly bent, contract the rhomboids and pull the shoulder blades together and down (scapular retraction)
- Pull the arms back, keeping them close to the side of the body until the elbows are about straight down from the shoulders

Eccentric phase

- Slowly return the arms and lats back to the original position, keeping the scapulae retracted

How to spot

- Spotter should be beside lifter in a kneeling lunge position
- Monitor spinal, scapular and arm positioning. Ensure that natural arch in lower back is not compromised

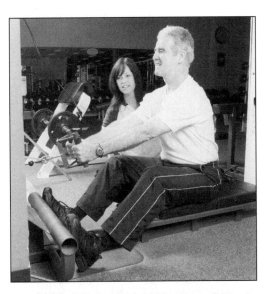

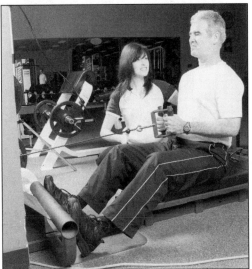

Variations

- Cable lat row (wide pronated grip)

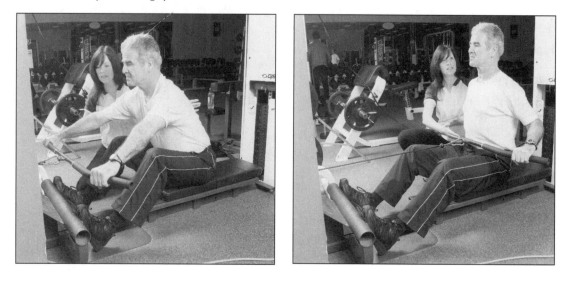

- Cable lat row (single arm)
- Tubing lat row (standing)

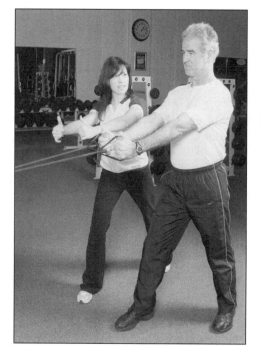
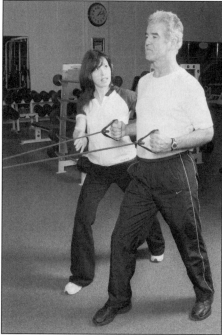

BARBELL LAT ROW (BENT OVER)

Movement—Scapular retraction, shoulder extension, elbow flexion
Primary muscles worked—Latissimus dorsi, teres major, rhomboids, mid-trapezius, posterior deltoid, biceps group

How to perform

Starting position

- Hold barbell with a pronated grip, hands wider than shoulder width
- Lean forward about 45 degrees, keeping the back and neck in a neutral position at all times
- Knees should be slightly bent and feet shoulder-width apart

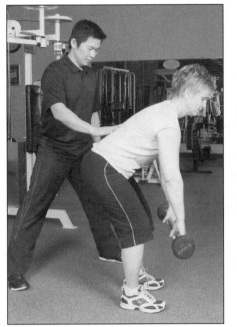
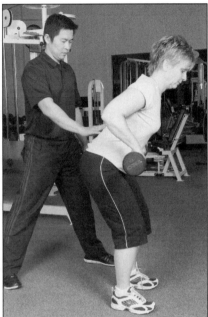

Concentric phase

- Pull the bar into lower sternum until elbows make a 90 degree angle
- Scapulae should be in a retracted position

Eccentric phase

- Lower the weight back to the starting position

How to spot

- Spotter should be monitoring body alignment from all angles while also being prepared to assist with the barbell if needed

Variations

- T-bar lat row (standing)

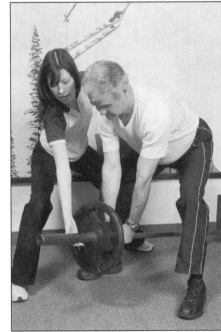
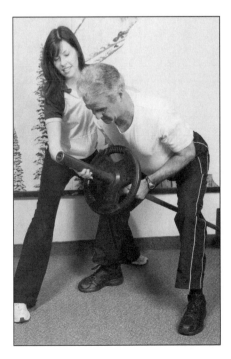

- Dumbbell lat row (one arm on bench)

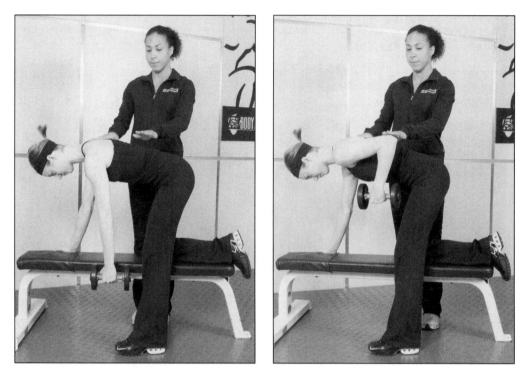

- Tubing lat row (standing)

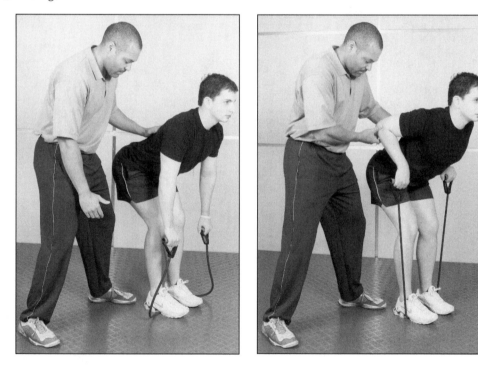

DUMBBELL TRAP SHRUG (SEATED)

Movement—Scapular elevation
Primary muscles worked—Levator scapulae, upper trapezius, mid-trapezius, rhomboids

How to perform

Starting position

- Sit with feet firmly on the ground
- Scapulae should be retracted
- Dumbbells will be at the lifter's side, palms facing inward
- Elbows should be extended but not locked

Concentric phase

- Pull the arms up by contracting the upper trapezius and levator scapulae

Eccentric phase

- Lower weight to starting position

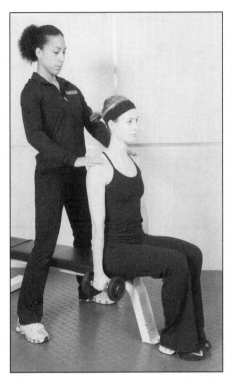
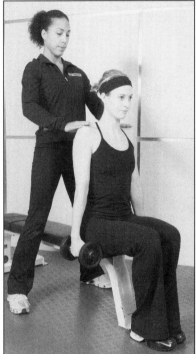

How to Spot

- Spotter should monitor the lifter's alignment while spotting from the side and behind

Variations

- Dumbbell trap shrug (standing, forward lean)

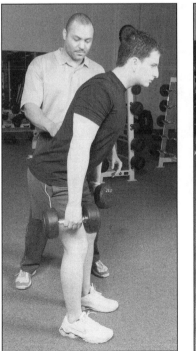
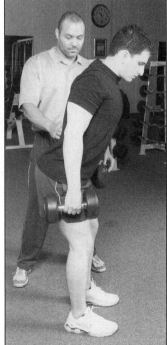

• Barbell trap shrug (standing)

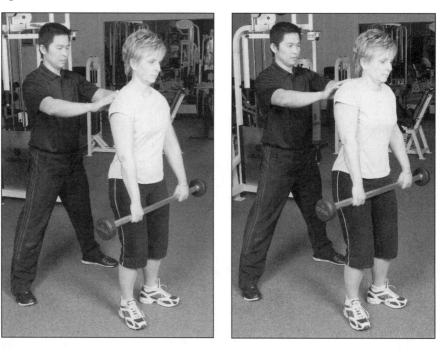

• Cable trap shrug (seated)

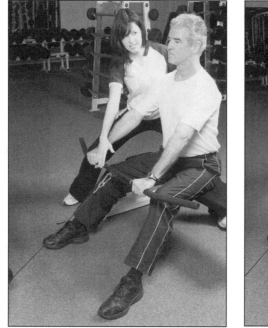
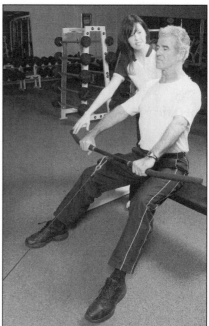

SHOULDERS

DUMBBELL SHOULDER PRESS (SEATED)

Movement—Shoulder flexion, elbow extension
Primary muscles worked—Anterior deltoids, pectoralis major, triceps group, trapezius

How to perform

Starting position

- Sit with feet firmly on the ground and knees at about 90 degrees, with a natural arch in the back
- Bring the arms up and out to the side with the upper arm parallel to the floor and elbows at about 90 degrees

Concentric phase

- Press the arms up and over the head until they are directly over the shoulders
- Attempt to elevate the shoulder blades as they rotate upward while maintaining proper posture

Eccentric phase

- Lower the weight back to the starting position while maintaining posture

How to spot

- Spotter should be directly behind lifter, spotting at the elbow but prepared to assist at wrist if lifter becomes unstable

Variations

- Barbell shoulder press (standing, anterior)

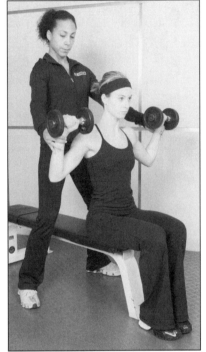
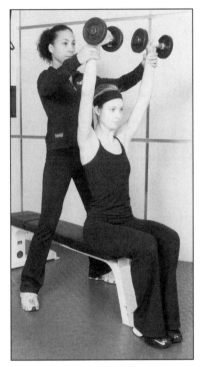
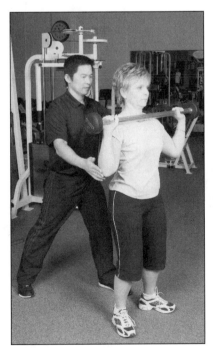
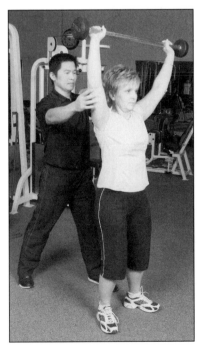

• Machine shoulder press (seated)

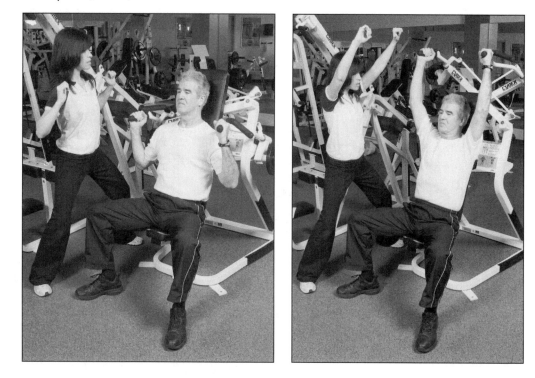

• Tubing shoulder press (standing, single arm)

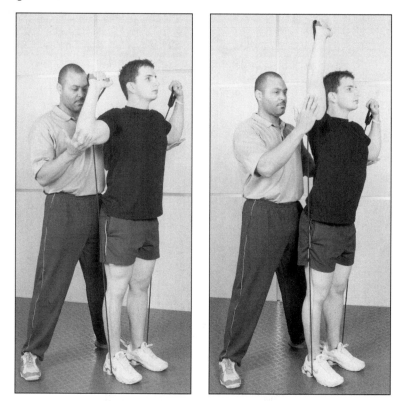

DUMBBELL SHOULDER RAISE (SEATED, LATERAL)

Movement—Shoulder abduction
Primary muscles worked—Deltoid (lateral head), trapezius

How to perform

Starting position

- Sit with feet firmly on the ground
- Dumbbells should be toward outer part of the upper leg, palms facing inward
- Elbows at approximately 90 degrees

Concentric phase

- Lift dumbbells by abducting the shoulder, while keeping 90 degree angle at elbow
- Lift weight until dumbbell and elbow are parallel to the ground and in line with one another

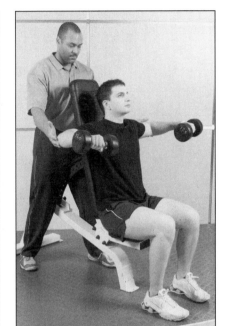

Eccentric phase

- Lower weight to starting position

How to spot

- Spotter should be situated behind lifter with arms close to upper arm or elbow of the lifter

Variations

- Dumbbell shoulder raise (prone, posterior)

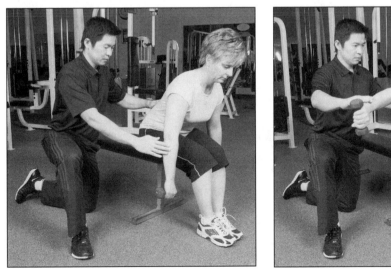
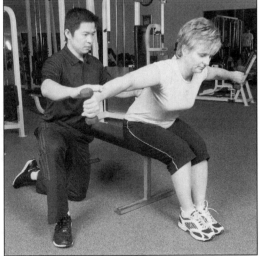

- Cable shoulder raise (standing, lateral, single arm)

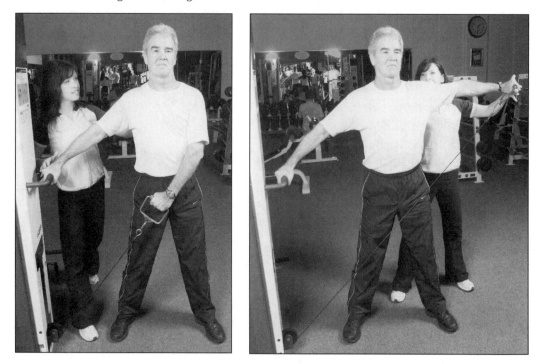

- Tubing shoulder raise (standing, anterior)

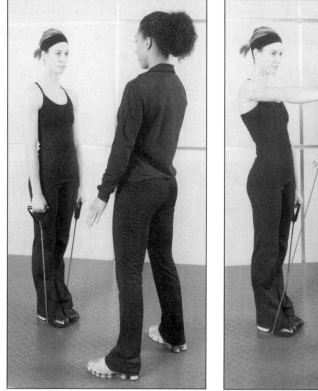
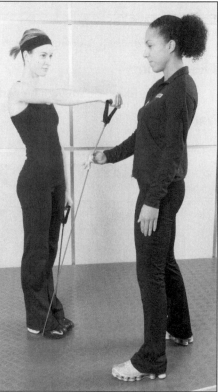

TUBING ROTATOR CUFF EXTERNAL ROTATION (STANDING)

Movement—Shoulder external rotation
Primary muscles worked—Infraspinatus, teres minor, posterior deltoid

How to perform

Starting position

- Stand in good posture with tubing at elbow height
- Grip the handle and flex elbow at 90 degrees

Concentric phase

- Rotate the shoulder, pulling the arm out and across the body, while keeping the elbow fixed
- Continue pulling the arm out, keeping the wrist neutral and elbow in tight against the torso

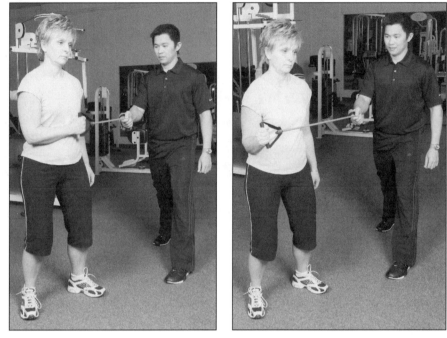

Eccentric phase

- Return tubing to starting position while maintaining posture and elbow flexion at 90 degrees

How to spot

- Spot on forearm while monitoring proper positioning

Variations

- Dumbbell rotator cuff external rotation (semi-prone)

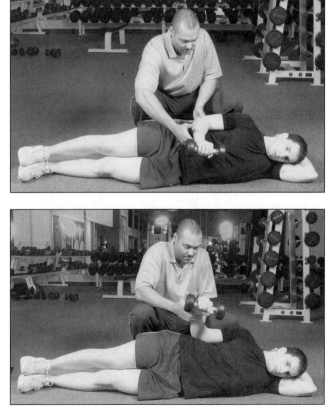

- Cable rotator cuff external rotation (supine)

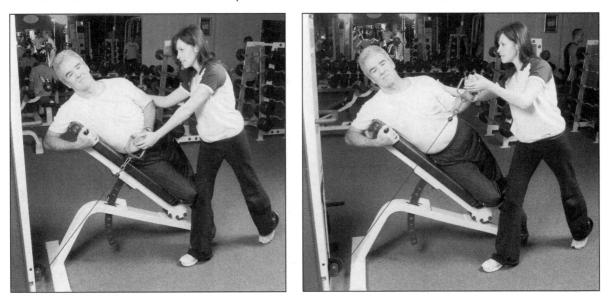

- Manual rotator cuff external rotation (standing)

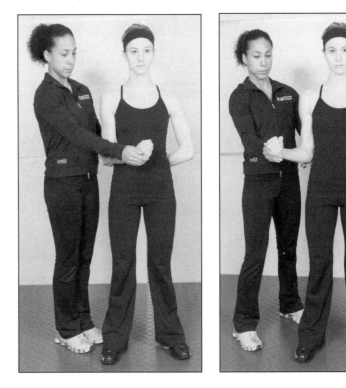

TUBING ROTATOR CUFF INTERNAL ROTATION (STANDING)

Movement—Shoulder internal rotation
Primary muscles worked—Subscapularis, anterior deltoid, pectoralis major, teres major

How to perform

Starting position

- Stand with good posture, with tubing at elbow height
- Grip on to the handle and flex elbow at 90 degrees

Concentric phase

- Rotate the shoulder, pulling the arm out and across the body while keeping the elbow fixed
- Continue pulling the arm out, keeping the wrist neutral and elbow in tight against the torso

Eccentric phase

- Return tubing to starting position, while maintaining posture and elbow flexion at 90 degrees

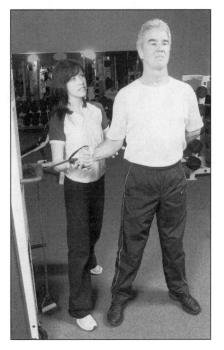
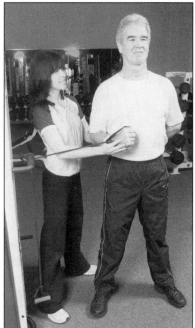

How to spot

- Spot on forearm while monitoring proper positioning

Variations

- Cable rotator cuff internal rotation (standing)

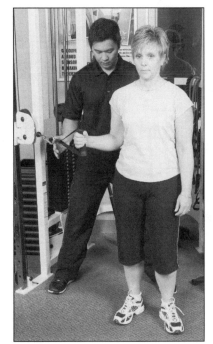
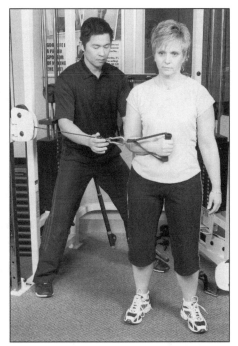

- Cable rotator cuff internal rotation (supine)

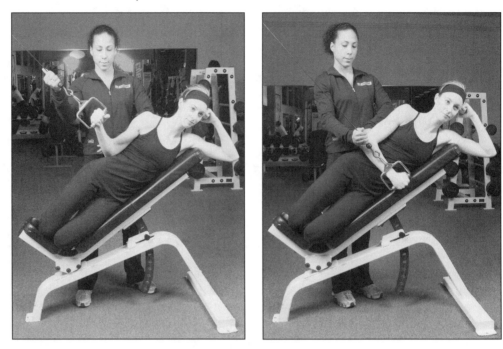

- Manual rotator cuff internal rotation (standing)

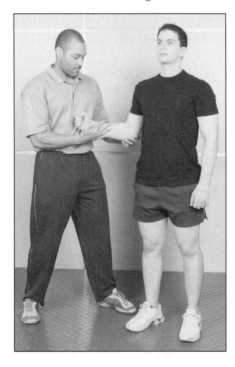 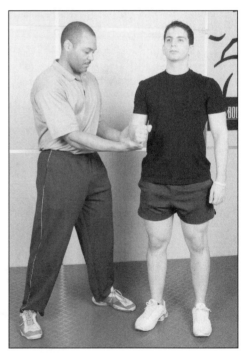

BICEPS

BARBELL BICEPS CURL (STANDING, SUPINATED GRIP)

Movement—Elbow flexion
Primary muscles worked—Biceps group, wrist flexors

How to perform

Starting position

- Grasp barbell with a common supinated grip
- While standing, maintain neutral spine, knees should be slightly flexed and scapulae should be retracted and depressed

Concentric phase

- Curl the bar up until elbows are fully flexed and barbell is in front of chest, keeping the elbows fixed against the torso

Eccentric phase

- Lower the bar to starting position until elbows are slightly bent

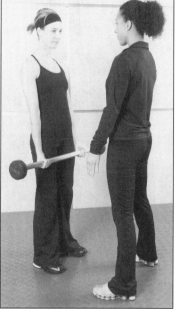
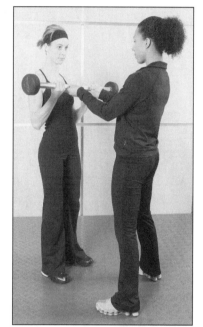

How to spot

- Trainer should be directly in front of lifter and spotting at the bar, inside of the lifter's hands
- Watch for proper alignment and posture throughout the movement

Variations

- E-Z bar biceps curl (standing)

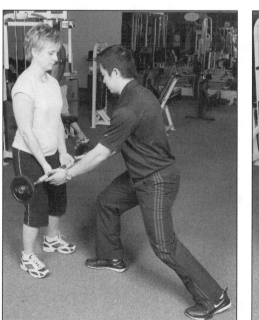
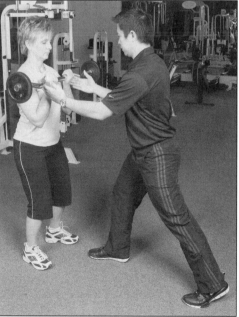

- Cable biceps curl (standing, straight bar)

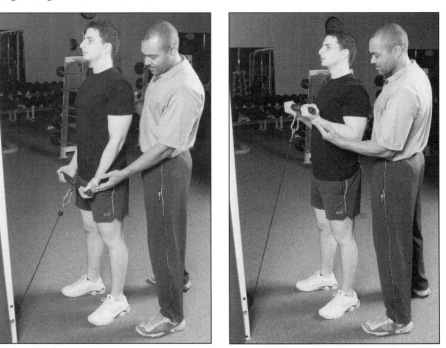

- Machine preacher biceps curl

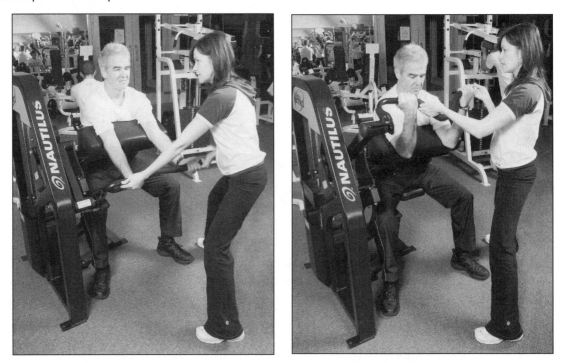

DUMBBELL BICEPS CURL (SEATED, WITH SUPINATION)

Movement—Elbow flexion and radioulnar supination
Primary muscles worked—Biceps group and wrist flexors

How to perform

Starting position

- Sit with feet firmly on the ground
- Grasp dumbbells with a pronated grip and hold them at your side with palms facing in
- Sit with an upright posture

Concentric phase

- Raise the dumbbells, while slowly supinating the wrist
- Lift the dumbbells until the elbows are fully flexed and the weight is in front of the anterior deltoid

Eccentric phase

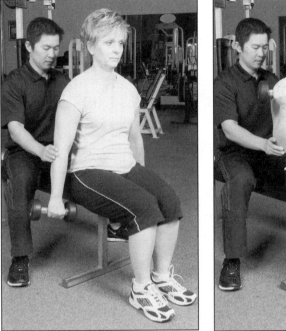
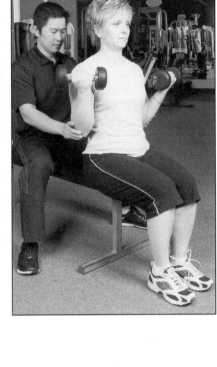

- Lower the weight back to the stating position so that the palms are facing inward

How to spot

- Trainer should spot in front of lifter as close to the weight as possible, without obstructing the lifter's movement

Variations

- Dumbbell biceps concentration curl (seated)

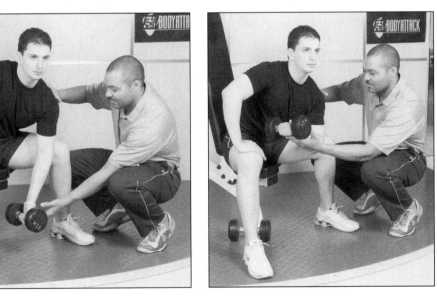

- Cable biceps single arm curl (standing)

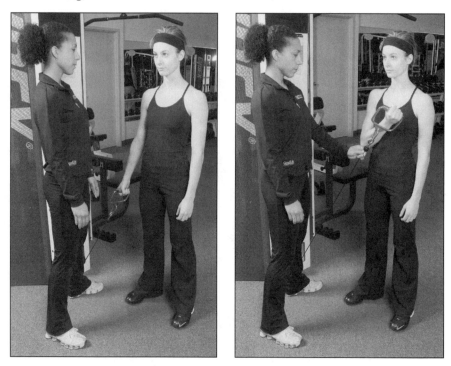

- Tubing biceps curl (standing)

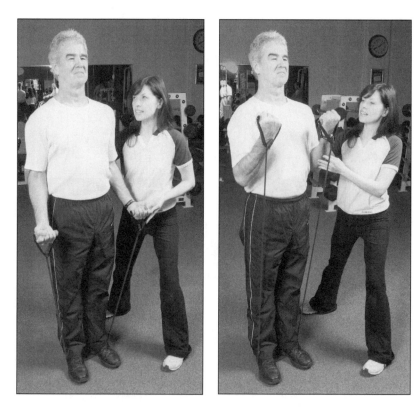

DUMBBELL BICEPS CURL (SEATED, HAMMER GRIP)

Movement—Elbow flexion
Primary muscles worked—Brachioradialis, biceps group

How to perform

Starting position

- Sit with feet firmly on the ground
- Grasp dumbbells so that the palms are facing in
- Elbows should be against the torso and at a 90 degree angle

Concentric phase

- Raise the dumbbells up until the elbows are fully flexed and weight is in front of anterior deltoid, ensuring that palms are facing in at all times

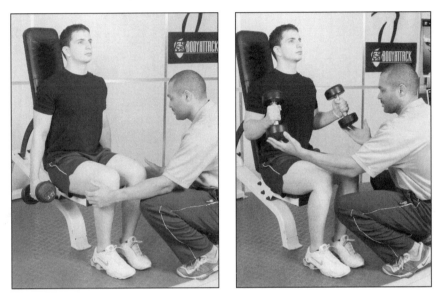

Eccentric phase

- Lower dumbbells back to starting position

How to spot

- Trainer will be in front of lifter spotting as close to the weight as possible, without obstructing the movement

Variations

- Tubing hammer curl (standing)

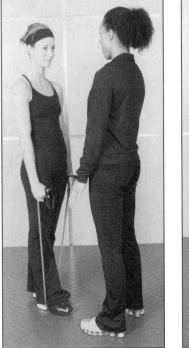
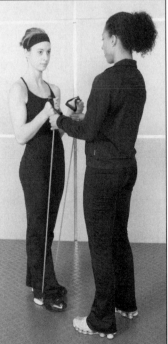

- Tubing biceps curl (standing, hammer grip)

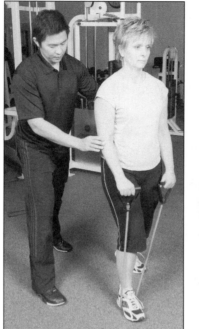
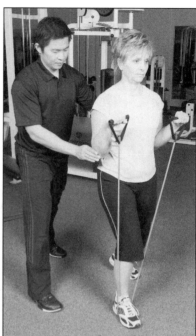

TRICEPS

CABLE TRICEPS EXTENSION (STANDING, V-BAR)

Movement—Elbow extension
Primary muscles worked—Triceps group

How to perform

Starting position

- Stand with feet shoulder-width apart and knees slightly flexed
- Grasp bar with a pronated grip so that elbows are against torso
- Forearms should be approximately parallel to the ground and elbows should be at 90 degrees

Concentric phase

- Push down, fully extending elbows but not locking them out

Eccentric phase

- Return bar back to starting position, finishing with approximately a 90 degree angle at the elbows
- Maintain upright posture throughout movement

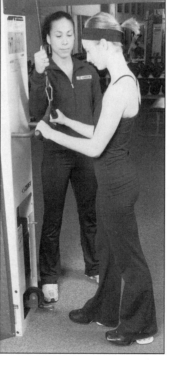
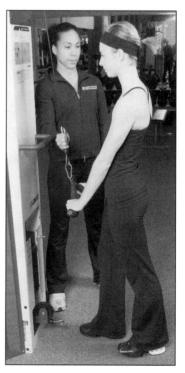

How to spot

- Trainer will spot from the side and behind
- Be aware of proper alignment and posture

Variations

- Dumbbell triceps kick-back (standing)

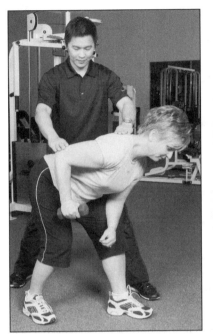
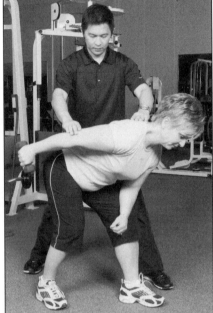

- Barbell triceps extension (standing, supinated grip, straight bar)

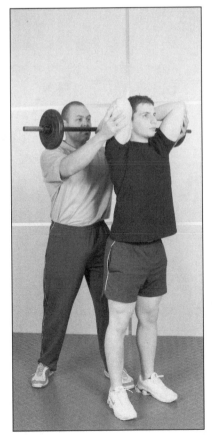
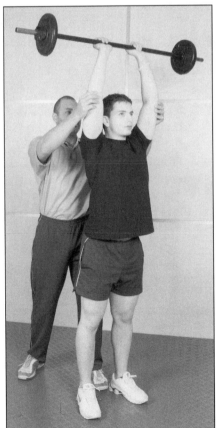

- Cable triceps extension (standing, rope)

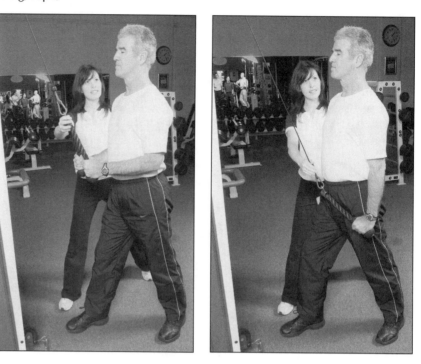

BARBELL TRICEPS EXTENSION (SUPINE)

Movement—Elbow extension
Primary muscles worked—Triceps group

How to perform

Starting position

- Lying supine on a bench, with both feet firmly on the ground, hold a barbell using a pronated grip over the front of the face

- Elbows should be aligned with wrists and shoulders. There may be variations in hand positioning based on individual factors (e.g., shoulder width, wrist flexibility, etc.)

- To start, lower barbell to the forehead or behind the head, depending on the experience level of your client

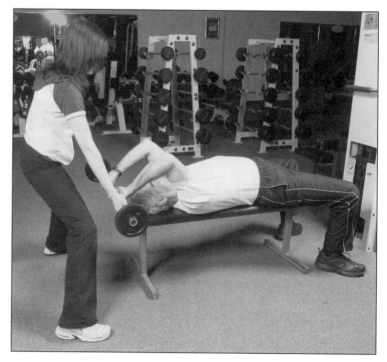

Concentric phase

- Lift barbell so that elbows are fully extended

Eccentric phase

- There should be no other movement at the shoulder or back

How to spot

- Spotter should be in a kneeling lunge position behind the head of the lifter

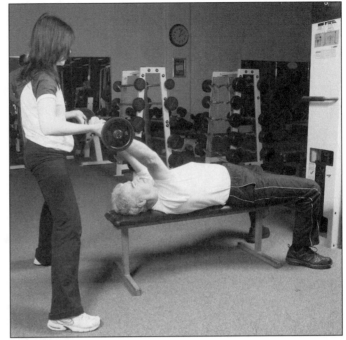

Variations

- Dumbbell triceps extension (supine)

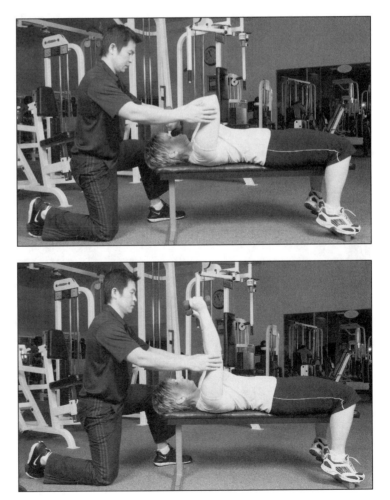

- Cable triceps extension (supine, rope)

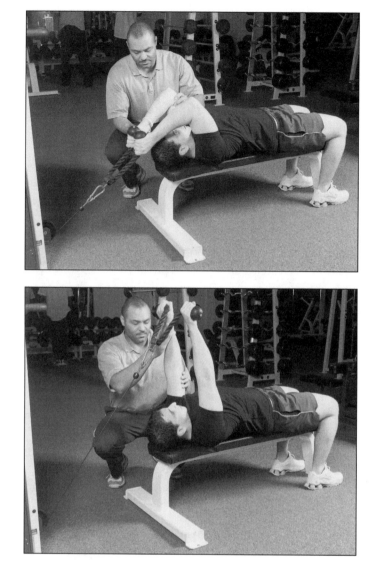

- Tubing triceps extension (supine)

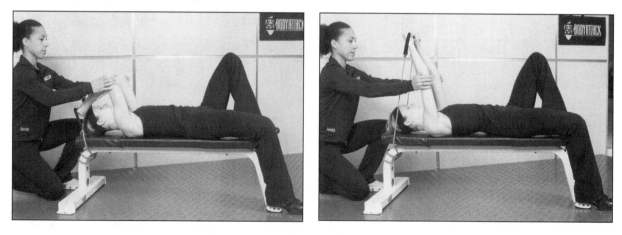

BENCH TRICEPS DIPS

Movement—Elbow flexion, scapular retraction
Primary muscles worked—Triceps group, pectoralis major, anterior deltoid

How to perform

Starting position

- Place the body so that the hands are on the edge of a bench and the legs are extended out in front, with heels on the ground and no flexion at the knee
- Lower the torso so that the upper arms are about parallel to the ground

Concentric phase

- Raise the torso by fully extending the elbows

Eccentric phase

- Lower the torso to starting position

How to spot

- Trainer will be at the side of the exerciser in a kneeling lunge position

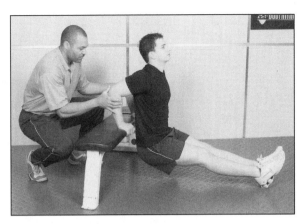

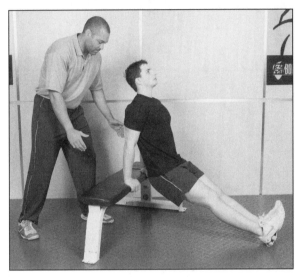

Variations

- Parallel bar triceps dips

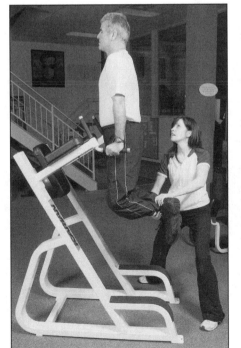

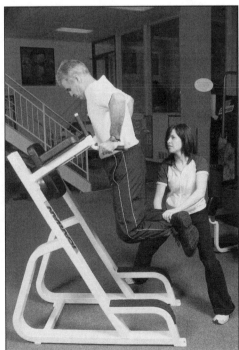

- Barbell triceps press (supine, narrow grip)

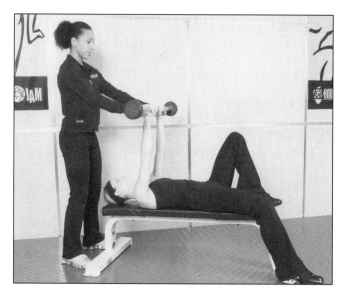

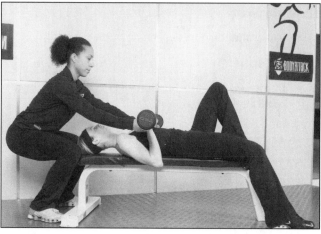

- Machine assisted triceps dips

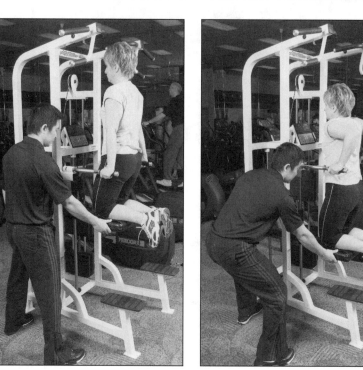

BARBELL TRICEPS EXTENSION (SEATED, OVERHEAD)

Movement—Elbow extension
Primary muscles worked—Triceps group

How to perform

Starting position

- Sit upright with feet firmly on the ground
- Grasp the bar above the head with an overhand grip and set elbows at approximately 90 degrees
- Elbows should be facing forward or slightly outward

Concentric phase

- Press the bar up until the elbows are fully extended

Eccentric phase

- Return bar to starting position

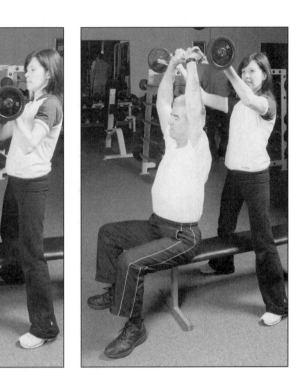

How to spot

- Trainer should be standing behind the lifter with hands at elbows but prepared to assist at bar if needed

Variations

- Dumbbell triceps extension (seated, overhead)

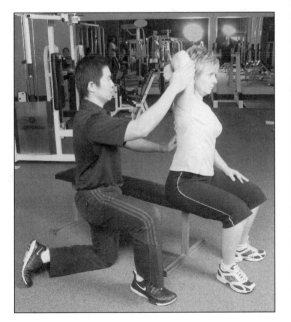

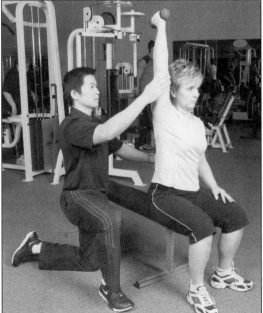

- Cable triceps extension (kneeling, rope)

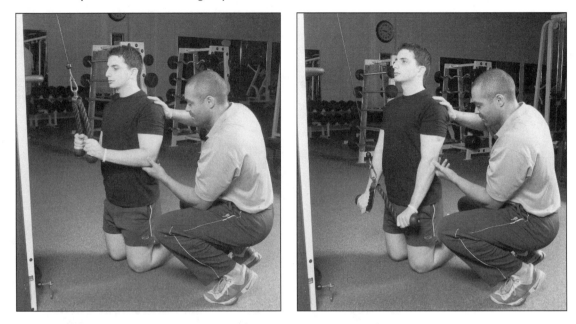

- Tubing triceps extension (standing, overhead)

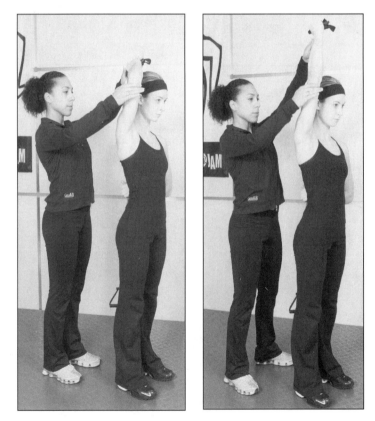

LOWER BODY

QUADRICEPS, HAMSTRINGS, AND GLUTES

BARBELL SQUAT

Movement—Hip extension, knee extension
Primary muscles worked—Hip extensors (glutes, hamstrings, hip adductors), quadriceps, spinal extensors

How to perform

Starting position

- Place the bar just above the scapluae with the hands placed comfortably on the bar and elbows pointed down
- Feet should be outside of shoulder width and angled out slightly
- Knees and hips should be slightly flexed, while the spine and neck are held in a neutral position

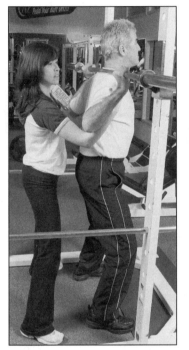
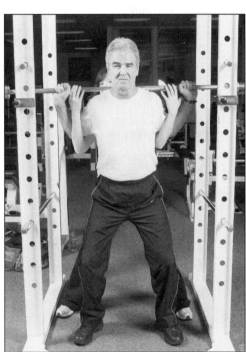

Eccentric phase

- Push the hips back, allow the knees to bend naturally and let the trunk lean forward slightly
- Lower the body until the upper legs are parallel to the ground or as far down as your client can comfortably go
- Maintain proper posture throughout movement
- Eyes should be forward throughout the movement
- Weight should be on the balls of the feet.
- Be careful that the knees do not come too far beyond the front of the toes

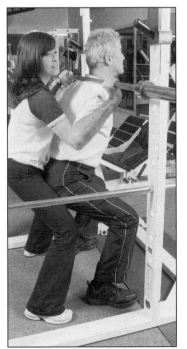
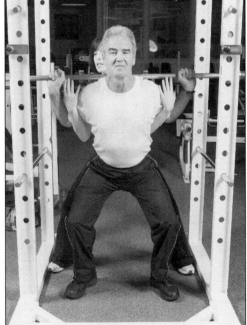

Concentric phase

- Return to the starting position by maintaining posture and pushing from the balls of the feet, keeping the eyes looking forward

How to spot

- Spotter should be behind exerciser with arm at lifter's torso
- Look for proper alignment, weight should be on balls of feet, knees should track over top of feet

Variations

- Barbell deadlift

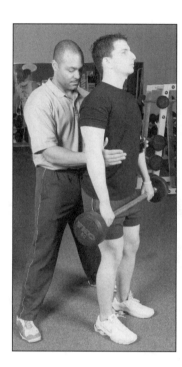 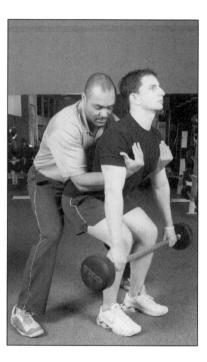

- Dumbbell lunge

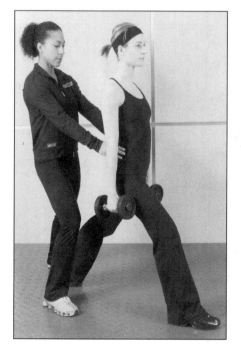 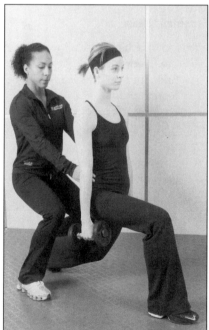

- Machine leg press

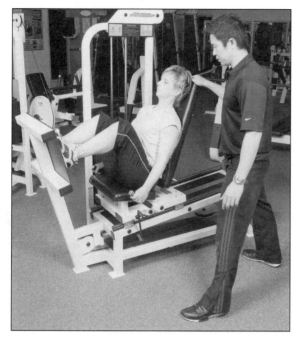
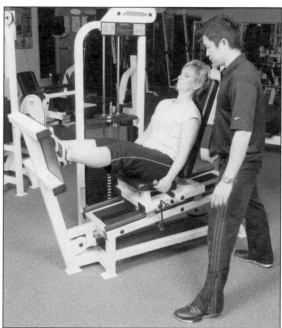

QUADRICEPS

MACHINE LEG EXTENSION

Movement—Knee extension
Primary muscles worked—Quadriceps

How to perform

Starting position

- Sit so that the knee joints are aligned with the axis of the machine
- Lower back should be firm against the seat
- Pad should be pressing against lower shins
- Sit upright, with a natural arch in lower back

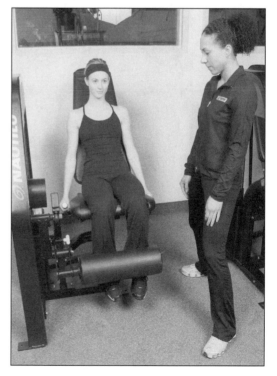

Concentric phase

- Raise the pad up until the legs are almost fully extended, while maintaining good posture throughout the movement

Eccentric phase

- Lower the legs to the starting position

How to spot

- Trainer should spot at the pad in a kneeling lunge position
- Knees should not lock out

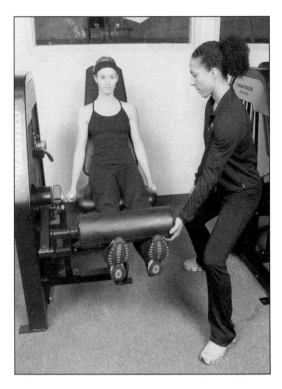

Variations

- Tubing leg extension
- Cable hip flexion
- Machine hip flexion

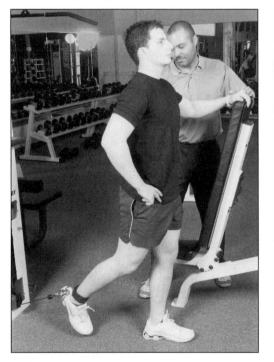

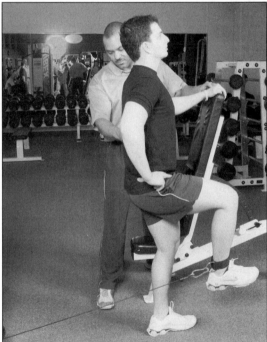

HAMSTRINGS

MACHINE LEG CURL (PRONE)

Movement—Knee flexion
Primary muscles worked—Hamstrings

How to perform

Starting position

- Lie prone on bench so that knee joints are in line with axis of machine and pad is below the gastrocnemius but above the Achilles tendon
- Position trunk and neck in proper posture

Concentric phase

- Press the pelvis against the bench and raise the weight until the knees form approximately a 90 degree angle

Eccentric phase

- Lower the weight to the starting position

How to spot

- Trainer should be at the side spotting on the pad, watching for proper alignment and ready to assist with weight

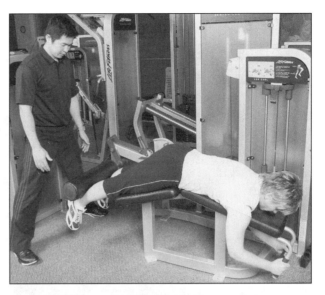

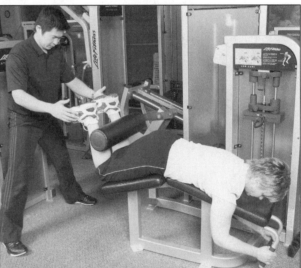

Variations

- Machine leg curl (seated)

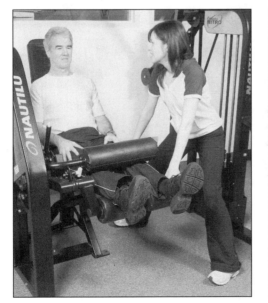

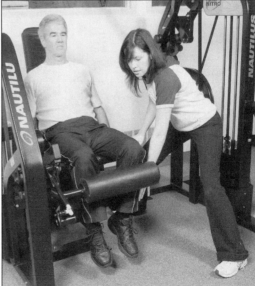

- Cable hip extension (standing)

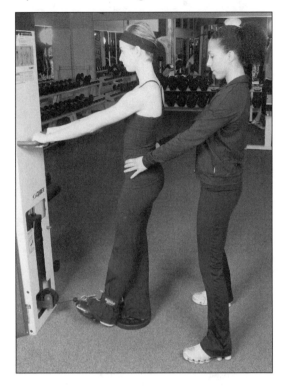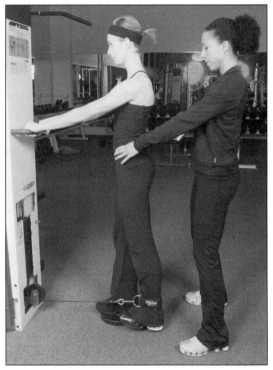

- Dumbbell stiffed legged deadlift

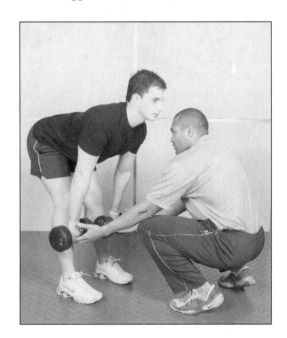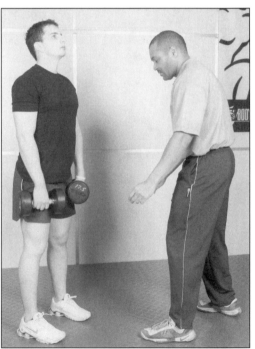

CABLE HIP ADDUCTION (STANDING)

Movement—Hip adduction
Primary muscles worked—Hip adductors

How to perform

Starting position

- Strap one cable to the inside ankle and stand with the opposite foot straight ahead, aligned directly under the hip and with the knee slightly bent
- Begin with the moving leg about 45 degrees out from the body and the inside hand resting lightly on the bar for balance
- Maintain good posture and keep pelvis level throughout the movement

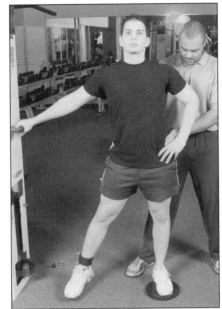 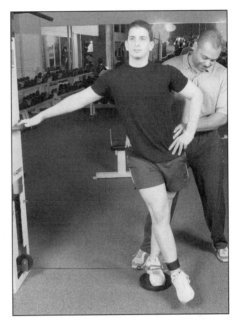

Concentric phase

- Pull the leg across the body

Eccentric phase

- Return weight to starting position

How to spot

- Trainer should be directly behind exerciser in a standing position with hands monitoring pelvis

Variations

- Machine hip adduction (seated)

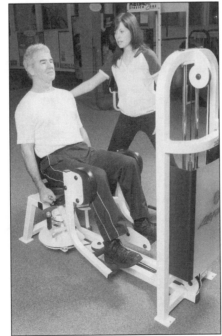 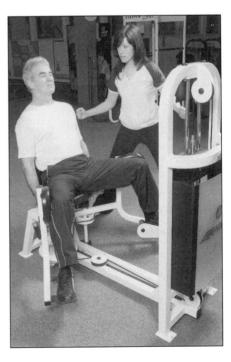

- Tubing hip adduction (standing)

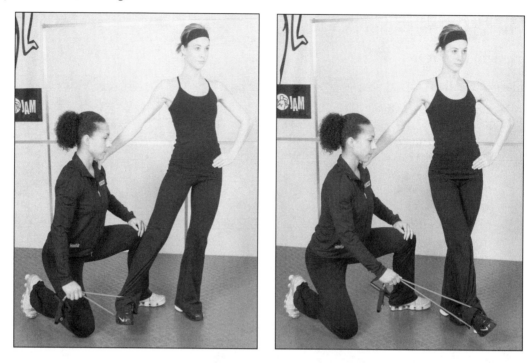

- Hip adduction (semi-prone)

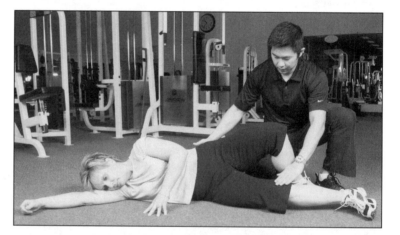

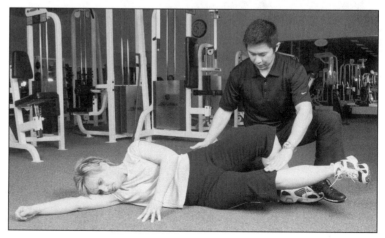

CABLE HIP ABDUCTION (STANDING)

Movement—Hip abduction
Primary muscles worked—Hip abductors

How to perform

Starting position

- Strap one cable to the outside ankle and stand with the opposite foot straight ahead, knee slightly bent
- Position the outside leg slightly across the body and in front of the stationary leg, while placing the hand closest to the machine on the handle

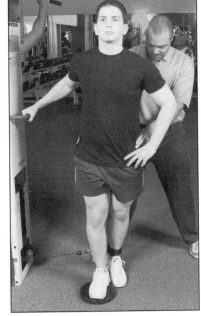
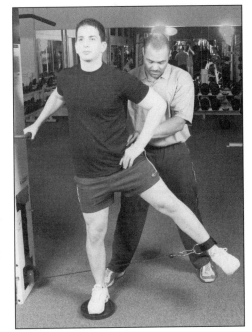

Concentric phase

- Pull the leg across and out from the body as far as possible, while maintaining good posture and pelvic position

Eccentric phase

- Lower the weight back to the starting position

How to spot

- Trainer should be behind the exerciser with hands at hips monitoring level of pelvis and overall alignment

Variations

- Machine hip abduction (seated)

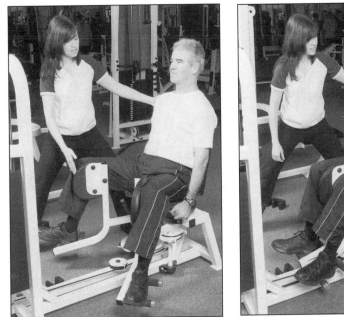
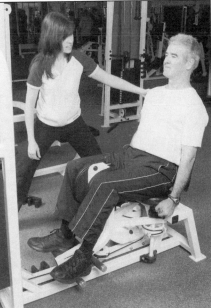

- Tubing hip abduction (standing)

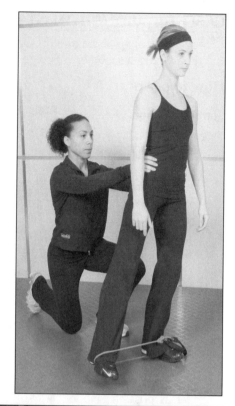

- Hip abduction (semi-prone)

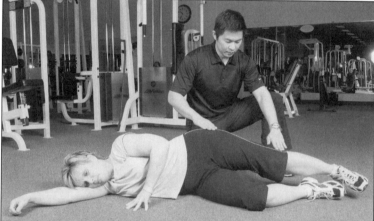

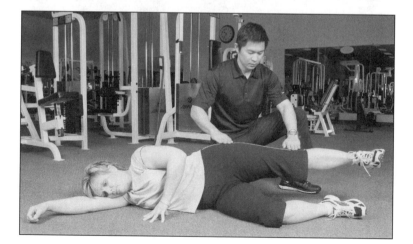

GASTROCNEMIUS AND SOLEUS

DUMBBELL HEEL RAISE (STANDING)

Movement—Plantar flexion
Primary muscles worked—Gastrocnemius and soleus

How to perform

Starting position

- Stand with toes on the edge of the platform
- Hold dumbbell in one hand with opposite hand holding bar of machine for support
- Begin with slight knee bend and heels close to floor

Concentric phase

- Raise up by extending the ankles, keeping the weight over the balls of the feet
- Extend the ankles as far as possible, while maintaining good posture

Eccentric phase

- Lower the body down to the starting position

How to spot

- Trainer should be beside exerciser monitoring movement

Variations

- Machine heel raise (standing)

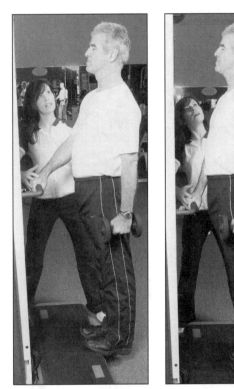

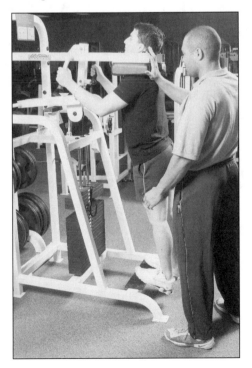

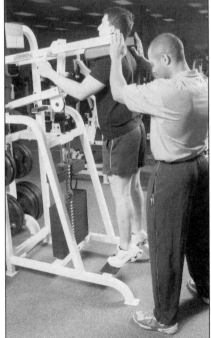

- Machine heel raise (seated)

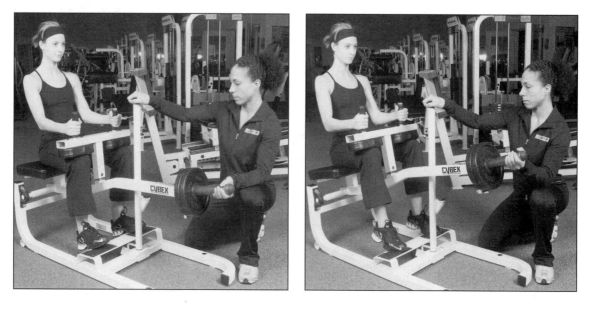

- Smith machine heel raise (standing)

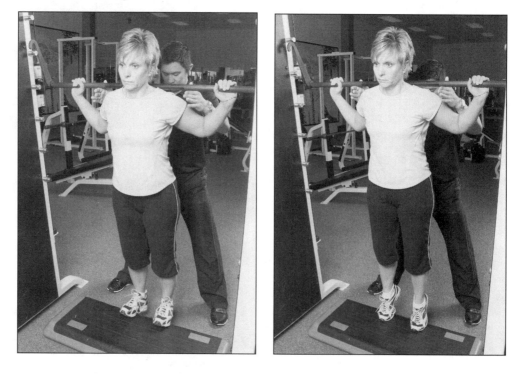

CORE EXERCISES

LOWER BACK

BACK EXTENSION (PRONE, UPPER BODY)

Movement—Trunk extensors
Primary muscles worked—Erector spinae

How to perform

Starting position

- Prone position on the floor with hands next to ears on the floor, elbows at torso and head slightly off the ground

Concentric phase

- Move up slowly by lifting the upper torso off the ground and retracting the scapulae
- Extend off the floor, without hyperextending the lower back
- Maintain head alignment throughout movement

Eccentric phase

- Lower body to start position

How to spot

- Trainer should be in a kneeling lunge position next to the lifter with their hand on the lower back monitoring the movement

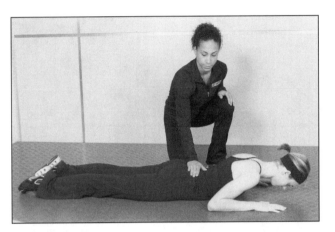

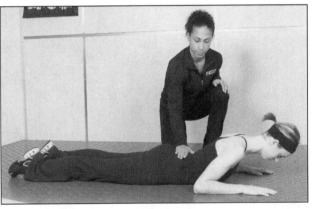

Variations

- Roman chair back extension (prone, upper body)

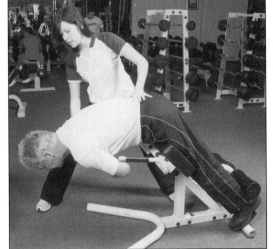

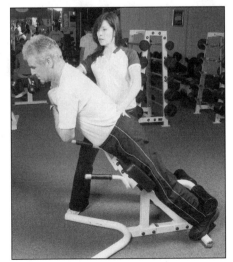

- Machine back extension (seated)

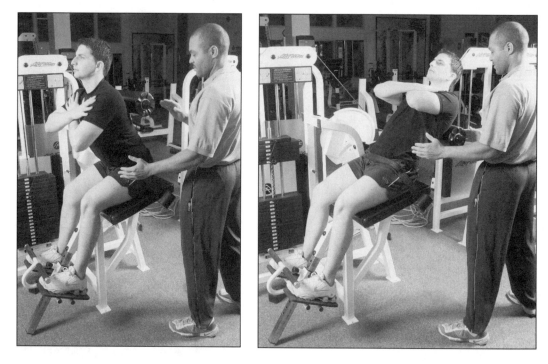

- Stability ball back extension

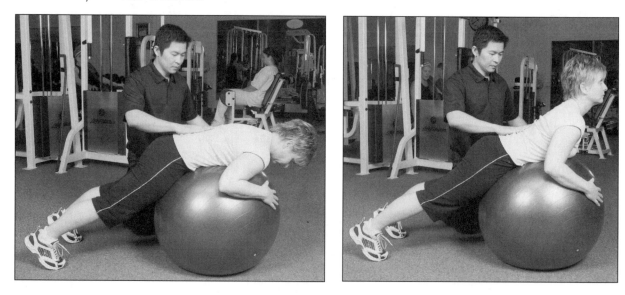

OBLIQUES

SHOULDER TO KNEE CURL-UP

Movement—Spinal flexion and rotation
Primary muscles worked—Rectus abdominis and obliques

How to perform

Starting position

- In a supine position, with 1 leg flat on the floor and the other leg at a 90 degree angle at the knee, place both hands behind the head

Concentric phase

- Bring the opposite elbow to the opposing knee by flexing the torso and pulling the ribs toward the pelvis
- Keep the neck in a neutral and relaxed position throughout the movement

Eccentric phase

- Return to starting position by lowering torso
- Continue movement by alternating sides

How to spot

- Trainer is in a kneeling lunge position next to the exerciser, monitoring alignment

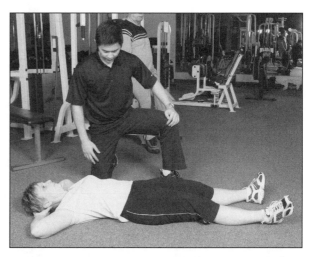

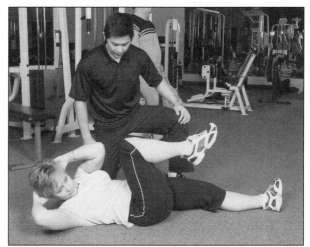

Variations

- Oblique lateral flexion (semi-prone)

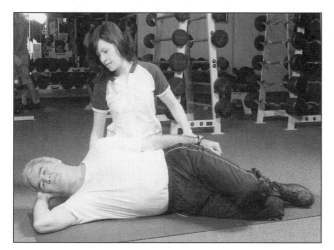

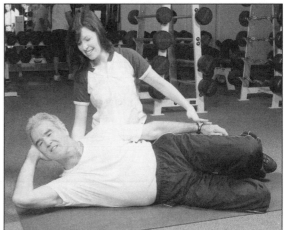

- Dumbbell oblique lateral flexion (standing)

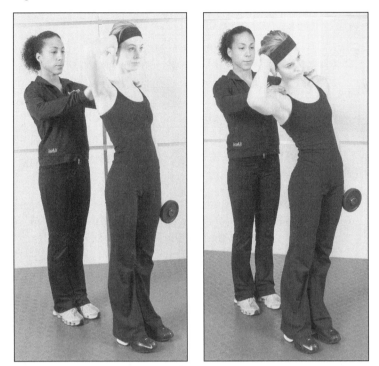

- Stability ball oblique lateral flexion (semi-prone)

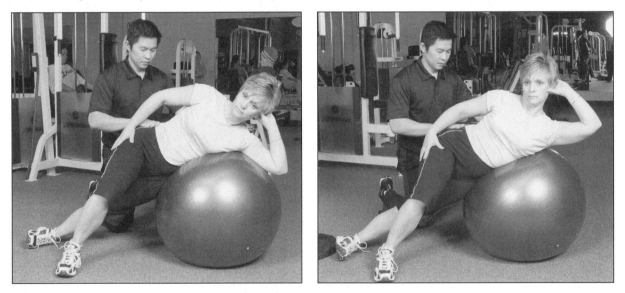

RECTUS ABDOMINIS

PARTIAL ABDOMINAL CURL-UP

Movement—Spinal flexion
Primary muscles worked—Rectus abdominis

How to perform

Starting position

- In a supine position, with arms fully extended along the torso, bend the knees so that the feet are flat on the floor

Concentric phase

- Curl the torso up by bringing the ribs toward the pelvis and moving the hands along the floor straight down toward the feet
- Curl the torso until the torso is fully flexed

Eccentric phase

- Return to starting position

How to spot

- Trainer is in a kneeling lunge position next to the exerciser

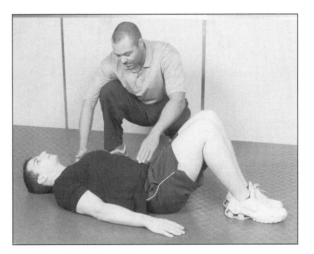

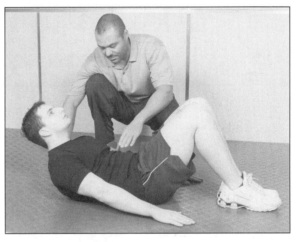

Variations

- Reverse abdominal curl

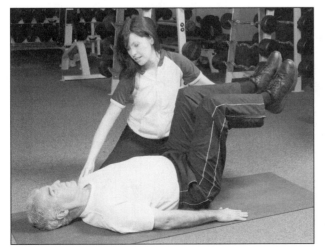

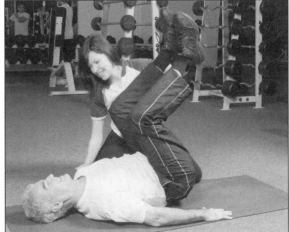

- Cable abdominal curl

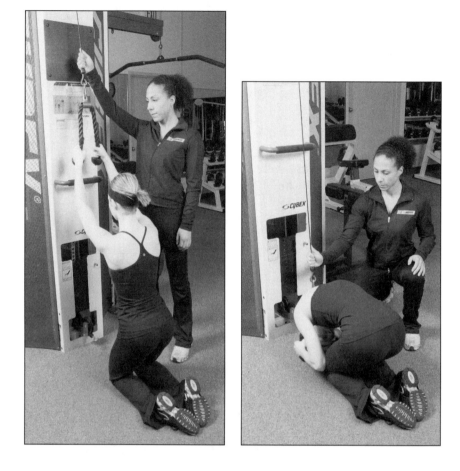

- Stability ball abdominal curl

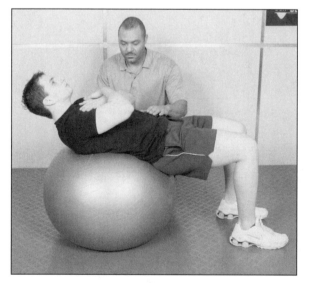 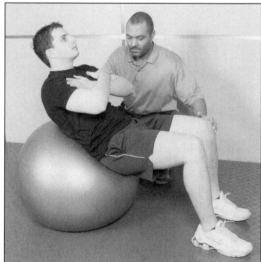

TRANSVERSE ABDOMINUS

PLANK (FROM ELBOWS)

Movement—Shoulder flexion, hip extension, spinal flexion
Primary muscles worked—Core, hip extensors, shoulder flexors, erector spinae

How to perform

Starting position

- In a prone position, with neck and back in proper alignment, place the elbows at a 90 degree angle along the torso
- Toes should be pointing down

Concentric phase

- Lift the upper and lower body up by pushing up from the elbows
- Maintain posture and alignment while holding body weight with elbows and toes

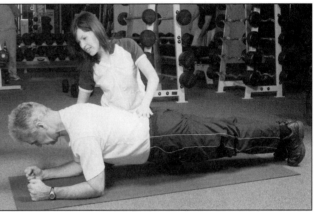

Eccentric phase

- Lower the body back to starting position

How to spot

- Trainer is in a kneeling lunge position next to the exerciser, watching for proper alignment

Variations

- Plank (from elbows, contralateral)

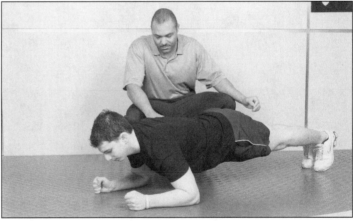

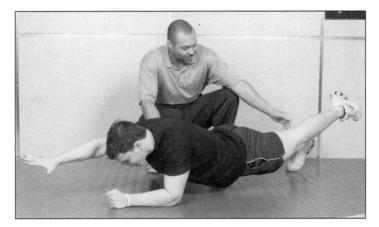

- Plank (semi-prone, from elbows)

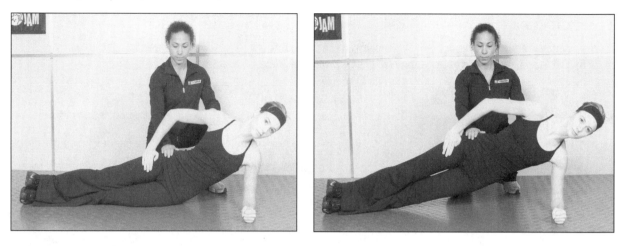

- V-sit

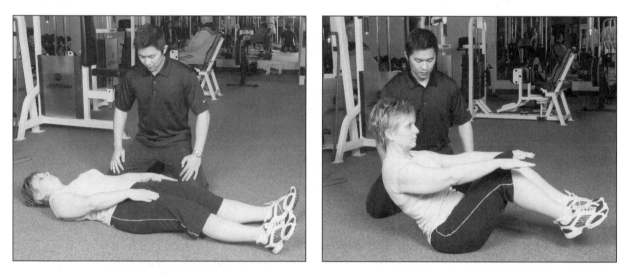

REFERENCES

Aaberg, E. 2007. *Resistance Training Instruction.* 2nd ed. Champaign, IL: Human Kinetics.

Delavier, F. 2006. *Strength Training Anatomy.* 2nd ed. Champaign, IL: Human Kinetics.

Golding, L.A., and Golding, S.M. 2003. *Fitness Professionals' Guide to Musculoskeletal Anatomy and Human Movement.* Monterey, California: Healthy Learning.

APPENDIX B

Stretches

Mike Bates, MBA

PECTORALS

CHEST EXPANSION

How to perform

- Hold elbows at shoulder height with the fingers near the ears
- Squeeze the shoulder blades together and pull the elbows back
- Hold the stretch for 10 to 30 seconds

Reprinted, by permission, from J. Blahnik, 2004, *Full-Body Flexibility,* (Champaign, IL: Human Kinetics), 50.

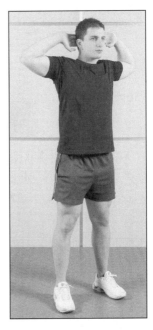

CHEST REACH-BACK AND TURN

How to perform

- Stand and raise the arm out to the side at shoulder height. Hold onto a stationary object, such as a door or cabinet. Slowly rotate the upper body away from the hand.
- Hold the stretch for 10 to 30 seconds.
- Repeat on the other arm.

Reprinted, by permission, from J. Blahnik, 2004, *Full-Body Flexibility,* (Champaign, IL: Human Kinetics), 49.

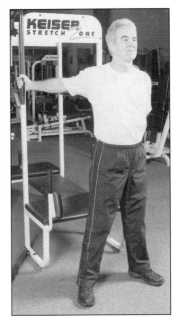

UPPER BACK

UPPER BACK SCOOP

How to perform

- Extend the legs straight in front with the knees slightly bent. Lean forward, reach for the back of the thighs, and round the upper back.
- Hold the stretch for 10 to 30 seconds.

Reprinted, by permission, from J. Blahnik, 2004, *Full-Body Flexibility*, (Champaign, IL: Human Kinetics), 53.

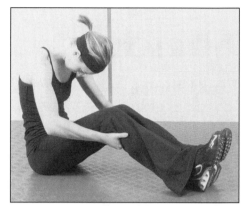

SIDE REACH

How to perform

- Stand with feet apart and knees slightly bent. Reach with one hand above the head and lean over to the opposite side.
- Hold the stretch for 10 to 30 seconds.
- Repeat on the other side.

Reprinted, by permission, from J. Blahnik, 2004, *Full-Body Flexibility*, (Champaign, IL: Human Kinetics), 59.

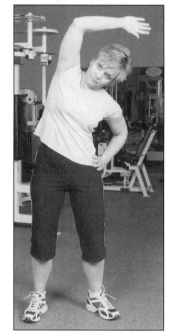

POLE REACH (LATISSIMUS DORSI STRETCH)

How to perform

- Stand with the feet apart. With one side of the body facing the wall, place both hands on the wall by leaning to the side.
- Hold the stretch for 10 to 30 seconds.
- Repeat on the other side.

Reprinted, by permission, from J. Blahnik, 2004, *Full-Body Flexibility*, (Champaign, IL: Human Kinetics), 60.

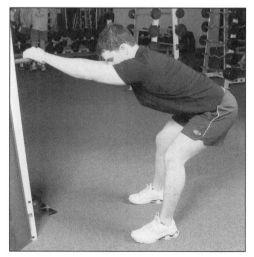

LOWER BACK

BACK SPINAL FLEXION (CAT STRETCH)

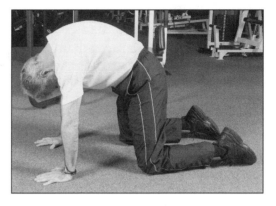

How to perform

- Kneel on the floor on the hands and knees
- Start: Pull in the abdominals to round the spine; tuck the chin into the chest
- Finish: Release the stretch by returning to kneeling in the all-fours position
- Repeat as a continuous, controlled, fluid sequence 10 to 12 times

Something to remember

- Keep the hips over the knees and shoulders over the hands

Reprinted, by permission, from J. Blahnik, 2004, *Full-Body Flexibility*, (Champaign, IL: Human Kinetics), 58.

SEATED TWIST

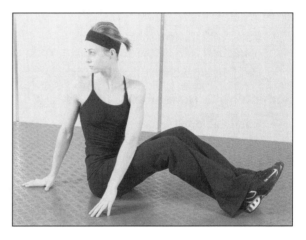

How to perform

- Sitting on the floor, extend the legs straight out in front with the knees slightly bent. Place one hand on the floor behind the body and the other across the thigh. Twist the upper body to one side.
- Hold the stretch for 10 to 30 seconds.
- Repeat on the other side.

Something to remember

- Sit up tall; don't round the spine.

Reprinted, by permission, from J. Blahnik, 2004, *Full-Body Flexibility*, (Champaign, IL: Human Kinetics), 62.

ABDOMINALS

BACK SPINAL EXTENSION (COBRA STRETCH)

How to perform

- Lie on the floor chest down with the hands near the shoulders. Lift the chest and ribs off the floor as far as comfortably possible by pushing with the hands.
- Hold the stretch for 10 to 30 seconds.

Something to remember

- Don't extend beyond the point that's comfortable for the lower back.
- Keep the head up and eyes ahead.

Reprinted, by permission, from J. Blahnik, 2004, *Full-Body Flexibility*, (Champaign, IL: Human Kinetics), 64.

LYING ARCH

How to perform

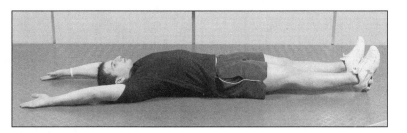

- Lie on the floor faceup with the arms extended above the head. Reach as far away from the body as comfortably possible while gently arching the lower back and lifting the ribs and chest toward the ceiling.
- Hold the stretch for 10 to 30 seconds.
- Don't extend beyond the point that's comfortable for the lower back.

Reprinted, by permission, from J. Blahnik, 2004, *Full-Body Flexibility,* (Champaign, IL: Human Kinetics), 66.

SHOULDERS

ARMS BEHIND AND OPEN

How to perform

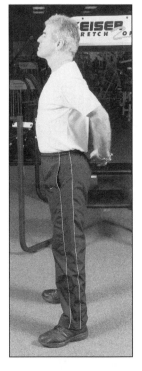

- Stand with the feet shoulder-width apart. Clasp the hands together in the small of the back and lift the arms upward.
- Hold the stretch for 10 to 30 seconds.

Something to remember

- Stand tall; don't round the spine.

Reprinted, by permission, from J. Blahnik, 2004, *Full-Body Flexibility,* (Champaign, IL: Human Kinetics), 26.

ARM STRAIGHT ACROSS

How to perform

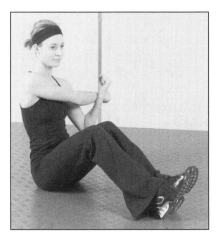

- Sit with feet shoulder-width apart. Bring one arm across the body at chest height and hold it in place with the opposite arm.
- Hold the stretch for 10 to 30 seconds.
- Repeat on the other arm.

Something to remember

- Don't round the spine.

Reprinted, by permission, from J. Blahnik, 2004, *Full-Body Flexibility,* (Champaign, IL: Human Kinetics), 31.

BICEPS

PRONATED HAND REACH-BACK AND TURN

How to perform

- Stand and raise the arm out to the side at shoulder height. Place the back of the hand (thumb down) against a stationary object, such as a wall or door. Slowly rotate the upper body away from the hand.
- Hold the stretch for 10 to 30 seconds.
- Repeat on the other arm.

Something to remember

- Slightly bend the elbow.

Reprinted, by permission, from J. Blahnik, 2004, *Full-Body Flexibility,* (Champaign, IL: Human Kinetics), 34.

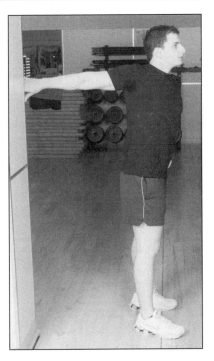

TRICEPS

ELBOW BEND AND PUSH

How to perform

- Stand or sit tall. Lift one arm above the head. Bend the elbow and place the hand between the shoulder blades. Use the other hand to gently push the elbow back.
- Hold the stretch for 10 to 30 seconds.
- Repeat on the other arm.

Something to remember

- Keep the chin up.

Reprinted, by permission, from J. Blahnik, 2004, *Full-Body Flexibility,* (Champaign, IL: Human Kinetics), 36.

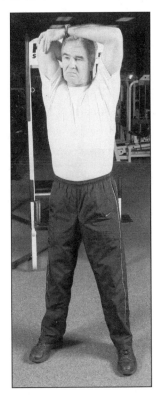

WRIST

WRIST FLEX AND EXTEND

How to perform

- Stand or sit with one hand in front of the body at shoulder height, palm facing down. Use the other hand to pull on the back of the hand, bringing the palm down toward the body. Return to setup position. Pull the hand up toward the body, bring the back of the hand up.
- Hold each stretch for 10 to 30 seconds.
- Repeat on the other hand.

Something to remember

- Don't round the spine.

Reprinted, by permission, from J. Blahnik, 2004, *Full-Body Flexibility*, (Champaign, IL: Human Kinetics), 39.

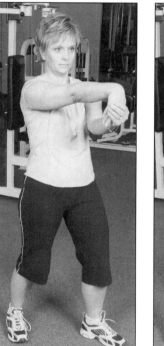
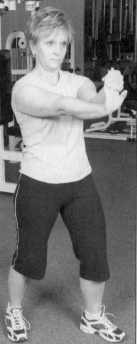

NECK

ARM REACH-BEHIND HEAD TILT

How to perform

- Stand with the feet apart and the arms next to the body. Slowly drop the head to one side. Reach behind and pull down on the wrist of the opposite arm.
- Hold the stretch for 10 to 30 seconds.
- Repeat on the other side.

Something to remember

- Stand tall; look straight ahead.

Reprinted, by permission, from J. Blahnik, 2004, *Full-Body Flexibility*, (Champaign, IL: Human Kinetics), 22.

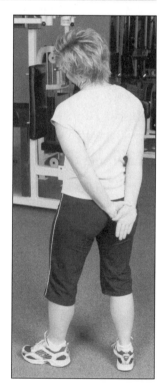

CHIN DIAGONAL DROP

How to perform

- Stand or sit tall
- Start: Drop the chin diagonally toward the armpit as far as comfortably possible while lifting the back of the head toward the ceiling.
- Finish: Release the stretch by lifting the head to neutral position and repeat on the other side.
- Repeat as a continuous, controlled, fluid sequence 10 to 12 times.

Something to remember

- Stand or sit tall; don't round the spine.

Reprinted, by permission, from J. Blahnik, 2004, *Full-Body Flexibility*, (Champaign, IL: Human Kinetics), 21.

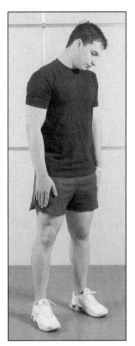

HIP FLEXORS

KNEELING LUNGE

How to perform

- Kneel on one leg. Step out with the front foot and gently press the hips forward.
- Place the hands on the front thigh for support, if necessary.
- Keep body weight distributed between both legs.
- Hold the stretch for 10 to 30 seconds.
- Repeat on the other leg.

Something to remember

- Don't extend the front knee beyond the toes.

Reprinted, by permission, from J. Blahnik, 2004, *Full-Body Flexibility*, (Champaign, IL: Human Kinetics), 82.

GLUTEALS

SEATED FIGURE

How to perform

- Sit with one foot across the thigh of the opposite leg in the figure 4 position. Move the chest toward the legs, pivoting at the hip. Use the arms to support the back, if necessary.
- Hold the stretch for 10 to 30 seconds.
- Repeat on the other leg.

Reprinted, by permission, from J. Blahnik, 2004, *Full-Body Flexibility*, (Champaign, IL: Human Kinetics), 72.

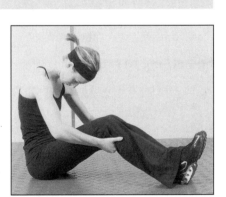

LYING KNEE HUG

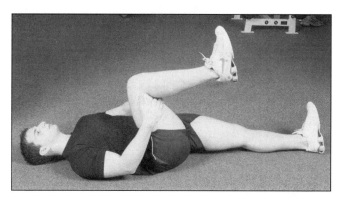

How to perform

- Lie with feet together. Bring one knee forward and up toward the chest.
- Start: Place the hands around the thigh and pull the knee into the chest.
- Finish: Release the stretch by putting the foot on the floor.
- Repeat as a continuous, controlled, fluid sequence 10 to 12 times, alternating legs.

Something to remember

- Don't round or arch the spine.

Reprinted, by permission, from J. Blahnik, 2004, *Full-Body Flexibility*, (Champaign, IL: Human Kinetics), 76.

ADDUCTORS

SEATED BUTTERFLY

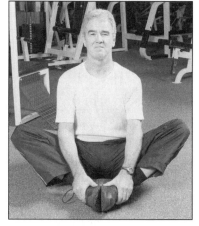

How to perform

- Sit on the floor with the soles of the feet together. Place the forearms or elbows on the inner thighs; bring the chest slightly toward the legs. Pivot from the hips and push the thighs toward the floor.
- Hold the stretch for 10 to 30 seconds.

Something to remember

- Don't round the spine.

Reprinted, by permission, from J. Blahnik, 2004, *Full-Body Flexibility*, (Champaign, IL: Human Kinetics), 86.

SIDE LUNGE

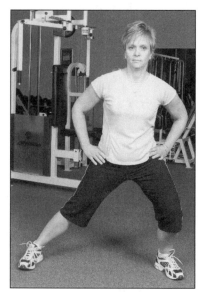

How to perform

- Stand with feet wide apart. Bend one knee and lunge to the same side, keeping the other leg straight.
- Don't round the spine.
- Hold the stretch for 10 to 30 seconds.
- Repeat on the other side.

Something to remember

- Don't extend the bent knee beyond the toes.
- Keep the upper body tall.

Reprinted, by permission, from J. Blahnik, 2004, *Full-Body Flexibility*, (Champaign, IL: Human Kinetics), 87.

ABDUCTORS

LYING LEG CROSSOVER

How to perform

- Lie on your back with your legs extended.
- Flex one knee, raise it to your chest, and grasp it with the opposite hand.
- Exhale and pull your knee across your body to the floor, keeping your elbows, head, and shoulders flat on the floor.

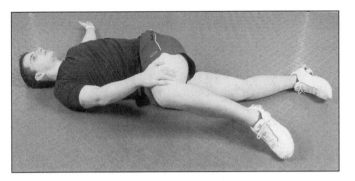

Reprinted, by permission, from M.J. Alter, 1998, *Sport Stretches,* 2nd ed. (Champaign, IL: Human Kinetics), 143.

QUADRICEPS

KNEE BEND

How to perform

- Stand with feet together. Bend one knee and hold the ankle with the same-side hand; pull the heel toward the gluteals.
- Hold the stretch for 10 to 30 seconds.
- Repeat on the other leg.
- Touch a wall or hold onto something for balance, if necessary.

Something to remember

- Hold the knees close together.

Reprinted, by permission, from J. Blahnik, 2004, *Full-Body Flexibility,* (Champaign, IL: Human Kinetics), 96.

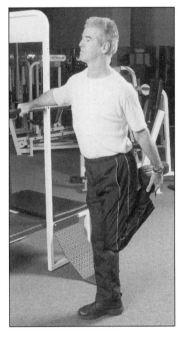

HURDLER STRETCH

How to perform

- Lie on your side, flex one knee, and raise your heel toward your buttocks.
- Exhale, grasp your raised ankle, and pull your heel toward your buttocks without overcompressing the knee.

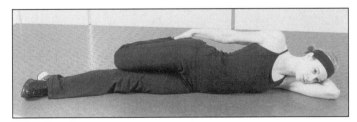

Something to remember

- To maximize the stretch, make sure the medial sides of your legs touch each other as your pelvis rotates backward (visualize pulling your tailbone between your legs).
- Do not arch your lower back or twist your pelvis.

Reprinted, by permission, from M.J. Alter, 1998, *Sport Stretch,* 2nd ed. (Champaign, IL: Human Kinetics), 129.

HAMSTRINGS

SEATED HIP HINGE

How to perform

- Sit on the floor with one leg straight and the other bent at the knee with the heel touching the inside of the opposite thigh.
- Lower the outside of the thigh and calf of the bent leg onto the floor.
- Exhale, keep the extended leg straight, and lower your upper torso onto your thigh.

Something to remember

- Try contracting your quadriceps to alleviate tension in your hamstrings.

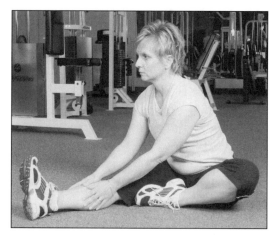

Reprinted, by permission, from M.J. Alter, 1998, *Sport Stretch,* 2nd ed. (Champaign, IL: Human Kinetics), 102.

LEG UP

How to perform

- Stand with feet together facing a bench or the back of a chair. Raise one leg and rest it on top of a bench or the back of the chair. Stand tall and straighten the knee.
- Hold the stretch for 10 to 30 seconds.
- Repeat on the other leg.
- Touch a wall or hold onto something for balance, if necessary.

Something to remember

- Don't lock the knee.

Reprinted, by permission, from J. Blahnik, 2004, *Full-Body Flexibility,* (Champaign, IL: Human Kinetics), 105.

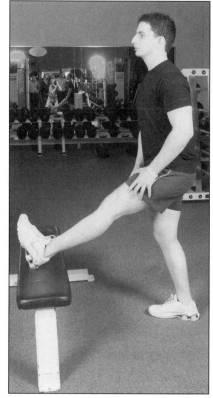

GASTROCNEMIUS

HEEL DROP

How to perform

- Place the ball of one foot on the edge of a step or curb. Push the heel down, keeping the knee straight. Place the other foot slightly in front.
- Hold the stretch for 10 to 30 seconds.
- Repeat on the other foot.
- Hold onto something for balance, if necessary.

Reprinted, by permission, from J. Blahnik, 2004, *Full-Body Flexibility,* (Champaign, IL: Human Kinetics), 112.

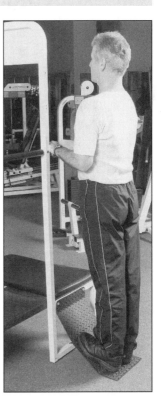

ACHILLES-SOLEUS

THINKER POSE

How to perform

- Kneel down on one knee and sit back on the heel. Place the opposite foot next to the knee, keeping the heel on the floor.
- Use the arms for balance.
- Hold the stretch for 10 to 30 seconds.
- Repeat on the other leg.

Something to remember

- Don't sit down too hard on the heel.

Reprinted, by permission, from J. Blahnik, 2004, *Full-Body Flexibility,* (Champaign, IL: Human Kinetics), 118.

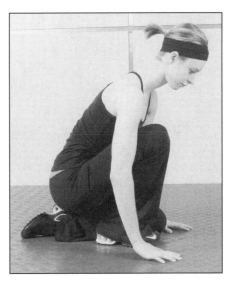

TIBIALIS ANTERIOR

TOE DROP

How to perform

- Place the top of one foot against the edge of a curb or step. Place the other foot in front. Press the back leg forward while pointing the toes.
- Hold the stretch for 10 to 30 seconds.
- Repeat on the other leg.
- Touch a wall or hold onto something for balance, if necessary.

Reprinted, by permission, from J. Blahnik, 2004, *Full-Body Flexibility,* (Champaign, IL: Human Kinetics), 123.

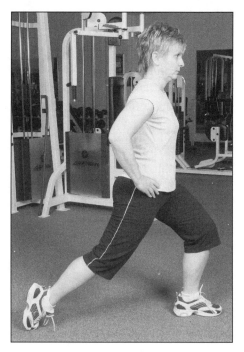

APPENDIX C

Fitness Norms for Health and Performance

CARDIOVASCULAR PROFILES

Table C. 1 **Resting and Maximal Heart Rates in Men and Women**

	Men					Women				
%	**20-29 Y**	**30-39 Y**	**40-49 Y**	**50-59 Y**	**60+ Y**	**20-29 Y**	**30-39 Y**	**40-49 Y**	**50-59 Y**	**60+ Y**
Resting heart rates (beats/min)										
90	50	50	50	50	52	55	55	55	55	52
80	54	55	54	55	55	59	58	60	60	57
70	58	58	58	58	58	60	62	62	61	60
60	60	60	60	60	60	63	65	64	64	62
50	63	63	62	63	62	65	68	66	67	64
40	66	65	65	65	65	70	70	70	69	66
30	70	68	69	68	68	72	74	72	72	72
20	72	72	72	72	72	75	76	76	75	74
10	80	77	78	77	77	84	82	80	83	79
n	358	1,538	1,826	1,046	267	115	280	260	162	43
$\bar{X}$	64	63	64	63	63	67	68	68	68	65
SD	12.5	11.0	11.5	11.0	10.4	11.2	11.5	10.7	11.7	9.6
Maximal heart rates (beats/min)										
90	205	200	196	188	184	203	196	192	185	176
80	200	198	191	183	175	198	192	186	180	165
70	199	194	188	180	170	194	189	183	176	160
60	197	191	185	176	165	190	185	180	173	155
50	194	189	182	173	162	188	184	177	170	153
40	192	186	180	170	159	186	182	173	167	150
30	188	183	176	166	152	182	180	170	162	145
20	183	180	171	160	145	180	176	166	160	140
10	179	174	164	150	131	172	170	158	152	126
n	371	1,632	1,898	1,087	249	119	309	286	169	46
$\bar{X}$	192	188	181	171	159	188	183	175	169	151
SD	12.2	11.7	13.3	15.9	19.5	11.8	14.8	14.8	14.5	17.5

Reprinted, by permission, from J. Hoffman, 2006, *Norms for fitness, performance, and health* (Champaign, IL: Human Kinetics), 121.

Data from the US Department of Health and Human Services.

ANTHROPOMETRY AND BODY COMPOSITION

Table C.2   **Waist-to-Hip Ratio Norms for Men and Women**

| | Risk for heart disease | | | | | | | |
| | Low | | Moderate | | High | | Very high | |
AGE (Y)	MEN	WOMEN	MEN	WOMEN	MEN	WOMEN	MEN	WOMEN
20-29	<0.83	<0.71	0.83-0.88	0.71-0.77	0.89-0.94	0.78-0.82	>0.94	>0.82
30-39	<0.84	<0.72	0.84-0.91	0.72-0.78	0.92-0.96	0.79-0.84	>0 .96	>0.84
40-49	<0 .88	<0.73	0.88-0.95	0.73-0.79	0.96-1.00	0.80-0.87	>1.00	>0.87
50-59	<0.90	<0.74	0.90-0.96	0.74-0.81	0.97-1.02	0.82-0.88	>1.02	>0.88
60-69	<0.91	<0.76	0.91-0.98	0.76-0.83	0.99-1.03	0.84-0.90	>1.03	>0.90

Adapted from G.A. Bray and D.S. Gray, 1988, "Obesity part I—Pathogenesis," *Western Journal of Medicine* 149:432.

MUSCULAR STRENGTH

Table C.3   **Descriptive Data for the Handgrip Dynamometer (in kg)**

POPULATION	GENDER	DOMINANT HAND	NONDOMINANT HAND	SOURCE
Baseball				
13 y	M	26.1 ± 6.6		Unpublished data
14 y	M	32.3 ± 7.2		Unpublished data
15 y	M	37.3 ± 6.7		Unpublished data
16 y	M	40.7 ± 6.5		Unpublished data
17 y	M	43.4 ± 7.3		Unpublished data
NAIA	M	45.2 ± 8.4	45.6 ± 6.8	Unpublished data
NCAA DII	M	57.0 ± 6.7		Hughes, Lyons, and Mayo 2004
Boxing				
Middleweight Italian amateurs	M	58.2 ± 6.9		Guidetti, Musulin, and Baldari 2002
Softball				
Masters	F	37.3 ± 6.9	38.4 ± 6.0	Terbizan et al. 1996
Tennis				
Ranked junior players (11.6 ± 0.6 y)	M	22.0 ± 5.8	18.4 ± 5.1	Roetart et al. 1992
Collegiate	F	36.6 ± 4.0	33.3 ± 2.2	Kraemer et al. 2003
Competitive (30.2 ± 5.8 y)	M	27.7 ± 2.7	22.2 ± 2.8	Ellenbecker 1991

Reprinted, by permission, from J. Hoffman, 2006, *Norms for fitness, performance, and health* (Champaign, IL: Human Kinetics), 28.

Table C.4 Percentile Ranks for Handgrip Strength (kg) in Recreationally Active Children

% RANK	7-8 Y RIGHT HAND	7-8 Y LEFT HAND	9-10 Y RIGHT HAND	9-10 Y LEFT HAND	11-12 Y RIGHT HAND	11-12 Y LEFT HAND
90	19.5	20.0	22.0	22.0	29.7	27.5
80	18.0	18.5	21.5	20.0	27.3	24.6
70	17.5	17.8	20.0	19.1	24.9	22.5
60	17.0	16.0	20.0	18.4	22.2	22.0
50	16.0	15.5	19.0	18.0	22.0	20.0
40	15.0	14.5	18.0	17.0	21.5	19.0
30	13.5	13.0	17.0	16.0	21.0	19.0
20	13.5	12.0	16.0	15.5	20.0	17.4
10	12.0	12.0	15.0	15.0	18.0	16.4
$\bar{X}$	16.0	15.5	18.9	18.0	23.0	21.2
SD	3.2	3.0	3.0	2.7	3.9	4.2
N	54	54	102	102	46	46

Reprinted, by permission, from J. Hoffman, 2006, *Norms for fitness, performance, and health* (Champaign, IL: Human Kinetics), 29.

Table C.5 Normative Values of Dominant Grip Strength (kg) in Adults

	20-29 Y M	20-29 Y F	30-39 Y M	30-39 Y F	40-49 Y M	40-49 Y F	50-59 Y M	50-59 Y F	60-69 Y M	60-69 Y F
Excellent	>54	>36	>53	>36	>51	>35	>49	>33	>49	>33
Good	51-54	33-36	50-53	34-36	48-51	33-35	46-49	31-33	46-49	31-33
Average	43-50	26-32	43-49	28-33	41-47	27-32	39-45	25-30	39-45	25-30
Fair	39-42	22-25	39-42	25-27	37-40	24-26	35-38	22-24	35-38	22-24
Poor	<39	<22	<39	<25	<37	<24	<35	<22	<35	<22

Adapted, by permission, from L.R. Gettman, 1993, Fitness testing. In *ACSM's resource manual for guidelines for exercise testing and prescription*, 2nd ed., edited by J.L. Durstine, et al. (Philadelphia, PA: Lippincott, Williams & Wilkins), 229-246.

MUSCULAR ENDURANCE

Table C.6   Push-Up Norms for Men and Women

| | Age (Y) | | | | | | | | | |
| | 20-29 | | 30-39 | | 40-49 | | 50-59 | | 60+ | |
PERCENTILE	M	F	M	F	M	F	M	F	M	F
90	57	42	46	36	36	28	30	25	26	17
80	47	36	39	31	30	24	25	21	23	15
70	41	32	34	28	26	20	21	19	21	14
60	37	30	30	24	24	18	19	17	18	12
50	33	26	27	21	21	15	15	13	15	8
40	29	23	24	19	18	13	13	12	10	5
30	26	20	20	15	15	10	10	9	8	3
20	22	17	17	11	11	6	9	6	6	2
10	18	12	13	8	9	2	6	1	4	0

Modified push-ups were used for women. Data are reported as total number of repetitions completed until exhaustion.

Adapted from D.C. Nieman, 1999, *Exercise testing & prescription: A health related approach*, 4th ed (Mountain View, CA: Mayfield Publishing), with permission of The McGraw-Hill Companies.

Table C.7   Percentiles by Age and Gender for Partial Curl-Up

| | Age (Y) | | | | | | | | | |
| | 20-29 | | 30-39 | | 40-49 | | 50-59 | | 60-69 | |
PERCENTILE	M	F	M	F	M	F	M	F	M	F
90	75	70	75	55	75	50	74	48	53	50
80	56	45	69	43	75	42	60	30	33	30
70	41	37	46	34	67	33	45	23	26	24
60	31	32	36	28	51	28	35	16	19	19
50	27	27	31	21	39	25	27	9	16	13
40	23	21	26	15	31	20	23	2	9	9
30	20	17	19	12	26	14	19	0	6	3
20	13	12	13	0	21	5	13	0	0	0
10	4	5	0	0	13	0	0	0	0	0

Reprinted, by permission, from American College of Sports Medicine, 2000, *ACSM's guidelines for exercise testing and prescription*, 6th ed. (Philadelphia, PA: Lippincott, Williams & Wilkins), 86. Data from *Canadian Standardized Test of Fitness and Operations Manual*, 3rd ed., Public Health Agency of Canada, 1986.

Table C.8 YMCA Norms for the Sit-Up Test in Adults

PERCENTILE	18-25 Y M	18-25 Y F	26-35 Y M	26-35 Y F	36-45 Y M	36-45 Y F	46-55 Y M	46-55 Y F	56-65 Y M	56-65 Y F	>65 Y M	>65 Y F
90	77	68	62	54	60	54	61	48	56	44	50	34
80	66	61	56	46	52	44	53	40	49	38	40	32
70	57	57	52	41	45	38	51	36	46	32	35	29
60	52	51	44	37	43	35	44	33	41	27	31	26
50	46	44	38	34	36	31	39	31	36	24	27	22
40	41	38	36	32	32	28	33	28	32	22	24	20
30	37	34	33	28	29	23	29	25	28	18	22	16
20	33	32	30	24	25	20	24	21	24	12	19	11
10	27	25	21	20	21	16	16	13	20	8	12	9

Values represent number of repetitions.

Reprinted from J.T. Cramer and J.W. Coburn, 2004, Fitness testing protocols and norms. In *NSCA's essentials of personal training,* edited by R.W. Earle and T.R. Baechle (Champaign, IL: Human Kinetics), 258; adapted from *YMCA fitness testing and assessment manual,* 4th edition, 2000.

FLEXIBILITY

Table C.9 Percentile Ranks for the Sit-and-Reach Test (cm)

% RANK	Age (Y) 20-29 M	20-29 F	30-39 M	30-39 F	40-49 M	40-49 F	50-59 M	50-59 F	60-69 M	60-69 F
90	39	40	37	39	34	37	35	37	32	34
80	35	37	34	36	31	33	29	34	27	31
70	33	35	31	34	27	32	26	32	23	28
60	30	33	29	32	25	30	24	29	21	27
50	28	31	26	30	22	28	22	27	19	25
40	26	29	24	28	20	26	19	26	15	23
30	23	26	21	25	17	23	15	23	13	21
20	20	23	18	22	13	21	12	20	11	20
10	15	19	14	18	9	16	9	16	8	15

Reprinted, by permission, from V.H. Heyward, 2002, *Advanced fitness assessment & exercise prescription,* 4th ed. (Champaign, IL: Human Kinetics), 236; from the *Canadian Standardized Test of Fitness (CSTF) Operations Manual,* 3rd ed., Public Health Agency of Canada, 1986. Adapted and reproduced with permission of the Minister of Public Works and Government Services, Canada, 2006.

Table C.10   Percentile Ranks for the Modified Sit-and-Reach Test

	Females							
	<18 Y		19-35 Y		36-49 Y		>50 Y	
% RANK	IN.	CM	IN.	CM	IN.	CM	IN.	CM
99	22.6	57.4	21.0	53.3	19.8	50.3	17.2	43.7
95	19.5	49.5	19.3	49.0	19.2	48.8	15.7	39.9
90	18.7	47.5	17.9	45.5	17.4	44.2	15.0	38.1
80	17.8	45.2	16.7	42.4	16.2	41.1	14.2	36.1
70	16.5	41.9	16.2	41.1	15.2	38.6	13.6	34.5
60	16.0	40.6	15.8	40.1	14.5	36.8	12.3	31.2
50	15.2	38.6	14.8	37.6	13.5	34.3	11.1	28.2
40	14.5	36.8	14.5	36.8	12.8	32.5	10.1	25.7
30	13.7	34.8	13.7	34.8	12.2	31.0	9.2	23.4
20	12.6	32.0	12.6	32.0	11.0	27.9	8.3	21.1
10	11.4	29.0	10.1	25.7	9.7	24.6	7.5	19.1

	Males							
	<18 Y		19-35 Y		36-49 Y		>50 Y	
% RANK	IN.	CM	IN.	CM	IN.	CM	IN.	CM
99	20.1	51.1	24.7	62.7	18.9	48.0	16.2	41.1
95	19.6	49.8	18.9	48.0	18.2	46.2	15.8	40.1
90	18.2	46.2	17.2	43.7	16.1	40.9	15.0	38.1
80	17.8	45.2	17.0	43.2	14.6	37.1	13.3	33.8
70	16.0	40.6	15.8	40.1	13.9	35.3	12.3	31.2
60	15.2	38.6	15.0	38.1	13.4	34.0	11.5	29.2
50	14.5	36.8	14.4	36.6	12.6	32.0	10.2	25.9
40	14.0	35.6	13.5	34.3	11.6	29.5	9.7	24.6
30	13.4	34.0	13.0	33.0	10.8	27.4	9.3	23.6
20	11.8	30.0	11.6	29.5	9.9	25.1	8.8	22.4
10	9.5	24.1	9.2	23.4	8.3	21.1	7.8	19.8

ENERGY EXPENDITURES

Table C.11 Energy Expenditures for Various Sports and Activities

DANCING	LB	99	110	121	132	143	154	165	176	187	198	209	220	231	242	253	264
	KG	45	50	55	60	65	70	75	80	85	90	95	100	105	110	115	120
	METS																
Aerobic, general	6.5	5.1	5.7	6.3	6.8	7.4	8.0	8.5	9.1	9.7	10.2	10.8	11.4	11.9	12.5	13.1	13.7
Aerobic, high impact	7.0	5.5	6.1	6.7	7.4	8.0	8.6	9.2	9.8	10.4	11.0	11.6	12.3	12.9	13.5	14.1	14.7
Aerobic, low impact	5.0	3.9	4.4	4.8	5.3	5.7	6.1	6.6	7.0	7.4	7.9	8.3	8.8	9.2	9.6	10.1	10.5
Aerobic, step with 10-12 in. (25.4-30.5 cm) step	10.0	7.9	8.8	9.6	10.5	11.4	12.3	13.1	14.0	14.9	15.8	16.6	17.5	18.4	19.3	20.1	21.0
Aerobic, step with 6-8 in. (15.2-20.3 cm) step	8.5	6.7	7.4	8.2	8.9	9.7	10.4	11.2	11.9	12.6	13.4	14.1	14.9	15.6	16.4	17.1	17.9
Ballet or modern	4.8	3.8	4.2	4.6	5.0	5.5	5.9	6.3	6.7	7.1	7.6	8.0	8.4	8.8	9.2	9.7	10.1
Ballroom, fast (disco, folk, square)	4.5	3.5	3.9	4.3	4.7	5.1	5.5	5.9	6.3	6.7	7.1	7.5	7.9	8.3	8.7	9.1	9.5
Ballroom, slow	3.0	2.4	2.6	2.9	3.2	3.4	3.7	3.9	4.2	4.5	4.7	5.0	5.3	5.5	5.8	6.0	6.3
General	4.5	3.5	3.9	4.3	4.7	5.1	5.5	5.9	6.3	6.7	7.1	7.5	7.9	8.3	8.7	9.1	9.5

(continued)

Table C.11 *(continued)*

EXERCISE	METS	99	110	121	132	143	154	165	176	187	198	209	220	231	242	253	264
	KG	45	50	55	60	65	70	75	80	85	90	95	100	105	110	115	120
BMX or mountain biking	8.5	6.7	7.4	8.2	8.9	9.7	10.4	11.2	11.9	12.6	13.4	14.1	14.9	15.6	16.4	17.1	17.9
General biking	8.0	6.3	7.0	7.7	8.4	9.1	9.8	10.5	11.2	11.9	12.6	13.3	14.0	14.7	15.4	16.1	16.8
<10 mph (16.09 km/h), leisure cycling	4.0	3.2	3.5	3.9	4.2	4.6	4.9	5.3	5.6	6.0	6.3	6.7	7.0	7.4	7.7	8.1	8.4
10-11.9 mph (16.09-19.15 km/h), leisure cycling, slow, light effort	6.0	4.7	5.3	5.8	6.3	6.8	7.4	7.9	8.4	8.9	9.5	10.0	10.5	11.0	11.6	12.1	12.6
12-13.9 mph (19.31-22.37 km/h), leisure cycling, moderate effort	8.0	6.3	7.0	7.7	8.4	9.1	9.8	10.5	11.2	11.9	12.6	13.3	14.0	14.7	15.4	16.1	16.8
14-15.9 mph (22.52-25.58 km/h), racing or leisure cycling, fast	10.0	7.9	8.8	9.6	10.5	11.4	12.3	13.1	14.0	14.9	15.8	16.6	17.5	18.4	19.3	20.1	21.0
16-19 mph (25.73-30.6 km/h), racing, not drafting	12.0	9.5	10.5	11.6	12.6	13.7	14.7	15.8	16.8	17.9	18.9	20.0	21.0	22.1	23.1	24.2	25.2
>20 mph (32.2 km/h), racing, not drafting	16.0	12.6	14.0	15.4	16.8	18.2	19.6	21.0	22.4	23.8	25.2	26.6	28.0	29.4	30.8	32.2	33.6

Activity																	
Bicycling, stationary, general	7.0	5.5	6.1	6.7	7.4	8.0	8.6	9.2	9.8	10.4	11.0	11.6	12.3	12.9	13.5	14.1	14.7
Bicycling, stationary, 50 W, very light effort	3.0	2.4	2.6	2.9	3.2	3.4	3.7	3.9	4.2	4.5	4.7	5.0	5.3	5.5	5.8	6.0	6.3
Bicycling, stationary, 100 W, light effort	5.5	4.3	4.8	5.3	5.8	6.3	6.7	7.2	7.7	8.2	8.7	9.1	9.6	10.1	10.6	11.1	11.6
Bicycling, stationary, 150 W, moderate effort	7.0	5.5	6.1	6.7	7.4	8.0	8.6	9.2	9.8	10.4	11.0	11.6	12.3	12.9	13.5	14.1	14.7
Bicycling, stationary, 200 W, vigorous effort	10.5	8.3	9.2	10.1	11.0	11.9	12.9	13.8	14.7	15.6	16.5	17.5	18.4	19.3	20.2	21.1	22.1
Bicycling, stationary, 250 W, very vigorous effort	12.5	9.8	10.9	12.0	13.1	14.2	15.3	16.4	17.5	18.6	19.7	20.8	21.9	23.0	24.1	25.2	26.3
Calisthenics (pushups, situps), heavy vigorous effort	8.0	6.3	7.0	7.7	8.4	9.1	9.8	10.5	11.2	11.9	12.6	13.3	14.0	14.7	15.4	16.1	16.8
Calisthenics, light or moderate effort	3.5	2.8	3.1	3.4	3.7	4.0	4.3	4.6	4.9	5.2	5.5	5.8	6.1	6.4	6.7	7.0	7.4
Circuit training	8.0	6.3	7.0	7.7	8.4	9.1	9.8	10.5	11.2	11.9	12.6	13.3	14.0	14.7	15.4	16.1	16.8
Powerlifting or bodybuilding	6.0	4.7	5.3	5.8	6.3	6.8	7.4	7.9	8.4	8.9	9.5	10.0	10.5	11.0	11.6	12.1	12.6
Rowing, stationary ergometer, general	7.0	5.5	6.1	6.7	7.4	8.0	8.6	9.2	9.8	10.4	11.0	11.6	12.3	12.9	13.5	14.1	14.7

(continued)

Table C.11 (continued)

EXERCISE	METS	99 / 45	110 / 50	121 / 55	132 / 60	143 / 65	154 / 70	165 / 75	176 / 80	187 / 85	198 / 90	209 / 95	220 / 100	231 / 105	242 / 110	253 / 115	264 / 120
Rowing, stationary, 50 W, light effort	3.5	2.8	3.1	3.4	3.7	4.0	4.3	4.6	4.9	5.2	5.5	5.8	6.1	6.4	6.7	7.0	7.4
Rowing, stationary, 100 W, moderate effort	7.0	5.5	6.1	6.7	7.4	8.0	8.6	9.2	9.8	10.4	11.0	11.6	12.3	12.9	13.5	14.1	14.7
Rowing, stationary, 150 W, vigorous effort	8.5	6.7	7.4	8.2	8.9	9.7	10.4	11.2	11.9	12.6	13.4	14.1	14.9	15.6	16.4	17.1	17.9
Rowing, stationary, 200 W, very vigorous effort	12.0	9.5	10.5	11.6	12.6	13.7	14.7	15.8	16.8	17.9	18.9	20.0	21.0	22.1	23.1	24.2	25.2
Ski machine, general	7.0	5.5	6.1	6.7	7.4	8.0	8.6	9.2	9.8	10.4	11.0	11.6	12.3	12.9	13.5	14.1	14.7
Slimnastics, jazzercise	6.0	4.7	5.3	5.8	6.3	6.8	7.4	7.9	8.4	8.9	9.5	10.0	10.5	11.0	11.6	12.1	12.6
Stretching	2.5	2.0	2.2	2.4	2.6	2.8	3.1	3.3	3.5	3.7	3.9	4.2	4.4	4.6	4.8	5.0	5.3
Teaching aerobic exercise class	6.0	4.7	5.3	5.8	6.3	6.8	7.4	7.9	8.4	8.9	9.5	10.0	10.5	11.0	11.6	12.1	12.6
Water aerobics, water calisthenics	4.0	3.2	3.5	3.9	4.2	4.6	4.9	5.3	5.6	6.0	6.3	6.7	7.0	7.4	7.7	8.1	8.4
Weightlifting	3.0	2.4	2.6	2.9	3.2	3.4	3.7	3.9	4.2	4.5	4.7	5.0	5.3	5.5	5.8	6.0	6.3

HOME ACTIVITIES	LB	99	110	121	132	143	154	165	176	187	198	209	220	231	242	253	264
	KG	45	50	55	60	65	70	75	80	85	90	95	100	105	110	115	120
	METS																
Carrying groceries upstairs	7.5	5.9	6.6	7.2	7.9	8.5	9.2	9.8	10.5	11.2	11.8	12.5	13.1	13.8	14.4	15.1	15.8
Cleaning, vigorous effort	3.0	2.4	2.6	2.9	3.2	3.4	3.7	3.9	4.2	4.5	4.7	5.0	5.3	5.5	5.8	6.0	6.3
Cooking	2.0	1.6	1.8	1.9	2.1	2.3	2.5	2.6	2.8	3.0	3.2	3.3	3.5	3.7	3.9	4.0	4.2
Household tasks, light effort	2.5	2.0	2.2	2.4	2.6	2.8	3.1	3.3	3.5	3.7	3.9	4.2	4.4	4.6	4.8	5.0	5.3
Household tasks, moderate effort	3.5	2.8	3.1	3.4	3.7	4.0	4.3	4.6	4.9	5.2	5.5	5.8	6.1	6.4	6.7	7.0	7.4
Household tasks, vigorous effort	4.0	3.2	3.5	3.9	4.2	4.6	4.9	5.3	5.6	6.0	6.3	6.7	7.0	7.4	7.7	8.1	8.4
Ironing	2.3	1.8	2.0	2.2	2.4	2.6	2.8	3.0	3.2	3.4	3.6	3.8	4.0	4.2	4.4	4.6	4.8
Mopping	3.5	2.8	3.1	3.4	3.7	4.0	4.3	4.6	4.9	5.2	5.5	5.8	6.1	6.4	6.7	7.0	7.4
Moving furniture	6.0	4.7	5.3	5.8	6.3	6.8	7.4	7.9	8.4	8.9	9.5	10.0	10.5	11	11.6	12.1	12.6
Scrubbing floors	3.8	3.0	3.3	3.7	4.0	4.3	4.7	5.0	5.3	5.7	6.0	6.3	6.7	7.0	7.3	7.6	8.0
Sweeping	3.3	2.6	2.9	3.2	3.5	3.8	4	4.3	4.6	4.9	5.2	5.5	5.8	6.1	6.4	6.6	6.9
Vacuuming	3.5	2.8	3.1	3.4	3.7	4.0	4.3	4.6	4.9	5.2	5.5	5.8	6.1	6.4	6.7	7.0	7.4
Washing dishes	2.3	1.8	2.0	2.2	2.4	2.6	2.8	3.0	3.2	3.4	3.6	3.8	4.0	4.2	4.4	4.6	4.8

(continued)

Table C.11 (continued)

HOME REPAIR	LB	99	110	121	132	143	154	165	176	187	198	209	220	231	242	253	264
	KG	45	50	55	60	65	70	75	80	85	90	95	100	105	110	115	120
	METS																
Automobile body work	4.0	3.2	3.5	3.9	4.2	4.6	4.9	5.3	5.6	6.0	6.3	6.7	7.0	7.4	7.7	8.1	8.4
Automobile repair	3.0	2.4	2.6	2.9	3.2	3.4	3.7	3.9	4.2	4.5	4.7	5.0	5.3	5.5	5.8	6.0	6.3
Carpentry, general, workshop	3.0	2.4	2.6	2.9	3.2	3.4	3.7	3.9	4.2	4.5	4.7	5.0	5.3	5.5	5.8	6.0	6.3
Carpentry, outside house	6.0	4.7	5.3	5.8	6.3	6.8	7.4	7.9	8.4	8.9	9.5	10.0	10.5	11.0	11.6	12.1	12.6
Carpentry, refinishing furniture	4.5	3.5	3.9	4.3	4.7	5.1	5.5	5.9	6.3	6.7	7.1	7.5	7.9	8.3	8.7	9.1	9.5
Carpentry, sawing hardwood	7.5	5.9	6.6	7.2	7.9	8.5	9.2	9.8	10.5	11.2	11.8	12.5	13.1	13.8	14.4	15.1	15.8
Caulking	5.0	3.9	4.4	4.8	5.3	5.7	6.1	6.6	7.0	7.4	7.9	8.3	8.8	9.2	9.6	10.1	10.5
Cleaning gutters	5.0	3.9	4.4	4.8	5.3	5.7	6.1	6.6	7.0	7.4	7.9	8.3	8.8	9.2	9.6	10.1	10.5
Hanging storm windows	5.0	3.9	4.4	4.8	5.3	5.7	6.1	6.6	7.0	7.4	7.9	8.3	8.8	9.2	9.6	10.1	10.5
Laying or removing carpet	4.5	3.5	3.9	4.3	4.7	5.1	5.5	5.9	6.3	6.7	7.1	7.5	7.9	8.3	8.7	9.1	9.5
Laying tile	4.5	3.5	3.9	4.3	4.7	5.1	5.5	5.9	6.3	6.7	7.1	7.5	7.9	8.3	8.7	9.1	9.5
Plastering, scraping, hanging sheetrock	3.0	2.4	2.6	2.9	3.2	3.4	3.7	3.9	4.2	4.5	4.7	5.0	5.3	5.5	5.8	6.0	6.3
Painting	4.5	3.5	3.9	4.3	4.7	5.1	5.5	5.9	6.3	6.7	7.1	7.5	7.9	8.3	8.7	9.1	9.5
Roofing	6.0	4.7	5.3	5.8	6.3	6.8	7.4	7.9	8.4	8.9	9.5	10.0	10.5	11.0	11.6	12.1	12.6
Sanding floors	4.5	3.5	3.9	4.3	4.7	5.1	5.5	5.9	6.3	6.7	7.1	7.5	7.9	8.3	8.7	9.1	9.5
Wiring, plumbing	3.0	2.4	2.6	2.9	3.2	3.4	3.7	3.9	4.2	4.5	4.7	5.0	5.3	5.5	5.8	6.0	6.3

LAWN AND GARDENING	LB	99	110	121	132	143	154	165	176	187	198	209	220	231	242	253	264
	KG	45	50	55	60	65	70	75	80	85	90	95	100	105	110	115	120
	METS																
Carrying or stacking lumber	5.0	3.9	4.4	4.8	5.3	5.7	6.1	6.6	7.0	7.4	7.9	8.3	8.8	9.2	9.6	10.1	10.5
Chopping wood	6.0	4.7	5.3	5.8	6.3	6.8	7.4	7.9	8.4	8.9	9.5	10	10.5	11.0	11.6	12.1	12.6
Clearing land	5.0	3.9	4.4	4.8	5.3	5.7	6.1	6.6	7.0	7.4	7.9	8.3	8.8	9.2	9.6	10.1	10.5
Digging sandbox	5.0	3.9	4.4	4.8	5.3	5.7	6.1	6.6	7.0	7.4	7.9	8.3	8.8	9.2	9.6	10.1	10.5
Fertilizing or seeding a lawn	2.5	2.0	2.2	2.4	2.6	2.8	3.1	3.3	3.5	3.7	3.9	4.2	4.4	4.6	4.8	5.0	5.3
Gardening with power tools	6.0	4.7	5.3	5.8	6.3	6.8	7.4	7.9	8.4	8.9	9.5	10.0	10.5	11.0	11.6	12.1	12.6
Gardening, general	4.0	3.2	3.5	3.9	4.2	4.6	4.9	5.3	5.6	6.0	6.3	6.7	7.0	7.4	7.7	8.1	8.4
Laying sod	5.0	3.9	4.4	4.8	5.3	5.7	6.1	6.6	7.0	7.4	7.9	8.3	8.8	9.2	9.6	10.1	10.5
Mowing lawn, general	5.5	4.3	4.8	5.3	5.8	6.3	6.7	7.2	7.7	8.2	8.7	9.1	9.6	10.1	10.6	11.1	11.6
Operating snow blower	4.5	3.5	3.9	4.3	4.7	5.1	5.5	5.9	6.3	6.7	7.1	7.5	7.9	8.3	8.7	9.1	9.5
Picking fruit	3.0	2.4	2.6	2.9	3.2	3.4	3.7	3.9	4.2	4.5	4.7	5.0	5.3	5.5	5.8	6.0	6.3
Planting	4.5	3.5	3.9	4.3	4.7	5.1	5.5	5.9	6.3	6.7	7.1	7.5	7.9	8.3	8.7	9.1	9.5
Raking lawn	4.3	3.4	3.8	4.1	4.5	4.9	5.3	5.6	6.0	6.4	6.8	7.1	7.5	7.9	8.3	8.7	9.0
Sacking grass, leaves	4.0	3.2	3.5	3.9	4.2	4.6	4.9	5.3	5.6	6.0	6.3	6.7	7.0	7.4	7.7	8.1	8.4
Trimming with power cutter	3.5	2.8	3.1	3.4	3.7	4.0	4.3	4.6	4.9	5.2	5.5	5.8	6.1	6.4	6.7	7.0	7.4
Trimming manually	4.5	3.5	3.9	4.3	4.7	5.1	5.5	5.9	6.3	6.7	7.1	7.5	7.9	8.3	8.7	9.1	9.5
Watering lawn	1.5	1.2	1.3	1.4	1.6	1.7	1.8	2.0	2.1	2.2	2.4	2.5	2.6	2.8	2.9	3.0	3.2

(continued)

277

Table C.11 *(continued)*

MUSIC PLAYING	LB	99	110	121	132	143	154	165	176	187	198	209	220	231	242	253	264
	KG	45	50	55	60	65	70	75	80	85	90	95	100	105	110	115	120
	METS																
Accordion	1.8	1.4	1.6	1.7	1.9	2.0	2.2	2.4	2.5	2.7	2.8	3.0	3.2	3.3	3.5	3.6	3.8
Cello	2.0	1.6	1.8	1.9	2.1	2.3	2.5	2.6	2.8	3.0	3.2	3.3	3.5	3.7	3.9	4.0	4.2
Conducting	2.5	2.0	2.2	2.4	2.6	2.8	3.1	3.3	3.5	3.7	3.9	4.2	4.4	4.6	4.8	5.0	5.3
Drums	4.0	3.2	3.5	3.9	4.2	4.6	4.9	5.3	5.6	6.0	6.3	6.7	7.0	7.4	7.7	8.1	8.4
Flute (sitting)	2.0	1.6	1.8	1.9	2.1	2.3	2.5	2.6	2.8	3.0	3.2	3.3	3.5	3.7	3.9	4.0	4.2
Horn	2.0	1.6	1.8	1.9	2.1	2.3	2.5	2.6	2.8	3.0	3.2	3.3	3.5	3.7	3.9	4.0	4.2
Piano or organ	2.5	2.0	2.2	2.4	2.6	2.8	3.1	3.3	3.5	3.7	3.9	4.2	4.4	4.6	4.8	5.0	5.3
Trombone	3.5	2.8	3.1	3.4	3.7	4.0	4.3	4.6	4.9	5.2	5.5	5.8	6.1	6.4	6.7	7.0	7.4
Trumpet	2.5	2.0	2.2	2.4	2.6	2.8	3.1	3.3	3.5	3.7	3.9	4.2	4.4	4.6	4.8	5.0	5.3
Violin	2.5	2.0	2.2	2.4	2.6	2.8	3.1	3.3	3.5	3.7	3.9	4.2	4.4	4.6	4.8	5.0	5.3
Woodwind	2.0	1.6	1.8	1.9	2.1	2.3	2.5	2.6	2.8	3.0	3.2	3.3	3.5	3.7	3.9	4.0	4.2
Guitar, classical, folk (sitting)	2.0	1.6	1.8	1.9	2.1	2.3	2.5	2.6	2.8	3.0	3.2	3.3	3.5	3.7	3.9	4.0	4.2
Guitar, rock 'n' roll (standing)	3.0	2.4	2.6	2.9	3.2	3.4	3.7	3.9	4.2	4.5	4.7	5.0	5.3	5.5	5.8	6.0	6.3
Marching band	4.0	3.2	3.5	3.9	4.2	4.6	4.9	5.3	5.6	6.0	6.3	6.7	7.0	7.4	7.7	8.1	8.4

OCCUPATION	METS	LB 99 / KG 45	110 / 50	121 / 55	132 / 60	143 / 65	154 / 70	165 / 75	176 / 80	187 / 85	198 / 90	209 / 95	220 / 100	231 / 105	242 / 110	253 / 115	264 / 120
Baking, moderate effort	4.0	3.2	3.5	3.9	4.2	4.6	4.9	5.3	5.6	6.0	6.3	6.7	7.0	7.4	7.7	8.1	8.4
Baking, light effort	2.5	2.0	2.2	2.4	2.6	2.8	3.1	3.3	3.5	3.7	3.9	4.2	4.4	4.6	4.8	5.0	5.3
Book binding	2.3	1.8	2.0	2.2	2.4	2.6	2.8	3.0	3.2	3.4	3.6	3.8	4.0	4.2	4.4	4.6	4.8
Building roads	6.0	4.7	5.3	5.8	6.3	6.8	7.4	7.9	8.4	8.9	9.5	10.0	10.5	11.0	11.6	12.1	12.6
Carpentry, general	3.5	2.8	3.1	3.4	3.7	4.0	4.3	4.6	4.9	5.2	5.5	5.8	6.1	6.4	6.7	7.0	7.4
Carrying heavy loads	8.0	6.3	7.0	7.7	8.4	9.1	9.8	10.5	11.2	11.9	12.6	13.3	14.0	14.7	15.4	16.1	16.8
Carrying moderate loads (16-40 lb or 7.3-18.1 kg)	8.0	6.3	7.0	7.7	8.4	9.1	9.8	10.5	11.2	11.9	12.6	13.3	14.0	14.7	15.4	16.1	16.8
Chambermaid, making bed (nursing)	2.5	2.0	2.2	2.4	2.6	2.8	3.1	3.3	3.5	3.7	3.9	4.2	4.4	4.6	4.8	5.0	5.3
Coal mining, general	6.0	4.7	5.3	5.8	6.3	6.8	7.4	7.9	8.4	8.9	9.5	10.0	10.5	11.0	11.6	12.1	12.6
Construction, outside, remodeling	5.5	4.3	4.8	5.3	5.8	6.3	6.7	7.2	7.7	8.2	8.7	9.1	9.6	10.1	10.6	11.1	11.6
Custodial work	3.5	2.8	3.1	3.4	3.7	4.0	4.3	4.6	4.9	5.2	5.5	5.8	6.1	6.4	6.7	7.0	7.4
Electrical work, plumbing	3.5	2.8	3.1	3.4	3.7	4.0	4.3	4.6	4.9	5.2	5.5	5.8	6.1	6.4	6.7	7.0	7.4
Farming, vigorous effort	8.0	6.3	7.0	7.7	8.4	9.1	9.8	10.5	11.2	11.9	12.6	13.3	14.0	14.7	15.4	16.1	16.8

(continued)

Table C.11 *(continued)*

OCCUPATION	LB	99	110	121	132	143	154	165	176	187	198	209	220	231	242	253	264
	KG	45	50	55	60	65	70	75	80	85	90	95	100	105	110	115	120
	METS																
Farming, driving tractor	2.5	2.0	2.2	2.4	2.6	2.8	3.1	3.3	3.5	3.7	3.9	4.2	4.4	4.6	4.8	5.0	5.3
Farming, feeding	4.0	3.2	3.5	3.9	4.2	4.6	4.9	5.3	5.6	6.0	6.3	6.7	7.0	7.4	7.7	8.1	8.4
Farming, forking straw bales	8.0	6.3	7.0	7.7	8.4	9.1	9.8	10.5	11.2	11.9	12.6	13.3	14.0	14.7	15.4	16.1	16.8
Farming, milking by hand	3.0	2.4	2.6	2.9	3.2	3.4	3.7	3.9	4.2	4.5	4.7	5.0	5.3	5.5	5.8	6.0	6.3
Farming, shoveling grain	5.5	4.3	4.8	5.3	5.8	6.3	6.7	7.2	7.7	8.2	8.7	9.1	9.6	10.1	10.6	11.1	11.6
Firefighter, general	12.0	9.5	10.5	11.6	12.6	13.7	14.7	15.8	16.8	17.9	18.9	20.0	21.0	22.1	23.1	24.2	25.2
Forestry, chopping, fast	17.0	13.4	14.9	16.4	17.9	19.3	20.8	22.3	23.8	25.3	26.8	28.3	29.8	31.2	32.7	34.2	35.7
Forestry, chopping, slow	5.0	3.9	4.4	4.8	5.3	5.7	6.1	6.6	7.0	7.4	7.9	8.3	8.8	9.2	9.6	10.1	10.5
Forestry, barking trees	7.0	5.5	6.1	6.7	7.4	8.0	8.6	9.2	9.8	10.4	11.0	11.6	12.3	12.9	13.5	14.1	14.7
Forestry, carrying logs	11.0	8.7	9.6	10.6	11.6	12.5	13.5	14.4	15.4	16.4	17.3	18.3	19.3	20.2	21.2	22.1	23.1
Forestry, felling trees	8.0	6.3	7.0	7.7	8.4	9.1	9.8	10.5	11.2	11.9	12.6	13.3	14.0	14.7	15.4	16.1	16.8
Forestry, general	8.0	6.3	7.0	7.7	8.4	9.1	9.8	10.5	11.2	11.9	12.6	13.3	14.0	14.7	15.4	16.1	16.8
Forestry, hoeing	5.0	3.9	4.4	4.8	5.3	5.7	6.1	6.6	7.0	7.4	7.9	8.3	8.8	9.2	9.6	10.1	10.5
Forestry, planting	6.0	4.7	5.3	5.8	6.3	6.8	7.4	7.9	8.4	8.9	9.5	10.0	10.5	11.0	11.6	12.1	12.6

OCCUPATION	LB	99	110	121	132	143	154	165	176	187	198	209	220	231	242	253	264
	KG	45	50	55	60	65	70	75	80	85	90	95	100	105	110	115	120
	METS																
Forestry, hand sawing	7.0	5.5	6.1	6.7	7.4	8.0	8.6	9.2	9.8	10.4	11.0	11.6	12.3	12.9	13.5	14.1	14.7
Forestry, power sawing	4.5	3.5	3.9	4.3	4.7	5.1	5.5	5.9	6.3	6.7	7.1	7.5	7.9	8.3	8.7	9.1	9.5
Forestry, trimming trees	9.0	7.1	7.9	8.7	9.5	10.2	11.0	11.8	12.6	13.4	14.2	15.0	15.8	16.5	17.3	18.1	18.9
Forestry, weeding	4.0	3.2	3.5	3.9	4.2	4.6	4.9	5.3	5.6	6.0	6.3	6.7	7.0	7.4	7.7	8.1	8.4
Locksmith	3.5	2.8	3.1	3.4	3.7	4.0	4.3	4.6	4.9	5.2	5.5	5.8	6.1	6.4	6.7	7.0	7.4
Machine tooling, machining	2.5	2.0	2.2	2.4	2.6	2.8	3.1	3.3	3.5	3.7	3.9	4.2	4.4	4.6	4.8	5.0	5.3
Machine tooling, tapping and drilling	4.0	3.2	3.5	3.9	4.2	4.6	4.9	5.3	5.6	6.0	6.3	6.7	7.0	7.4	7.7	8.1	8.4
Machine tooling, welding	3.0	2.4	2.6	2.9	3.2	3.4	3.7	3.9	4.2	4.5	4.7	5.0	5.3	5.5	5.8	6.0	6.3
Masonry	7.0	5.5	6.1	6.7	7.4	8.0	8.6	9.2	9.8	10.4	11.0	11.6	12.3	12.9	13.5	14.1	14.7
Masseur, masseuse	4.0	3.2	3.5	3.9	4.2	4.6	4.9	5.3	5.6	6.0	6.3	6.7	7.0	7.4	7.7	8.1	8.4
Operating heavy duty equipment	2.5	2.0	2.2	2.4	2.6	2.8	3.1	3.3	3.5	3.7	3.9	4.2	4.4	4.6	4.8	5.0	5.3
Orange grove work	4.5	3.5	3.9	4.3	4.7	5.1	5.5	5.9	6.3	6.7	7.1	7.5	7.9	8.3	8.7	9.1	9.5
Printing (standing)	2.3	1.8	2.0	2.2	2.4	2.6	2.8	3.0	3.2	3.4	3.6	3.8	4.0	4.2	4.4	4.6	4.8
Shoveling, digging ditches	8.5	6.7	7.4	8.2	8.9	9.7	10.4	11.2	11.9	12.6	13.4	14.1	14.9	15.6	16.4	17.1	17.9

(continued)

Table C.11 (continued)

OCCUPATION	LB	99	110	121	132	143	154	165	176	187	198	209	220	231	242	253	264
	KG	45	50	55	60	65	70	75	80	85	90	95	100	105	110	115	120
	METS																
Shoveling, >16 lb/min (7.3 kg/min)	9.0	7.1	7.9	8.7	9.5	10.2	11.0	11.8	12.6	13.4	14.2	15.0	15.8	16.5	17.3	18.1	18.9
Shoveling, <10 lb/min (4.5 kg/min)	6.0	4.7	5.3	5.8	6.3	6.8	7.4	7.9	8.4	8.9	9.5	10.0	10.5	11.0	11.6	12.1	12.6
Shoveling, 10-15 lb/min (4.5-6.8 kg/min)	7.0	5.5	6.1	6.7	7.4	8.0	8.6	9.2	9.8	10.4	11.0	11.6	12.3	12.9	13.5	14.1	14.7
Standing, light (bartender, store clerk)	2.3	1.8	2.0	2.2	2.4	2.6	2.8	3.0	3.2	3.4	3.6	3.8	4.0	4.2	4.4	4.6	4.8
Steel mill, general	8.0	6.3	7.0	7.7	8.4	9.1	9.8	10.5	11.2	11.9	12.6	13.3	14.0	14.7	15.4	16.1	16.8
Tailoring, general	2.5	2.0	2.2	2.4	2.6	2.8	3.1	3.3	3.5	3.7	3.9	4.2	4.4	4.6	4.8	5.0	5.3
Using heavy power tools (jackhammers)	6.0	4.7	5.3	5.8	6.3	6.8	7.4	7.9	8.4	8.9	9.5	10.0	10.5	11.0	11.6	12.1	12.6
Using heavy tools (not power)	8.0	6.3	7.0	7.7	8.4	9.1	9.8	10.5	11.2	11.9	12.6	13.3	14.0	14.7	15.4	16.1	16.8
Teaching physical education	4.0	3.2	3.5	3.9	4.2	4.6	4.9	5.3	5.6	6.0	6.3	6.7	7.0	7.4	7.7	8.1	8.4

RUNNING	LB	99	110	121	132	143	154	165	176	187	198	209	220	231	242	253	264
	KG	45	50	55	60	65	70	75	80	85	90	95	100	105	110	115	120
	METS																
Jogging, general	7.0	5.5	6.1	6.7	7.4	8.0	8.6	9.2	9.8	10.4	11.0	11.6	12.3	12.9	13.5	14.1	14.7
Jogging, on a minitrampoline	4.5	3.5	3.9	4.3	4.7	5.1	5.5	5.9	6.3	6.7	7.1	7.5	7.9	8.3	8.7	9.1	9.5
Running, 5 mph (8.0 km/h or 12 min/mi)	8.0	6.3	7.0	7.7	8.4	9.1	9.8	10.5	11.2	11.9	12.6	13.3	14.0	14.7	15.4	16.1	16.8
Running, 5.2 mph (8.37 km/h or 11.5 min/mi)	9.0	7.1	7.9	8.7	9.5	10.2	11.0	11.8	12.6	13.4	14.2	15.0	15.8	16.5	17.3	18.1	18.9
Running, 6 mph (9.6 km/h or 10 min/mi)	10.0	7.9	8.8	9.6	10.5	11.4	12.3	13.1	14.0	14.9	15.8	16.6	17.5	18.4	19.3	20.1	21.0
Running, 6.7 mph (10.78 km/h or 9 min/mi)	11.0	8.7	9.6	10.6	11.6	12.5	13.5	14.4	15.4	16.4	17.3	18.3	19.3	20.2	21.2	22.1	23.1
Running, 7 mph (11.3 km/h or 8.5 min/mi)	11.5	9.1	10.1	11.1	12.1	13.1	14.1	15.1	16.1	17.1	18.1	19.1	20.1	21.1	22.1	23.1	24.2
Running, 7.5 mph (12.07 km/h or 8 min/mi)	12.5	9.8	10.9	12.0	13.1	14.2	15.3	16.4	17.5	18.6	19.7	20.8	21.9	23.0	24.1	25.2	26.3
Running, 8 mph (12.8 km/h or 7.5 min/mi)	13.5	10.6	11.8	13.0	14.2	15.4	16.5	17.7	18.9	20.1	21.3	22.4	23.6	24.8	26.0	27.2	28.4

(continued)

Table C.11 (continued)

RUNNING	LB	99	110	121	132	143	154	165	176	187	198	209	220	231	242	253	264
	KG	45	50	55	60	65	70	75	80	85	90	95	100	105	110	115	120
	METS																
Running, 8.6 mph (13.84 km/h or 7 min/mi)	14.0	11.0	12.3	13.5	14.7	15.9	17.2	18.4	19.6	20.8	22.1	23.3	24.5	25.7	27.0	28.2	29.4
Running, 9 mph (14.5 km/h or 6.5 min/mi)	15.0	11.8	13.1	14.4	15.8	17.1	18.4	19.7	21.0	22.3	23.6	24.9	26.3	27.6	28.9	30.2	31.5
Running, 10 mph (16.1 km/h or 6 min/mi)	16.0	12.6	14.0	15.4	16.8	18.2	19.6	21.0	22.4	23.8	25.2	26.6	28.0	29.4	30.8	32.2	33.6
Running, 10.9 mph (17.54 km/h or 5.5 min/mi)	18.0	14.2	15.8	17.3	18.9	20.5	22.1	23.6	25.2	26.8	28.4	29.9	31.5	33.1	34.7	36.2	37.8
Running, cross country	9.0	7.1	7.9	8.7	9.5	10.2	11.0	11.8	12.6	13.4	14.2	15.0	15.8	16.5	17.3	18.1	18.9
Running, stairs	15.0	11.8	13.1	14.4	15.8	17.1	18.4	19.7	21.0	22.3	23.6	24.9	26.3	27.6	28.9	30.2	31.5
Running, track practice	10.0	7.9	8.8	9.6	10.5	11.4	12.3	13.1	14.0	14.9	15.8	16.6	17.5	18.4	19.3	20.1	21.0

SPORTS	LB	99	110	121	132	143	154	165	176	187	198	209	220	231	242	253	264
	KG	45	50	55	60	65	70	75	80	85	90	95	100	105	110	115	120
	METS																
Archery (non-hunting)	3.5	2.8	3.1	3.4	3.7	4.0	4.3	4.6	4.9	5.2	5.5	5.8	6.1	6.4	6.7	7.0	7.4
Badminton, competitive	7.0	5.5	6.1	6.7	7.4	8.0	8.6	9.2	9.8	10.4	11.0	11.6	12.3	12.9	13.5	14.1	14.7
Badminton, recreational	4.5	3.5	3.9	4.3	4.7	5.1	5.5	5.9	6.3	6.7	7.1	7.5	7.9	8.3	8.7	9.1	9.5
Basketball, game	8.0	6.3	7.0	7.7	8.4	9.1	9.8	10.5	11.2	11.9	12.6	13.3	14.0	14.7	15.4	16.1	16.8
Basketball, officiating	7.0	5.5	6.1	6.7	7.4	8.0	8.6	9.2	9.8	10.4	11.0	11.6	12.3	12.9	13.5	14.1	14.7
Basketball, shooting baskets	4.5	3.5	3.9	4.3	4.7	5.1	5.5	5.9	6.3	6.7	7.1	7.5	7.9	8.3	8.7	9.1	9.5
Basketball, wheelchair	6.5	5.1	5.7	6.3	6.8	7.4	8.0	8.5	9.1	9.7	10.2	10.8	11.4	11.9	12.5	13.1	13.7
Billiards	2.5	2.0	2.2	2.4	2.6	2.8	3.1	3.3	3.5	3.7	3.9	4.2	4.4	4.6	4.8	5.0	5.3
Bowling	3.0	2.4	2.6	2.9	3.2	3.4	3.7	3.9	4.2	4.5	4.7	5.0	5.3	5.5	5.8	6.0	6.3
Boxing, punching bag	6.0	4.7	5.3	5.8	6.3	6.8	7.4	7.9	8.4	8.9	9.5	10.0	10.5	11.0	11.6	12.1	12.6
Boxing, sparring	9.0	7.1	7.9	8.7	9.5	10.2	11.0	11.8	12.6	13.4	14.2	15.0	15.8	16.5	17.3	18.1	18.9
Coaching	4.0	3.2	3.5	3.9	4.2	4.6	4.9	5.3	5.6	6.0	6.3	6.7	7.0	7.4	7.7	8.1	8.4
Cricket	5.0	3.9	4.4	4.8	5.3	5.7	6.1	6.6	7.0	7.4	7.9	8.3	8.8	9.2	9.6	10.1	10.5
Croquet	2.5	2.0	2.2	2.4	2.6	2.8	3.1	3.3	3.5	3.7	3.9	4.2	4.4	4.6	4.8	5.0	5.3
Curling	4.0	3.2	3.5	3.9	4.2	4.6	4.9	5.3	5.6	6.0	6.3	6.7	7.0	7.4	7.7	8.1	8.4

(continued)

Table C.11 (continued)

SPORTS	METS	99 / 45	110 / 50	121 / 55	132 / 60	143 / 65	154 / 70	165 / 75	176 / 80	187 / 85	198 / 90	209 / 95	220 / 100	231 / 105	242 / 110	253 / 115	264 / 120
Darts	2.5	2.0	2.2	2.4	2.6	2.8	3.1	3.3	3.5	3.7	3.9	4.2	4.4	4.6	4.8	5.0	5.3
Fencing	6.0	4.7	5.3	5.8	6.3	6.8	7.4	7.9	8.4	8.9	9.5	10.0	10.5	11.0	11.6	12.1	12.6
Football, competitive	9.0	7.1	7.9	8.7	9.5	10.2	11.0	11.8	12.6	13.4	14.2	15.0	15.8	16.5	17.3	18.1	18.9
Football, touch, flag	8.0	6.3	7.0	7.7	8.4	9.1	9.8	10.5	11.2	11.9	12.6	13.3	14.0	14.7	15.4	16.1	16.8
Football or baseball, playing catch	2.5	2.0	2.2	2.4	2.6	2.8	3.1	3.3	3.5	3.7	3.9	4.2	4.4	4.6	4.8	5.0	5.3
Frisbee, catch	3.0	2.4	2.6	2.9	3.2	3.4	3.7	3.9	4.2	4.5	4.7	5.0	5.3	5.5	5.8	6.0	6.3
Frisbee, ultimate	8.0	6.3	7.0	7.7	8.4	9.1	9.8	10.5	11.2	11.9	12.6	13.3	14.0	14.7	15.4	16.1	16.8
Golf	4.5	3.5	3.9	4.3	4.7	5.1	5.5	5.9	6.3	6.7	7.1	7.5	7.9	8.3	8.7	9.1	9.5
Golf, miniature, driving range	3.0	2.4	2.6	2.9	3.2	3.4	3.7	3.9	4.2	4.5	4.7	5.0	5.3	5.5	5.8	6.0	6.3
Gymnastics	4.0	3.2	3.5	3.9	4.2	4.6	4.9	5.3	5.6	6.0	6.3	6.7	7.0	7.4	7.7	8.1	8.4
Handball	12.0	9.5	10.5	11.6	12.6	13.7	14.7	15.8	16.8	17.9	18.9	20.0	21.0	22.1	23.1	24.2	25.2
Handball, team	8.0	6.3	7.0	7.7	8.4	9.1	9.8	10.5	11.2	11.9	12.6	13.3	14.0	14.7	15.4	16.1	16.8
Hang gliding	3.5	2.8	3.1	3.4	3.7	4.0	4.3	4.6	4.9	5.2	5.5	5.8	6.1	6.4	6.7	7.0	7.4
Hockey, field	8.0	6.3	7.0	7.7	8.4	9.1	9.8	10.5	11.2	11.9	12.6	13.3	14.0	14.7	15.4	16.1	16.8
Hockey, ice	8.0	6.3	7.0	7.7	8.4	9.1	9.8	10.5	11.2	11.9	12.6	13.3	14.0	14.7	15.4	16.1	16.8

SPORTS	LB	99	110	121	132	143	154	165	176	187	198	209	220	231	242	253	264
	KG	45	50	55	60	65	70	75	80	85	90	95	100	105	110	115	120
	METS																
Horseback riding	4.0	3.2	3.5	3.9	4.2	4.6	4.9	5.3	5.6	6.0	6.3	6.7	7.0	7.4	7.7	8.1	8.4
In-line skating	12.5	9.8	10.9	12.0	13.1	14.2	15.3	16.4	17.5	18.6	19.7	20.8	21.9	23.0	24.1	25.2	26.3
Kickball	7.0	5.5	6.1	6.7	7.4	8.0	8.6	9.2	9.8	10.4	11.0	11.6	12.3	12.9	13.5	14.1	14.7
Lacrosse	8.0	6.3	7.0	7.7	8.4	9.1	9.8	10.5	11.2	11.9	12.6	13.3	14.0	14.7	15.4	16.1	16.8
Martial arts	10.0	7.9	8.8	9.6	10.5	11.4	12.3	13.1	14.0	14.9	15.8	16.6	17.5	18.4	19.3	20.1	21.0
Motor cross	4.0	3.2	3.5	3.9	4.2	4.6	4.9	5.3	5.6	6.0	6.3	6.7	7.0	7.4	7.7	8.1	8.4
Orienteering	9.0	7.1	7.9	8.7	9.5	10.2	11.0	11.8	12.6	13.4	14.2	15.0	15.8	16.5	17.3	18.1	18.9
Paddleball, recreational	6.0	4.7	5.3	5.8	6.3	6.8	7.4	7.9	8.4	8.9	9.5	10.0	10.5	11.0	11.6	12.1	12.6
Paddleball, competitive	10.0	7.9	8.8	9.6	10.5	11.4	12.3	13.1	14.0	14.9	15.8	16.6	17.5	18.4	19.3	20.1	21.0
Polo	8.0	6.3	7.0	7.7	8.4	9.1	9.8	10.5	11.2	11.9	12.6	13.3	14.0	14.7	15.4	16.1	16.8
Racquetball, recreational	7.0	5.5	6.1	6.7	7.4	8.0	8.6	9.2	9.8	10.4	11.0	11.6	12.3	12.9	13.5	14.1	14.7
Racquetball, competitive	10.0	7.9	8.8	9.6	10.5	11.4	12.3	13.1	14.0	14.9	15.8	16.6	17.5	18.4	19.3	20.1	21.0
Rappelling	8.0	6.3	7.0	7.7	8.4	9.1	9.8	10.5	11.2	11.9	12.6	13.3	14.0	14.7	15.4	16.1	16.8
Rock climbing	11.0	8.7	9.6	10.6	11.6	12.5	13.5	14.4	15.4	16.4	17.3	18.3	19.3	20.2	21.2	22.1	23.1
Rope jumping, fast	12.0	9.5	10.5	11.6	12.6	13.7	14.7	15.8	16.8	17.9	18.9	20.0	21.0	22.1	23.1	24.2	25.2
Rope jumping, moderate	10.0	7.9	8.8	9.6	10.5	11.4	12.3	13.1	14.0	14.9	15.8	16.6	17.5	18.4	19.3	20.1	21.0

(continued)

Table C.11 *(continued)*

SPORTS	LB	99	110	121	132	143	154	165	176	187	198	209	220	231	242	253	264
	KG	45	50	55	60	65	70	75	80	85	90	95	100	105	110	115	120
	METS																
Rope jumping, slow	8.0	6.3	7.0	7.7	8.4	9.1	9.8	10.5	11.2	11.9	12.6	13.3	14.0	14.7	15.4	16.1	16.8
Rugby	10.0	7.9	8.8	9.6	10.5	11.4	12.3	13.1	14.0	14.9	15.8	16.6	17.5	18.4	19.3	20.1	21.0
Shuffleboard	3.0	2.4	2.6	2.9	3.2	3.4	3.7	3.9	4.2	4.5	4.7	5.0	5.3	5.5	5.8	6.0	6.3
Skateboarding	5.0	3.9	4.4	4.8	5.3	5.7	6.1	6.6	7.0	7.4	7.9	8.3	8.8	9.2	9.6	10.1	10.5
Skating, roller	7.0	5.5	6.1	6.7	7.4	8.0	8.6	9.2	9.8	10.4	11.0	11.6	12.3	12.9	13.5	14.1	14.7
Skydiving	3.5	2.8	3.1	3.4	3.7	4.0	4.3	4.6	4.9	5.2	5.5	5.8	6.1	6.4	6.7	7.0	7.4
Soccer, competitive	10.0	7.9	8.8	9.6	10.5	11.4	12.3	13.1	14.0	14.9	15.8	16.6	17.5	18.4	19.3	20.1	21.0
Soccer, recreational	7.0	5.5	6.1	6.7	7.4	8.0	8.6	9.2	9.8	10.4	11.0	11.6	12.3	12.9	13.5	14.1	14.7
Softball or baseball	5.0	3.9	4.4	4.8	5.3	5.7	6.1	6.6	7.0	7.4	7.9	8.3	8.8	9.2	9.6	10.1	10.5
Softball, pitching	6.0	4.7	5.3	5.8	6.3	6.8	7.4	7.9	8.4	8.9	9.5	10.0	10.5	11.0	11.6	12.1	12.6
Squash	12.0	9.5	10.5	11.6	12.6	13.7	14.7	15.8	16.8	17.9	18.9	20.0	21.0	22.1	23.1	24.2	25.2
Table tennis, ping pong	4.0	3.2	3.5	3.9	4.2	4.6	4.9	5.3	5.6	6.0	6.3	6.7	7.0	7.4	7.7	8.1	8.4
Tai chi	4.0	3.2	3.5	3.9	4.2	4.6	4.9	5.3	5.6	6.0	6.3	6.7	7.0	7.4	7.7	8.1	8.4
Tennis, general	7.0	5.5	6.1	6.7	7.4	8.0	8.6	9.2	9.8	10.4	11.0	11.6	12.3	12.9	13.5	14.1	14.7
Tennis, doubles	6.0	4.7	5.3	5.8	6.3	6.8	7.4	7.9	8.4	8.9	9.5	10.0	10.5	11.0	11.6	12.1	12.6

SPORTS	LB	99	110	121	132	143	154	165	176	187	198	209	220	231	242	253	264
	KG	45	50	55	60	65	70	75	80	85	90	95	100	105	110	115	120
	METS																
Tennis, singles	8.0	6.3	7.0	7.7	8.4	9.1	9.8	10.5	11.2	11.9	12.6	13.3	14.0	14.7	15.4	16.1	16.8
Track and field, jumpers	6.0	4.7	5.3	5.8	6.3	6.8	7.4	7.9	8.4	8.9	9.5	10.0	10.5	11.0	11.6	12.1	12.6
Track and field, steeplechase, hurdles	10.0	7.9	8.8	9.6	10.5	11.4	12.3	13.1	14.0	14.9	15.8	16.6	17.5	18.4	19.3	20.1	21.0
Track and field, throwing	4.0	3.2	3.5	3.9	4.2	4.6	4.9	5.3	5.6	6.0	6.3	6.7	7.0	7.4	7.7	8.1	8.4
Trampoline	3.5	2.8	3.1	3.4	3.7	4.0	4.3	4.6	4.9	5.2	5.5	5.8	6.1	6.4	6.7	7.0	7.4
Volleyball	4.0	3.2	3.5	3.9	4.2	4.6	4.9	5.3	5.6	6.0	6.3	6.7	7.0	7.4	7.7	8.1	8.4
Volleyball, beach	8.0	6.3	7.0	7.7	8.4	9.1	9.8	10.5	11.2	11.9	12.6	13.3	14.0	14.7	15.4	16.1	16.8
Volleyball, competitive	8.0	6.3	7.0	7.7	8.4	9.1	9.8	10.5	11.2	11.9	12.6	13.3	14.0	14.7	15.4	16.1	16.8
Volleyball, recreational	3.0	2.4	2.6	2.9	3.2	3.4	3.7	3.9	4.2	4.5	4.7	5.0	5.3	5.5	5.8	6.0	6.3
Wallyball	7.0	5.5	6.1	6.7	7.4	8.0	8.6	9.2	9.8	10.4	11.0	11.6	12.3	12.9	13.5	14.1	14.7
Wrestling	6.0	4.7	5.3	5.8	6.3	6.8	7.4	7.9	8.4	8.9	9.5	10.0	10.5	11.0	11.6	12.1	12.6

(continued)

Table C.11 (continued)

WALKING	METS	99 / 45	110 / 50	121 / 55	132 / 60	143 / 65	154 / 70	165 / 75	176 / 80	187 / 85	198 / 90	209 / 95	220 / 100	231 / 105	242 / 110	253 / 115	264 / 120
Backpacking	7.0	5.5	6.1	6.7	7.4	8.0	8.6	9.2	9.8	10.4	11.0	11.6	12.3	12.9	13.5	14.1	14.7
Carrying 1-15 lb (0.5-6.8 kg) load	5.0	3.9	4.4	4.8	5.3	5.7	6.1	6.6	7.0	7.4	7.9	8.3	8.8	9.2	9.6	10.1	10.5
Carrying 16-24 lb (7.3-10.9 kg) load	6.0	4.7	5.3	5.8	6.3	6.8	7.4	7.9	8.4	8.9	9.5	10.0	10.5	11.0	11.6	12.1	12.6
Carrying 25-49 lb (11.3-22.2 kg) load	8.0	6.3	7.0	7.7	8.4	9.1	9.8	10.5	11.2	11.9	12.6	13.3	14.0	14.7	15.4	16.1	16.8
Carrying 50-74 lb (22.7-33.6 kg) load	10.0	7.9	8.8	9.6	10.5	11.4	12.3	13.1	14.0	14.9	15.8	16.6	17.5	18.4	19.3	20.1	21.0
Carrying 74+ lb (33.6 kg) load	12.0	9.5	10.5	11.6	12.6	13.7	14.7	15.8	16.8	17.9	18.9	20.0	21.0	22.1	23.1	24.2	25.2
Climbing hills with 0-9 lb (0-4.1 kg) load	7.0	5.5	6.1	6.7	7.4	8.0	8.6	9.2	9.8	10.4	11.0	11.6	12.3	12.9	13.5	14.1	14.7
Climbing hills with 10-20 lb (4.5-9.1 kg) load	7.5	5.9	6.6	7.2	7.9	8.5	9.2	9.8	10.5	11.2	11.8	12.5	13.1	13.8	14.4	15.1	15.8
Climbing hills with 21-42 lb (9.5-19.1 kg) load	8.0	6.3	7.0	7.7	8.4	9.1	9.8	10.5	11.2	11.9	12.6	13.3	14.0	14.7	15.4	16.1	16.8
Climbing hills with 42+ lb (19.1+ kg) load	9.0	7.1	7.9	8.7	9.5	10.2	11.0	11.8	12.6	13.4	14.2	15.0	15.8	16.5	17.3	18.1	18.9

WALKING	LB / METS	99 / 45	110 / 50	121 / 55	132 / 60	143 / 65	154 / 70	165 / 75	176 / 80	187 / 85	198 / 90	209 / 95	220 / 100	231 / 105	242 / 110	253 / 115	264 / 120
Hiking, cross country	6.0	4.7	5.3	5.8	6.3	6.8	7.4	7.9	8.4	8.9	9.5	10.0	10.5	11.0	11.6	12.1	12.6
Marching rapidly	6.5	5.1	5.7	6.3	6.8	7.4	8.0	8.5	9.1	9.7	10.2	10.8	11.4	11.9	12.5	13.1	13.7
Racewalking	6.5	5.1	5.7	6.3	6.8	7.4	8.0	8.5	9.1	9.7	10.2	10.8	11.4	11.9	12.5	13.1	13.7
Rock or mountain climbing	8.0	6.3	7.0	7.7	8.4	9.1	9.8	10.5	11.2	11.9	12.6	13.3	14.0	14.7	15.4	16.1	16.8
Walking, <2.0 mph (3.22 km/h)	2.0	1.6	1.8	1.9	2.1	2.3	2.5	2.6	2.8	3.0	3.2	3.3	3.5	3.7	3.9	4.0	4.2
Walking, 2.0 mph (3.22 km/h), level	2.5	2.0	2.2	2.4	2.6	2.8	3.1	3.3	3.5	3.7	3.9	4.2	4.4	4.6	4.8	5.0	5.3
Walking, 2.5 mph (4.02 km/h)	2.8	2.2	2.5	2.7	2.9	3.2	3.4	3.7	3.9	4.2	4.4	4.7	4.9	5.1	5.4	5.6	5.9
Walking, 3.0 mph (4.83 km/h)	3.3	2.6	2.9	3.2	3.5	3.8	4.0	4.3	4.6	4.9	5.2	5.5	5.8	6.1	6.4	6.6	6.9
Walking, 3.5 mph (5.63 km/h)	3.8	3.0	3.3	3.7	4.0	4.3	4.7	5.0	5.3	5.7	6.0	6.3	6.7	7.0	7.3	7.6	8.0
Walking, 3.5 mph (5.63 km/h), uphill	6.0	4.7	5.3	5.8	6.3	6.8	7.4	7.9	8.4	8.9	9.5	10.0	10.5	11.0	11.6	12.1	12.6

(continued)

Table C.11 (continued)

WALKING	LB	99	110	121	132	143	154	165	176	187	198	209	220	231	242	253	264
	KG	45	50	55	60	65	70	75	80	85	90	95	100	105	110	115	120
	METS																
Walking, 4.0 mph (6.44 km/h)	5.0	3.9	4.4	4.8	5.3	5.7	6.1	6.6	7.0	7.4	7.9	8.3	8.8	9.2	9.6	10.1	10.5
Walking, 4.5 mph (7.24 km/h)	6.3	5.0	5.5	6.1	6.6	7.2	7.7	8.3	8.8	9.4	9.9	10.5	11.0	11.6	12.1	12.7	13.2
Walking, 5.0 mph (8.05 km/h)	8.0	6.3	7.0	7.7	8.4	9.1	9.8	10.5	11.2	11.9	12.6	13.3	14.0	14.7	15.4	16.1	16.8
Walking, for pleasure	3.5	2.8	3.1	3.4	3.7	4.0	4.3	4.6	4.9	5.2	5.5	5.8	6.1	6.4	6.7	7.0	7.4
Walking, household	2.0	1.6	1.8	1.9	2.1	2.3	2.5	2.6	2.8	3.0	3.2	3.3	3.5	3.7	3.9	4.0	4.2
Walking, grass track	5.0	3.9	4.4	4.8	5.3	5.7	6.1	6.6	7.0	7.4	7.9	8.3	8.8	9.2	9.6	10.1	10.5
Walking the dog	3.0	2.4	2.6	2.9	3.2	3.4	3.7	3.9	4.2	4.5	4.7	5.0	5.3	5.5	5.8	6.0	6.3
Walking to work or class	4.0	3.2	3.5	3.9	4.2	4.6	4.9	5.3	5.6	6.0	6.3	6.7	7.0	7.4	7.7	8.1	8.4

WATER ACTIVITIES	LB	99	110	121	132	143	154	165	176	187	198	209	220	231	242	253	264
	KG	45	50	55	60	65	70	75	80	85	90	95	100	105	110	115	120
	METS																
Canoeing, on camping trip	4.0	3.2	3.5	3.9	4.2	4.6	4.9	5.3	5.6	6.0	6.3	6.7	7.0	7.4	7.7	8.1	8.4
Canoeing, rowing 2.0-3.9 mph (3.22-6.28 km/h), light effort	3.0	2.4	2.6	2.9	3.2	3.4	3.7	3.9	4.2	4.5	4.7	5.0	5.3	5.5	5.8	6.0	6.3
Canoeing, rowing 4.0-5.9 mph (6.44-9.49 km/h), moderate effort	7.0	5.5	6.1	6.7	7.4	8.0	8.6	9.2	9.8	10.4	11.0	11.6	12.3	12.9	13.5	14.1	14.7
Canoeing, rowing >6 mph (9.65 km/h)	12.0	9.5	10.5	11.6	12.6	13.7	14.7	15.8	16.8	17.9	18.9	20.0	21.0	22.1	23.1	24.2	25.2
Canoeing, rowing for pleasure	3.5	2.8	3.1	3.4	3.7	4.0	4.3	4.6	4.9	5.2	5.5	5.8	6.1	6.4	6.7	7.0	7.4
Canoeing, rowing for competition or crew	12.0	9.5	10.5	11.6	12.6	13.7	14.7	15.8	16.8	17.9	18.9	20.0	21.0	22.1	23.1	24.2	25.2
Diving, springboard	3.0	2.4	2.6	2.9	3.2	3.4	3.7	3.9	4.2	4.5	4.7	5.0	5.3	5.5	5.8	6.0	6.3
Kayaking	5.0	3.9	4.4	4.8	5.3	5.7	6.1	6.6	7.0	7.4	7.9	8.3	8.8	9.2	9.6	10.1	10.5
Paddleboating	4.0	3.2	3.5	3.9	4.2	4.6	4.9	5.3	5.6	6.0	6.3	6.7	7.0	7.4	7.7	8.1	8.4
Sailing, wind-surfing	3.0	2.4	2.6	2.9	3.2	3.4	3.7	3.9	4.2	4.5	4.7	5.0	5.3	5.5	5.8	6.0	6.3

(continued)

Table C.11 (continued)

WATER ACTIVITIES	LB	99	110	121	132	143	154	165	176	187	198	209	220	231	242	253	264
	KG	45	50	55	60	65	70	75	80	85	90	95	100	105	110	115	120
	METS																
Sailing, in competition	5.0	3.9	4.4	4.8	5.3	5.7	6.1	6.6	7.0	7.4	7.9	8.3	8.8	9.2	9.6	10.1	10.5
Sailing	3.0	2.4	2.6	2.9	3.2	3.4	3.7	3.9	4.2	4.5	4.7	5.0	5.3	5.5	5.8	6.0	6.3
Skiing, water	6.0	4.7	5.3	5.8	6.3	6.8	7.4	7.9	8.4	8.9	9.5	10.0	10.5	11.0	11.6	12.1	12.6
Skimobiling	7.0	5.5	6.1	6.7	7.4	8.0	8.6	9.2	9.8	10.4	11.0	11.6	12.3	12.9	13.5	14.1	14.7
Skin diving, scuba diving	7.0	5.5	6.1	6.7	7.4	8.0	8.6	9.2	9.8	10.4	11.0	11.6	12.3	12.9	13.5	14.1	14.7
Snorkeling	5.0	3.9	4.4	4.8	5.3	5.7	6.1	6.6	7.0	7.4	7.9	8.3	8.8	9.2	9.6	10.1	10.5
Surfing, body or board	3.0	2.4	2.6	2.9	3.2	3.4	3.7	3.9	4.2	4.5	4.7	5.0	5.3	5.5	5.8	6.0	6.3
Swimming laps, freestyle	10.0	7.9	8.8	9.6	10.5	11.4	12.3	13.1	14.0	14.9	15.8	16.6	17.5	18.4	19.3	20.1	21.0
Swimming, backstroke	7.0	5.5	6.1	6.7	7.4	8.0	8.6	9.2	9.8	10.4	11.0	11.6	12.3	12.9	13.5	14.1	14.7
Swimming, breaststroke	10.0	7.9	8.8	9.6	10.5	11.4	12.3	13.1	14.0	14.9	15.8	16.6	17.5	18.4	19.3	20.1	21.0
Swimming, butterfly	11.0	8.7	9.6	10.6	11.6	12.5	13.5	14.4	15.4	16.4	17.3	18.3	19.3	20.2	21.2	22.1	23.1
Swimming, crawl, fast (75 yd/min or 68.6 m/min)	11.0	8.7	9.6	10.6	11.6	12.5	13.5	14.4	15.4	16.4	17.3	18.3	19.3	20.2	21.2	22.1	23.1
Swimming, crawl, slow (50 yd/min or 45.7 m/min)	8.0	6.3	7.0	7.7	8.4	9.1	9.8	10.5	11.2	11.9	12.6	13.3	14.0	14.7	15.4	16.1	16.8

294

WATER ACTIVITIES	LB	99	110	121	132	143	154	165	176	187	198	209	220	231	242	253	264
	KG	45	50	55	60	65	70	75	80	85	90	95	100	105	110	115	120
	METS																
Swimming, leisurely, not lap	6.0	4.7	5.3	5.8	6.3	6.8	7.4	7.9	8.4	8.9	9.5	10.0	10.5	11.0	11.6	12.1	12.6
Swimming, sidestroke	8.0	6.3	7.0	7.7	8.4	9.1	9.8	10.5	11.2	11.9	12.6	13.3	14.0	14.7	15.4	16.1	16.8
Swimming, synchronized	8.0	6.3	7.0	7.7	8.4	9.1	9.8	10.5	11.2	11.9	12.6	13.3	14.0	14.7	15.4	16.1	16.8
Swimming, treading water	10.0	7.9	8.8	9.6	10.5	11.4	12.3	13.1	14.0	14.9	15.8	16.6	17.5	18.4	19.3	20.1	21.0
Water aerobics, water calisthenics	4.0	3.2	3.5	3.9	4.2	4.6	4.9	5.3	5.6	6.0	6.3	6.7	7.0	7.4	7.7	8.1	8.4
Water jogging	8.0	6.3	7.0	7.7	8.4	9.1	9.8	10.5	11.2	11.9	12.6	13.3	14.0	14.7	15.4	16.1	16.8
Water polo	10.0	7.9	8.8	9.6	10.5	11.4	12.3	13.1	14.0	14.9	15.8	16.6	17.5	18.4	19.3	20.1	21.0
Water volleyball	3.0	2.4	2.6	2.9	3.2	3.4	3.7	3.9	4.2	4.5	4.7	5.0	5.3	5.5	5.8	6.0	6.3
White-water rafting, kayaking	5.0	3.9	4.4	4.8	5.3	5.7	6.1	6.6	7.0	7.4	7.9	8.3	8.8	9.2	9.6	10.1	10.5

WINTER ACTIVITIES	LB	99	110	121	132	143	154	165	176	187	198	209	220	231	242	253	264
	KG	45	50	55	60	65	70	75	80	85	90	95	100	105	110	115	120
	METS																
Skating, ice, 9 mph (14.5 km/h) or less	5.0	3.9	4.4	4.8	5.3	5.7	6.1	6.6	7.0	7.4	7.9	8.3	8.8	9.2	9.6	10.1	10.5
Skating, ice	7.0	5.5	6.1	6.7	7.4	8.0	8.6	9.2	9.8	10.4	11.0	11.6	12.3	12.9	13.5	14.1	14.7
Skating, ice, >9 mph (14.5 km/h)	9.0	7.1	7.9	8.7	9.5	10.2	11.0	11.8	12.6	13.4	14.2	15.0	15.8	16.5	17.3	18.1	18.9

(continued)

Table C.11 (continued)

WINTER ACTIVITIES	LB	99	110	121	132	143	154	165	176	187	198	209	220	231	242	253	264
	KG	45	50	55	60	65	70	75	80	85	90	95	100	105	110	115	120
	METS																
Skating, speed, competitive	15.0	11.8	13.1	14.4	15.8	17.1	18.4	19.7	21.0	22.3	23.6	24.9	26.3	27.6	28.9	30.2	31.5
Ski jumping	7.0	5.5	6.1	6.7	7.4	8.0	8.6	9.2	9.8	10.4	11.0	11.6	12.3	12.9	13.5	14.1	14.7
Skiing, cross country, 2.5 mph (4.02 km/h)	7.0	5.5	6.1	6.7	7.4	8.0	8.6	9.2	9.8	10.4	11.0	11.6	12.3	12.9	13.5	14.1	14.7
Skiing, cross country, 4.0 mph (6.44km/h)	8.0	6.3	7.0	7.7	8.4	9.1	9.8	10.5	11.2	11.9	12.6	13.3	14.0	14.7	15.4	16.1	16.8
Skiing, cross country, 5.0-7.9 mph (8.05-12.71 km/h)	9.0	7.1	7.9	8.7	9.5	10.2	11.0	11.8	12.6	13.4	14.2	15.0	15.8	16.5	17.3	18.1	18.9
Skiing, cross country, >8.0 mph (12.8 km/h)	14.0	11.0	12.3	13.5	14.7	15.9	17.2	18.4	19.6	20.8	22.1	23.3	24.5	25.7	27.0	28.2	29.4
Skiing, cross country, uphill	16.5	13.0	14.4	15.9	17.3	18.8	20.2	21.7	23.1	24.5	26.0	27.4	28.9	30.3	31.8	33.2	34.7
Skiing, down-hill, light effort	5.0	3.9	4.4	4.8	5.3	5.7	6.1	6.6	7.0	7.4	7.9	8.3	8.8	9.2	9.6	10.1	10.5
Skiing, down-hill, moderate effort	6.0	4.7	5.3	5.8	6.3	6.8	7.4	7.9	8.4	8.9	9.5	10.0	10.5	11.0	11.6	12.1	12.6

Reprinted, by permission, from J. Hoffman, 2006, *Norms for fitness, performance, and health* (Champaign, IL: Human Kinetics), 153-163.

Adapted, by permission, from Ainsworth et al., 2000, "Compendium of physical activities: An update of activity codes and MET intensities," *Medicine and Science in Sports and Exercise* 32: S498-504.

CALORIC VALUES

Table C.12   **Hints on Estimating the Amount of Food Consumed**

FOOD	SERVING	ESTIMATED SIZE
Breads and grains	1/2 cup cereal, pasta, or rice	Volume of cupcake wrapper or half a baseball
	4 oz (113 g) bagel (large)	Diameter of a compact disc
	Medium piece of cornbread	Medium bar of soap
Fruits and vegetables	Medium piece of fruit	Tennis ball
	1/4 cup of dried fruit	Golf ball or handful for average adult
	1/2 cup of fruit or vegetable	Half of a baseball
	1 cup of broccoli	Light bulb
	1/2 cup	6 asparagus spears, 7 or 8 baby carrots
Meat, fish, and poultry	1 oz (28 g)	3 tbsp. meat or poultry
	2 oz (57 g)	Small chicken drumstick or thigh
	3 oz (85 g)	Adult's hand, small chicken breast, or medium pork chop
Cheese	1 oz (28 g)	Average person's thumb, 2 dominoes, or 4 dice

Adapted from USDA (United States Department of Agriculture) 2002, "Nutritive value of foods," *Home and Garden Bulletin* No. 72. (Washington, DC: US Government Printing Office).

BIBLIOGRAPHY

Chapter 1 Principles of Fitness, Health, and Wellness Concepts

American College of Sports Medicine. 2005. *ACSM's guidelines for exercise testing and prescription*, 7th ed. Philadelphia, PA: Lippincott, Williams and Wilkins.

Brooks, D. 2004. *The complete book of personal training.* Champaign, IL: Human Kinetics.

Canada's Physical Activity Guides for Helath: Adults, older adults, children and youth. http://www.phac-aspc.gc.ca/pau-uap/paguide/index.html.

Greenberg, J.S., G.B. Dintiman, and B.M. Oakes. 2004. *Physical fitness and wellness*, 3rd ed. Champaign, IL: Human Kinetics.

Zaryski, C., and D.J. Smith. 2005. Training principles and issues for ultra-endurance athletes. *Current Sports Medicine Reports* 4: 165-170.

Chapter 2 Nutrition Concepts for Personal Trainers

Armstrong, L. 2000. *Performing in extreme environments.* Champaign, IL: Human Kinetics.

Benardot, D. 2006. *Advanced sports nutrition.* Champaign, IL: Human Kinetics.

Brooks, D. 2004. *The complete book of personal training.* Champaign, IL: Human Kinetics.

Canada's Guide to Healthy Eating and Physical Activity. http://www.phac-aspc.gc.ca/guide/index_e.html

Centre for Nutrition Policy and Promotion. My Pyramid. http://www.cnpp.usda.gov/

Enig, M. 2000. *Know your fats: The complete primer for understanding the nutrition of fats, oils, and cholesterol.* Silver Spring, MD: Betheseda Press.

Thompson, J., M. Manore, and J. Sheeshka. 2007. *Nutrition: A functional approach*, Canadian Edition. Toronto, Ontario: Pearson Education Canada.

Chapter 3 Bioenergetics Concepts

Brooks, D. 2004. *The complete book of personal training.* Champaign, IL: Human Kinetics.

Griffin, J. 2006. *Client-centered exercise prescription*, 2nd ed. Champaign, IL: Human Kinetics.

Hoffman, J. 2002. *Physiological aspects of sport training and performance.* Champaign, IL: Human Kinetics.

McArdle, W., F. Katch, and V. Katch. 2007. *Exercise physiology: Energy, nutrition, and human performance*, 6th ed. Baltimore, MD: Lippincott, Williams and Wilkins.

National Strength and Conditioning Association. 2000. *Essentials of strength training and conditioning*, 2nd ed. Champaign, IL: Human Kinetics.

National Strength and Conditioning Association: Performance Training Journal. http://www.nsca-lift.org/Perform/backissues.asp

Sharkey, B., and S. Gaskill. 2006. *Sport physiology for coaches.* Champaign, IL: Human Kinetics.

Siff, M. 2003. *Supertraining.* Denver, CO: Supertraining Institute.

Twist Conditioning Inc. 2004. *Sport movement specialist certification course handouts.* North Vancouver, BC: Twist Conditioning Inc.

Whyte, G. 2006. *Physiology of training.* London, UK: Churchill Livingstone Elsevier.

Chapter 4 Cardiorespiratory Concepts

Canada's Physical Activity Guides for Health: Adults, older adults, children and youth. http://www.phac-aspc.gc.ca/pau-uap/paguide/index.html.

Centres for Disease Control and Prevention. Physical Activity for Everyone. http://www.cdc.gov/nccdphp/dnpa/physical/index.htm.

McArdle, W., F. Katch, and V. Katch. 2007. *Exercise physiology: Energy, nutrition, and human performance*, 6th ed. Baltimore, MD: Lippincott, Williams and Wilkins.

National Strength and Conditioning Association: Performance Training Journal. http://www.nsca-lift.org/Perform/backissues.asp.

Chapter 5 Skeletal Anatomy and Flexibility Concepts

Fu, F., and S. Lephart. 2000. *Proprioception and neuromuscular control in joint stability.* Champaign, IL: Human Kinetics.

National Strength and Conditioning Association. 2000. *Essentials of strength training and conditioning*, 2nd ed. Champaign, IL: Human Kinetics.

Siff, M. 2003. *Supertraining.* Denver, CO: Supertraining Institute.

Chapter 6 Muscular Concepts

ACSM Brochures: http://www.acsm.org/AM/Template. cfm?Section=Brochures2

Brooks, D. 2004. *The complete book of personal training.* Champaign, IL: Human Kinetics.

McArdle, W., F. Katch, and V. Katch. 2007. *Exercise physiology: Energy, nutrition, and human performance,* 6th ed. Baltimore, MD: Lippincott, Williams and Wilkins.

National Strength and Conditioning Association. 2000. *Essentials of strength training and conditioning,* 2nd ed. Champaign, IL: Human Kinetics.

National Strength and Conditioning Association: Performance Training Journal. http://www.nsca-lift.org/Perform/backissues.asp

Chapter 8 Preexercise Screening

ACSM Brochures: Pre-participation Physical Examinations: http://www.acsm.org/Content/ContentFolders/Publications/Brochures/prepart022702.pdf.

American College of Sports Medicine. 2003. *ACSM's exercise management for persons with chronic diseases and disabilities,* 2nd ed. Champaign, IL: Human Kinetics.

CSEP: PAR-Q, PARmedX: http://www.csep.ca/forms.asp

Delforge, G. 2002. *Musculoskeletal trauma - Implications for sports injury management.* Champaign, IL: Human Kinetics.

Health Screen (Release 1.0). Human Kinetics Software. Champaign, IL: Human Kinetics.

Houglum, P. 2005. *Therapeutic exercise for musculoskeletal injuries,* 2nd ed. Champaign, IL: Human Kinetics.

Loudon, J., S.L. Bell, and J.M. Johnston. 1998. *The clinical orthopedic assessment guide.* Champaign, IL: Human Kinetics.

Olds, T., and K. Norton. 1999. *Pre-exercise health screening guide.* Champaign, IL: Human Kinetics.

Whiting, W.C., and R.F. Zernicke. 1998. *Biomechanics of musculoskeletal injury.* Champaign, IL: Human Kinetics.

Chapter 9 Fitness Assessment

Brooks, D. 2004. *The complete book of personal training.* Champaign, IL: Human Kinetics.

CSEP. 2003. *The Canadian physical activity, fitness, and lifestyle approach.* Ottawa, Ontario: Canadian Society for Exercise Physiology.

Heyward, V. 2006. *Advanced fitness assessment and exercise prescription,* 5th ed. Champaign IL: Human Kinetics.

Hoffman, J. 2006. *Norms for fitness, performance, and health.* Champaign, IL: Human Kinetics.

Niemen, D. 2007. *Exercise testing and prescription: A health related approach,* 6th ed. Dubuque, Iowa: McGraw Hill.

Chapter 10 Program Desing Concepts

American College of Sports Medicine. 2005. *ACSM's guidelines for exercise testing and prescription,* 7th ed. Philadelphia, PA: Lippincott, Williams and Wilkins.

Bompa, T.O. 1999. *Periodization: Theory and methodology of training,* 4th ed. Champaign, IL: Human Kinetics.

Zaryski, C., and Smith, D.J. 2005. Training principles and issues for ultra-endurance athletes. *Current Sports Medicine Reports* 4: 165-170.

Chapter 11 Typical Personal Training Programs

Bompa, T.O. 1999. *Periodization: Theory and methodology of training,* 4th ed. Champaign, IL: Human Kinetics.

Brooks, D. 1998. *Program design for personal trainers: Bridging theory into application.* Champaign, IL: Human Kinetics.

National Strength and Conditioning Association. 2000. *Essentials of strength training and conditioning,* 2nd ed. Champaign, IL: Human Kinetics.

Wilmore, J.H., and D.L. Costill, 2004. *Physiology of sport and exercise,* 3rd ed. Champaign, IL: Human Kinetics.

Zaryski, C., and Smith, D.J. 2005. Training principles and issues for ultra-endurance athletes. *Current Sports Medicine Reports* 4:165-170.

Chapter 12 Psychology of Personal Training

Blair, S.N., A.L. Dunn, B.H. Marcus, R.A. Carpenter, and P. Jaret. 2001. *Active living every day.* Champaign, IL: Human Kinetics.

Gavin, J. 2005. *Lifestyle fitness coaching.* Champaign, IL: Human Kinetics.

Griffin, J.C. 2006. *Client-centered exercise prescription,* 2nd ed. Champaign, IL: Human Kinetics.

Howley, E.T., and B.D. Franks. 2003. *Health fitness instructor's handbook,* 4th ed. Champaign, IL: Human Kinetics.

Marcus, B.H., and L. Forsyth. 2003. *Motivating people to be physically active.* Champaign, IL: Human Kinetics.

Weinberg, R.S., and D. Gould. *Foundations of sport and exercise psychology,* 3rd ed. Champaign, IL: Human Kinetics.

Chapter 13 Business of Personal Training

Mullin, B.J., S. Hardy, and W.A. Sutton. 1999. *Sport marketing,* 2nd ed. Champaign, IL: Human Kinetics.

INDEX

Note: Page numbers followed by *f* or *t* indicate figures or tables, *ff* or *tt* indicate multiple figures or tables.

ABOUT CAN-FIT-PRO

Can-Fit-Pro

Can-Fit-Pro was established in 1993 to serve as a voice for all fitness professionals. Since then, Can-Fit-Pro has grown to become one of the largest providers of education in the fitness industry with over 14,000 members regularly influencing over 1,000,000 people. Can-Fit-Pro offers a comprehensive membership, certification opportunities and continuing education events.

Can-Fit-Pro recognizes that certification is the starting point in a fitness professional's career. Can-Fit-Pro's focus is to make the certification experience challenging and enjoyable while providing programming and resources that are affordable, accessible, and attainable. Can-Fit-Pro certification courses and exams are delivered by professional trainers (PRO Trainers) who are hand picked for their area of expertise. Can-Fit-Pro certification provides a foundation of competency through theory and practical knowledge to deliver a safe and effective fitness experience.

In addition to our certification and conference opportunities, Can-Fit-Pro offers a comprehensive Web site and annual membership that includes discounts to Can-Fit-Pro events, a full-color magazine and much more. Visit our Web site at www.canfitpro.com or call us today at 416-493-3515 or 800-667-5622 for certification information, course and exam dates, conference news, and more information on everything we offer!